Rheumatic Disorders

Summaries in Clinical Practice

Jeremiah A. Barondess, MD, Series Editor

Rheumatic Disorders

EDITED BY

Stephen A. Paget, M.D.
ASSOCIATE PROFESSOR OF CLINICAL MEDICINE, CORNELL UNIVERSITY MEDICAL COLLEGE, NEW YORK, NEW YORK

Theodore R. Fields, M.D.
ASSISTANT PROFESSOR OF MEDICINE, CORNELL UNIVERSITY MEDICAL COLLEGE, NEW YORK, NEW YORK

WITH 20 CONTRIBUTING AUTHORS

Andover Medical Publishers

Boston   London   Oxford   Singapore   Sydney   Toronto   Wellington

Andover Medical Publishers is an imprint of
Butterworth–Heinemann

Copyright © 1992 by Butterworth–Heinemann, a division
of Reed Publishing (USA) Inc. All rights reserved.

No part of this publication may be reproduced, stored in
a retrieval system, or transmitted, in any form or by any
means, electronic, mechanical, photocopying, recording,
or otherwise, without the prior written permission of the
publisher.

Every effort has been made to ensure that the drug dosage schedules within this text are accurate and conform to standards accepted at time of publication. However, as treatment recommendations vary in the light of continuing research and clinical experience, the reader is advised to verify drug dosage schedules herein with information found on product information sheets. This is especially true in cases of new or infrequently used drugs.

∞ Recognizing the importance of preserving what has been written, it is the policy of Butterworth–Heinemann to have the books it publishes printed on acid-free paper, and we exert our best efforts to that end.

Library of Congress Cataloging-in-Publication Data
Rheumatic disorders / [edited by] Stephen A. Paget,
　　Theodore R. Fields.
　　　　p. cm.
　　Includes bibliographical references and index.
　　ISBN 0-9626521-4-8 (casebound : alk. paper)
　　1. Rheumatism. 2. Arthritis. I. Paget, Stephen A. II. Fields,
Theodore R.
　　[DNLM: 1. Arthritis, Rheumatoid. 2. Rheumatic Diseases.
WE 344 R4715]
RC927.R4543　　1992
616.7'23—dc20
DNLM/DLC
for Library of Congress　　　　　　　　　　　　92-2770
　　　　　　　　　　　　　　　　　　　　　　　　　CIP

British Library Cataloguing in Publication Data
Paget, Stephen A.
　　Rheumatic Disorders
　　I. Title II. Fields, Theodore R.
　　616.7
　　ISBN 0-9626521-4-8

Butterworth–Heinemann
80 Montvale Avenue
Stoneham, MA 02180

10　9　8　7　6　5　4　3　2　1

Printed in the United States of America

Contents

Contributing Authors ix
Preface xi

1. **Introduction and Differential Diagnosis of Rheumatic Disorders** 1
   Charles L. Christian

   Scope of Rheumatic Disorders 1
   Elements of Differential Diagnosis 1
   Summary 6

2. **Origin and Clinical Relevance of Autoantibodies** 7
   Keith B. Elkon

   Autoantibodies 7
   Autoimmune Diseases 8
   Significance of Autoantibodies 8
   Diagnostic Value and Clinical Utility of Autoantibodies 9
   Autoantibodies and Tissue Injury 10
   Clues to the Origins of Autoimmunity 12
   Autoantibodies in Clinical Practice 13
   Summary 15

3. **Rheumatoid Arthritis** 19
   Nina Bhardwaj and Stephen A. Paget

   Epidemiology 20
   Etiology and Pathogenesis 20
   Diagnostic and Clinical Aspects 31
   Extra-Articular Manifestations 34
   Laboratory and Radiologic Manifestations 38
   Therapy 42
   Summary 53
   Appendix 3-1 Salicylates in the Treatment of Rheumatoid Arthritis 59
   Appendix 3-2 Profile of Nonsteroidal Anti-Inflammatory Drugs (NSAIDs) 60
   Appendix 3-3 Nonsalicylate Nonsteroidal Anti-Inflammatory Drugs (NSAIDs)
   in the Treatment of Rheumatoid Arthritis 63

		Appendix 3-4	Gold Salt Therapy in the Treatment of Rheumatoid Arthritis	65
		Appendix 3-5	Sulfasalazine Therapy in the Treatment of Rheumatoid Arthritis	70
		Appendix 3-6	D-Penicillamine Therapy in the Treatment of Rheumatoid Arthritis	72
		Appendix 3-7	Azathioprine Therapy in the Treatment of Rheumatoid Arthritis	74
		Appendix 3-8	Methotrexate Therapy in the Treatment of Rheumatoid Arthritis	76

4. **Septic Arthritis, Lyme Disease, and Prosthetic Joint Infection** 79
   Barry D. Brause

   Septic Arthritis 79
   Lyme Disease 82
   Prosthetic Joint Infection 86

5. **Osteoarthritis** 93
   Lee D. Kaufman and Leon Sokoloff

   Introduction 93
   Current Concepts of Pathogenesis 93
   Clinical Manifestations 97
   Types of Osteoarthritis 98
   Therapeutic Intervention: Evolving Concepts 106

6. **Reiter's Syndrome and Reactive Arthritis** 111
   Robert D. Inman

   Introduction 111
   Clinical Manifestations 111
   Current Concepts of Pathogenesis 112
   Differential Diagnosis 114
   Treatment 114
   Prognosis 115

7. **Vasculitis** 119
   Michael D. Lockshin

   Introduction 119
   Definitions 119
   Syndromes 121

8. **Crystal-Induced Inflammatory Joint Disease** 135
   Theodore R. Fields and Lawrence M. Ryan

   Introduction 135
   Pathophysiology 135
   Gout 139
   Pseudogout 146
   Basic Calcium Phosphate-Related Joint Inflammation 148

9. **Systemic Lupus Erythematosus**   151
   Robert P. Kimberly

   Introduction   151
   Etiology   151
   Epidemiology   152
   Pathogenesis   152
   Clinical Spectrum of Disease   154
   Approach to Management   157
   Course and Prognosis   160

10. **Dermatomyositis and Polymyositis**   161
    Lawrence J. Kagen

    Introduction   161
    Clinical Manifestations   161
    Pathogenesis   164
    Association with Malignant Disease   167
    Other Forms of Myositis   167
    Treatment   168
    Prognosis   169

11. **The Spectrum of Scleroderma**   175
    E. Carwile LeRoy

    Introduction   175
    Clinical Manifestations   175
    Pathogenesis   177
    Diagnosis and Management   179
    Conclusion   182

12. **Sjögren's Syndrome**   185
    Stuart S. Kassan and Haralampos M. Moutsopoulos

    Introduction   185
    Epidemiology   185
    Pathogenesis   186
    Clinical Manifestations   187
    Laboratory Tests   193
    Treatment   194

13. **Immunosuppressive Therapy in the Treatment of Joint and Connective Tissue Disorders**   201
    David P. Recker and John H. Klippel

    Introduction   201
    Indications for Immunosuppressives   201
    Immunosuppressive Drugs   202
    Cyclosporine   208

14. **Total Hip Replacement Arthroplasty in Patients with Inflammatory Arthritis**   213
Chitranjan S. Ranawat, Michael J. Maynard, and William F. Flynn, Jr.

     Inflammatory Hip Arthritis   213
     Clinical and Radiographic Features of Rheumatoid Arthritis   215
     Total Hip Replacement Arthroplasty   215

15. **Nonoperative Orthopedics**   223
Norman A. Johanson

     Introduction   223
     Neck   223
     Shoulder   224
     Elbow   225
     Hand and Wrist   226
     Lumbar Spine   227
     Hip   231
     Knee   233
     Foot and Ankle   235

Index   239

Contributing Authors

Nina Bhardwaj, M.D., Ph.D.
Assistant Professor, Rockefeller University, Cornell University Medical Center; Assistant Attending Physician of Rheumatology, Hospital for Special Surgery, New York, New York

Barry D. Brause, M.D., F.A.C.P.
Clinical Associate Professor of Medicine, Cornell University Medical Center; Associate Attending Physician, New York Hospital, Hospital for Special Surgery, New York, New York

Charles L. Christian, M.D.
Professor of Medicine, Cornell University Medical Center; Physician in Chief, Hospital for Special Surgery, New York, New York

Keith B. Elkon, M.D.
Associate Professor of Medicine, Hospital for Special Surgery, Cornell University Medical Center, New York, New York

Theodore R. Fields, M.D., F.A.C.P., F.A.C.R.
Assistant Professor of Medicine, Hospital for Special Surgery, New York Hospital, Cornell University Medical Center, New York, New York

William F. Flynn, Jr., M.D.
Fellow, Orthopedic Surgery, Hospital for Special Surgery, New York, New York

Robert D. Inman, M.D., F.R.C.P.C., F.A.C.P.
Director, Division of Rheumatology, The Toronto Western Hospital, Toronto, Ontario

Norman A. Johanson, M.D.
Associate Professor of Orthopedic Surgery, Temple University School of Medicine, St. Christopher's Hospital for Children, Shriners Hospital for Crippled Children, Philadelphia, Pennsylvania

Lawrence J. Kagen, M.D.
Professor of Medicine, Cornell University Medical Center; Attending Physician of Rheumatology, Hospital for Special Surgery, New York Hospital, New York, New York

Stuart S. Kassan, M.D., F.A.C.P.
Associate Clinical Professor of Medicine, University of Colorado Health Sciences Center, Denver, Colorado

Lee D. Kaufman, M.D., F.A.C.P.
Associate Professor of Medicine, Director of Clinical Rheumatology, Health Sciences Center, State University of New York at Stony Brook, Stony Brook, New York

Robert P. Kimberly, M.D.
Professor of Medicine, Cornell University Medical Center, Hospital for Special Surgery; Director, Biomedical Component, Cornell University Medical Center, New York, New York

John H. Klippel, M.D.
Clinical Director, Arthritis and Rheumatism Branch, National Institutes of Health, Bethesda, Maryland

E. Carwile LeRoy, M.D.
Professor of Medicine, Director, Division of Rheumatology, South Carolina Medical University, Charleston, South Carolina

Michael D. Lockshin, M.D.
Director, Extramural Programs, National Institutes of Health, Bethesda, Maryland

Michael J. Maynard, M.D.
Fellow, Orthopedic Surgery, Hospital for Special Surgery, New York, New York

Stephen A. Paget, M.D., F.A.C.P., F.A.C.R.
Associate Professor, Clinical Medicine, Hospital for Special Surgery, New York Hospital, Cornell University Medical Center, New York, New York

Haralampos M. Moutsopoulos, M.D., F.A.C.P.
Professor and Head of Medicine, Department of Internal Medicine, University of Ioannina School of Medicine, Ioannina, Greece

Chitranjan S. Ranawat, M.D.
Professor of Orthopedic Surgery, Cornell University Medical Center; Attending Orthopedic Surgeon, Hospital for Special Surgery, New York, New York

David P. Recker, M.D., F.A.C.R.
Senior Medical Advisor, Minority Council, House Appropriations–United States Congress, Washington, D.C.

Lawrence M. Ryan, M.D.
Professor of Medicine, Chief, Division of Rheumatology, Medical College of Wisconsin, Milwaukee, Wisconsin

Leon Sokoloff, M.D., M.A.C.R.
Professor Emeritus, Department of Pathology, Health Science Center, State University of New York at Stony Brook, Stony Brook, New York

Preface

This is an exciting time to have edited a book that updates rheumatology for the practicing physician. Great changes have taken place over the last ten years, and many of them are only beginning to reflect themselves in the practice of rheumatology.

We have tried to provide in-depth and practical reviews of the key areas in rheumatology, by physicians expert in both the basic science and the "nuts-and-bolts" aspects of their topics. Each contributor has given the practicing physician an up-to-date guideline for managing a disease, as well as a concise review of the scientific framework on which management is based.

The dramatic recent advances in immunology are reflected in Dr. Elkon's chapter on autoantibodies and in the pathophysiology sections of various chapters, such as those on rheumatoid arthritis and Sjögren's syndrome. Progress in immunogenetics is reflected in Dr. Inman's section on Reiter's syndrome and reactive arthritis. Drs. Klippel and Recker have helped us by updating the use of immunosuppressive therapy in the rheumatic diseases and expand on the limitations still inherent in this approach.

New developments in other areas of medicine have required that rheumatology keep pace. The wide use of cyclosporin A for kidney and heart transplant patients has produced a particularly difficult form of gout for rheumatologists to manage, and we have attempted to address this problem here. The development of synthetic biologics, many feel, may transform the future management of inflammatory disorders. In the pathophysiology section of the rheumatoid arthritis chapter, background material is provided that will allow the practicing physician to understand future developments in the use of biologics, such as monoclonal antibodies, in arthritis management.

We have tried to go beyond the "cookbook" approach to management and have encouraged our contributors to explain their management suggestions. Where there is controversy, our aim is to acknowledge it and then to allow our contributors to give their personal approaches. Subtleties in management are almost the rule in rheumatology. Dr. Kimberly has provided an overview of the complexities of corticosteroid management in lupus. Dr. Klippel's section reflects the complex decision making involved in starting immunosuppressive therapy.

Clinicians will find information here on the overall approach to rheumatic diseases, as well as specific information on individual disorders. Dr. Christian's chapter reviews the general approach to the patient with arthritis and connective tissue disorders. Dr. Elkon furnishes a background understanding of the great variety of autoantibody tests currently available. On the other hand, detailed presentations on individual disorders, such as Dr. LeRoy's chapter on scleroderma and Dr. Kagen's section on polymyositis and dermatomyositis, make up the bulk of our volume.

The rheumatologist's practice is in many ways intimately linked to that of the orthopedic surgeon. Dr. Johanson's section reminds us of the many nonoperative orthopedic issues that are dealt with on a daily basis by both the rheumatologist and the primary physician.

We would like to express our sincere thanks to Judith R. Javier-Reyes for her tireless organizational efforts and for keeping our contributors advised through all the phases of development of this book. Mr. John de Carville, our publisher, provided continuous support. We express our thanks to Peg Markow, Project Manager, for her excellent work in editorial production.

We hope that this book shares some of our enthusiasm for the evolving field of rheumatology with our readers. We have tried to give our readers a solid, practical approach to patients with rheumatic diseases. A great effort has also been made to provide our readers with the basic science information that will be required to understand new developments in therapy as they unfold.

Stephen Paget, M.D.
Theodore Fields, M.D.

Chapter 1

Introduction and Differential Diagnosis of Rheumatic Disorders

CHARLES L. CHRISTIAN, M.D.

Scope of Rheumatic Disorders

Over the past two decades, rheumatology has emerged as a distinct medical subspecialty. However, the discipline is firmly rooted in general medicine, and the differential diagnosis of musculoskeletal pain or dysfunction encompasses all of internal medicine and some elements of neurology and orthopedics. Pain in the trunk or extremities may be a manifestation of a primary rheumatic disorder, neuropathic conditions, vascular abnormalities, metabolic disease, or referral from visceral sites remote to the localization of symptoms. Even anatomically discrete problems, such as joint pain and swelling, may result from such diverse conditions as trauma, internal derangement, infection, metabolic disorder, neoplasia, or immunologic mechanisms. The causes of rheumatic disorders that are often classified as "connective tissue syndromes" are not known, but there is abundant evidence implicating immunologic mechanisms in the mediation of tissue injury and inflammation characteristic of the diseases.

The spectrum of rheumatic diseases has changed. This reflects diminished frequencies of some problems (acute rheumatic fever, neuropathic arthropathy), the emergence of new illnesses (Lyme disease, rheumatic complications of human immunodeficiency virus [HIV] infection), new concepts (crystal arthropathies, Kawasaki disease, hepatitis B arthritis/arteritis, diffuse fasciitis), and the recognition of several variant, mixed, or undifferentiated syndromes, some of which are associated with autoantibodies that are specific for discrete and defined cellular constituents (centeromeric proteins, nuclear ribonucleoprotein, phospholipids, ribosomal P protein, tRNA synthetases).

Elements of Differential Diagnosis

The differential diagnosis is based on the medical history, physical examination, and laboratory studies. The observation of a patient begins with the first encounter, analysis of gait, posture, general appearance and expression, performance of simple tasks, and so forth, but the formal physical examination should *not* begin before there is a careful and complete medical history. Reliance on the laboratory, before exploiting the power of the medical history and physical examination, is wasteful and results in many more errors than does the failure to "order the right tests." The number of specific diagnostic procedures in rheumatology is small.

Medical History

General Advice

1. Guide the interview but listen to the patient and don't hurry through a history form in rapid sequence.
2. Avoid asking leading questions in attempts to elicit historical items of considerable differential value, such as morning stiffness, Raynaud's phenomenon, symptoms of keratoconjunctivitis sicca, dysphagia, and so forth.
3. Explore leads as they emerge in the interview. For example, regarding musculoskeletal pain, what is the anatomic pattern? Is it migratory or sustained? Have there been objective signs of inflammation?

Is the discomfort sufficient to alter function? To what degree? What makes the discomfort worse or better? The level of symptomatic benefit from simple analgesic therapy provides some gradation of severity of pain. If there is a history of fever, inquire about magnitude, duration, and pattern of pyrexia, as well as associated rigor, and presence or absence of symptoms referable to genitourinary, respiratory, and gastrointestinal symptoms. If skin lesions have been observed, elicit additional information, such as distribution, presence or absence of pruritus, evidence of photosensitivity, and character of lesions. (The patient's observation can often indicate whether the lesions were papular, erythematous, purpuric, necrotic, vesicular, scaly, healing with or without residual change, and so forth.)
4. Note any historical items that should direct special attention in performance of the physical examination, for example, trauma, neurosensory symptoms, back pain, dysuria, headache, or ocular symptoms.

Historical Items of Interest

Mode of Onset. Did the symptoms begin abruptly or gradually? Was there associated trauma or participation in unusual physical activities?

Chronology. Diagnostic considerations for acute rheumatic syndromes are different, and generally broader, than those for chronic disease. Recent-onset synovitis, particularly if associated with fever or other evidence of sepsis, deserves prompt consideration of infectious causes. Episodic and remittent patterns of disease can occur with most rheumatic syndromes but are more common with gout, pseudogout, and nonarticular and traumatic syndromes. The clinical picture of acute rheumatoid arthritis may be identical to remittent forms of synovitis associated with suspected or proven viral syndromes, such as rubella, HB hepatitis, or mononucleosis.

Functional Alterations. The severity of disease and the extent of disability can often be better quantified from the medical history than from the physical examination. To what extent have activities of daily living, maintenance of vocation, or participation in sports been affected by the illness? Is the main source of disability fatigue, or pain, or weakness?

Aggravation or Amelioration of Symptoms. Detailed inquiry regarding activities that aggravate or lessen symptoms can be dramatically discriminating. Pain in the area of the hip and proximal lower extremity may be the result of lumbar radiculopathy, hip joint disease, bursitis, tendinitis, or arterial insufficiency. Radiculopathy pain tends to be maximal in sedentary attitudes, such as sitting, and may be relieved by ambulation. Trochanteric bursitis pain is aggravated by pressure, as when lying on the affected side. In patients with arterial insufficiency, the pattern of discomfort associated with ambulation is usually quite different from that associated with hip joint disease. Likewise, the relief or aggravation of pain in the upper extremity tends to be distinct for cervical radiculopathy, nonarticular rheumatic syndromes, and synovitis.

Demographic Characteristics. Certain syndromes (gout, Reiter's syndrome, ankylosing spondylitis) are more frequent in males, while others (systemic lupus erythematosus, systemic sclerosis, rheumatoid arthritis) are more common in females. Age is not very discriminating, although the frequency of degenerative syndromes increases with age. Sexual orientation and activity have statistical significance with regard to gonococcal disease, Reiter's syndrome, hepatitis B arthropathy, and HIV infection. Concomitant or antecedent drug use is potentially relevant. Examples include diuretics (gout), procainamide and hydralazine (drug-induced lupus), penicillin and other drugs (serum sickness), anticoagulants (hemarthrosis), and corticosteroids (avascular osteonecrosis, osteoporosis, myopathy).

Physical Examination

Only rarely is a complete general physical examination not required for a patient with musculoskeletal pain or disfunction. Physical findings, guided by the medical history, usually will indicate whether a problem is articular, periarticular, muscular, neurogenetic, or vascular. When joints are affected, the physical examination usually will discriminate between inflammatory and noninflammatory arthropathy. For example, monarticular patterns suggest infection, mechanical derangement, trauma, gout, chondrocalcinosis, and so forth, and there are "classic" anatomic patterns for syndromes such as psoriatic arthropathy, Reiter's syndrome, rheumatoid arthritis, osteoarthritis, and gout. Fever may be a manifestation of most of the connective tissue syndromes but this feature, particularly when associated with rigor, suggests sepsis. Skin lesions, if present, have high differential value and may be pathognomonic, as in Reiter's syndrome, systemic lupus erythematosus, dermatomyositis, psoriatic arthropathy, systemic pattern juvenile arthritis, gonococcal sepsis, Lyme disease, systemic sclerosis, and vasculitis.

Clinical Formulation

At the completion of the clinical evaluation, the diagnosis may be known and limited laboratory testing may be indicated in order to confirm the diagnosis. If a definite diagnosis is lacking, a strategy should have evolved regarding the most likely diagnosis and some important questions should be addressed:

1. How serious is the illness?
2. Are the rheumatic symptoms part of a more generalized disease?
3. Can subsequent diagnostic evaluation be staged, or is there a sense of urgency in obtaining a diagnosis?
4. Does the patient require immediate hospitalization?
5. How can the laboratory be employed most efficiently and economically in clarifying the problem?

Laboratory Studies

The number of rheumatic syndromes that can be proved by laboratory examination is small. In the great majority of cases, diagnosis derives from integration of clinical information with laboratory data that are supportive or confirmatory but not definitive.

Examples of laboratory procedures with high specificity include identification of urate and calcium pyrophosphate crystals in synovial fluids of patients with gout and chondrocalcinosis syndromes, respectively, isolation of bacterial forms in patients with pyarthrosis, early recognition of osteomyelitis and avascular osteonecrosis by radionuclide bone scans, documentation of vasculitis and myositis in biopsy specimens from patients with relevant syndromes, demonstration of arterial aneurysms by arteriography in patients with vasculitis syndromes, and verification of mechanical derangements by arthrography or arthroscopy.

With the exceptions noted above, biochemical, pathologic, immunologic, and radiographic studies have statistical, not definitive, relevance to the diagnosis of rheumatic disease. Examples are rheumatoid factors in rheumatoid arthritis, antinuclear antibodies and hypocomplementemia in systemic lupus erythematosus, hyperuricemia in gout, HLA-B27 typing in the spondyloarthropathies, and increased serum enzymes in myositis syndromes. These and other laboratory procedures, although lacking absolute specificity, may be decisive when interpreted in the light of clinical information. The presence of hypocomplementemia and antinuclear antibodies (particularly anti-dsDNA antibodies) can discriminate between systemic lupus erythematosus and polyarteritis in patients with arthritis and renal disease. The radiographic demonstration of hilar adenopathy in a patient with lower extremity arthritis and erythema nodosum helps identify patients with a generally benign form of sarcoidosis (Löfgren's syndrome).

Basic Laboratory Studies

The simplicity and low cost of the routine studies listed in Table 1-1 warrant their performance in most patients presenting with undiagnosed rheumatic symptoms. Some exceptions include individuals in otherwise good health presenting with painful Heberden's nodes, shoulder bursitis, tenosynovitis, or an obvious traumatic synovitis. The erythrocyte sedimentation rate tends to separate cases into the two broad categories of inflammatory and noninflammatory rheumatism, and the routine blood studies, urinalysis, and serum chemical profile can provide clues for further study regarding the presence of systemic disease. Including uric acid and serum enzymes in automated analysis allows detection of hyperuricemia and can help identify a relatively common clinical syndrome, hepatitis B arthropathy. (Salicylate therapy can spuriously elevate uric acid levels and liver enzymes.)

Synovial Fluid Analysis

Cytologic, bacteriologic, and polarized light microscopic analysis of joint fluid provides more discriminating and diagnostic information than other categories of tests. Synovial fluid leukocyte counts in excess of 50,000 per mm^3 suggest sepsis, but levels in that range can be seen in multiple forms of inflammatory arthropathy. The importance and the specificity of polarized light microscopy and bacteriologic studies are self-evident. Regarding arthrocentesis, (1) if a joint effusion is demonstrable in an undiagnosed patient with acute synovitis, the physician should tap it, for the opportunity might pass, and (2) for bacteriologic studies, the physician should not trust routine routing of the samples to the laboratory.

Immunologic Studies

The list of serologic procedures in Table 1-1 includes the majority of tests that are relatively standardized and available in most clinical settings. The presence of anti-ds DNA antibodies is the most specific serologic feature of systemic lupus erythematosus and

Table 1-1. Laboratory Studies in Differential Diagnosis of Rheumatoid Disorders

Procedure	Usefulness in Diagnosis
Basic Studies	
Complete blood count	Simple and inexpensive tests that have nonspecific relevance to inflammatory and/or systemic disease and that are appropriate for general health assessment.
Erythrocyte sedementation rate	
Urinalysis	
Stool guaiac	
Chemical profile (automated)	Myositis—enzyme elevation, gout—hyperuricemia, liver dysfunction—hepatitis arthropathy or vasculitis, metabolic bone disease—alkaline phosphatase and serum calcium.
Synovial Fluid Studies	
Complete blood count	Differentiation of noninflammatory from inflammatory and septic disease.
Polarized Light Microscopy	
Gram stain	High relevance and specificity for gout and pseudogout.
	High relevance and specifity for bacterial synovitis (other biologic specimens should be cultured)
Culture	
Immunologic Studies	
Rheumatoid factor test	80% positive for RA but also positive in other rheumatic and nonrheumatic illnesses.
Antinuclear antibodies (ANA)	90% positive in SLE but also positive in other rheumatic and nonrheumatic illnesses.
Anti-ds DNA antibodies	70% positive in active SLE; most specific serologic test for SLE, but occasionally positive in other rheumatic syndromes.
Anti-Sm	SLE 30% (high specificity).
Anti-Ro (SS-A)	Sjögren's syndrome (60%), also in SLE.
	Congenital SLE in children of Anti-Ro mothers.
Anti-La (SS-B)	Sjögren's syndrome (40%) also SLE
Anti-nuclear ribonucleoprotein (RNP)	Mixed or undifferentiated connective tissue syndrome.
Anti-Jo-1	Polymyositis (30%).
Anti-Scl-70	Diffuse systemic sclerosis
Anti-centromere	CREST, variant of systemic sclerosis.
Anti-histone	Drug-induced SLE.
Anti-phospholipids (cardiolipin)	Procoagulant complications (including spontaneous abortion) in SLE and related syndromes.
	Associated with lupus-type anticoagulant.
Serum complement (or components)	70% abnormal (reduced) in active SLE, also reduced in other syndromes.
STS (serologic test for syphilis)	20% positive in SLE (biologic false-positive Wassermann).
FTA (flourescent treponemal antibody)	Positive in syphilis, negative in SLE.
Antistreptolysin-O	80% positive in acute rheumatic fever and in uncomplicated beta-hemolytic streptoccal infection.
Mono test	Positive indicates recent Epstein-Barr virus infection.
HB antigen	Positive indicates recent infection or carrier state, relevant to preicteric hepatitis arthropathy and to HB-associated vasculitis.
Lyme agent (Borrelia burgdorferi)	Presence of antibody indicates past or current infection, high titer favors but does not prove active infection.
Serum or urine immunoelectrophoresis	Detection of monoclonal immunoglobulins, relevant to amyloid, cryoglobulinemia, lymphoma, and detection of immunodeficiency states.
HLA-B27 antigen	HLA antigen associated with increased risk of spondyloarthropathies; important epidemiologic tool, not a diagnostic test.
Immunoglobulin quantification	Detection of monoclonal immunoglobulins, relevant to amyloid, cryoglobulinemia, lymphoma, and detection of immunodeficiency states.
Cryoglobulins	Positive in "essential" cryogobulinemia, RA, SLE, vasculitis syndromes, and lymphoproliferative diseases.

Table 1-1. Laboratory Studies in Differential Diagnosis of Rheumatoid Disorders. *Continued*

Procedure	Usefulness in Diagnosis
Microbiologic Studies	
Culture for bacterial, fungal or biologic fluids and/or tissues	High relevance and specificity for infectious arthritis (gonococcal and mycobacterial species of relevant others), and bacterial endocarditis.
Pathologic Studies	
Muscle, skin, nerve biopsies	High degree of specificity for histopathologic diagnoses (myositis, vasculitis, panniculitis), and sarcoidosis.
Temporal artery biopsy	High degree of specificity for temporal arteritis if positive, does not exclude diagnosis if negative.
Synovial biopsy	Rarely diagnostic, but important in ruling in or out infection when that is suspect.
Other biopsies	Renal (glomerulonephritis), rectal (amyloidosis), lip (Sjögren's), lymph node (lymphoma), sarcoidosis
Radiographic Studies	
Chest radiograph	Relevant to Löfgren's syndrome (hilar adenopathy), Wegener's granulomatosis, pulmonary osteoarthropathy, interstitial pneumonitis, and pleural disease.
Joint(s) radiograph	Infrequently diagnostic except in chronic forms of arthritis and CPPD.
Gastrointestinal (barium) studies	Demonstration of esophageal and pharyngeal dysmotility (myositis and PSS), ulcerative colitis, and Crohn's disease (enteropathic arthropathy).
Radionuclide bone scan	Permits early diagnosis of osteomyelitis, avascular osteonecrosis, and osteoid osteoma.
Arthrography	Demonstration of mechanical disorders or ruptured bursa.
Arteriography	Documentation of vasculitis syndromes via demonstration of aneurysms.
Magnetic resonance imaging (MRI)	Emerging as the most definative technique for imaging neural lesions relative to vasculitis, myelopathy and radiculopathy. Also for demonstration of mechanical derangements of joints and early recognition of avascular osteonecrosis.
Other Studies	
Hematologic Bone marrow	Important in considering rheumatic manifestations of leukemia, lymphoma, metastatic cancer, plasma cell dyscrasias, and disseminated tuberculosis, and in exploring bases for cytopenias.
Coombs', haptoglobin, reticulocytes, serum iron, and TIBC	Consideration of hemochromatosis arthropathy, differentiation of iron deficiency anemia from anemia of chronic disease, and evaluation of the presence of a hemolytic anemia.
Coagulation profile	Identification of intravascular coagulation in SLE and vasculitis, and the presence of circulating anticoagulants.
EMG and Nerve Conduction Studies	Aid in diagnosis of neuropathic and myopathic syndromes.
Chemistries	
Thyroid chemistries	Diagnosis of hypothyroid arthralgia syndrome or myopathy.
Lipid studies	Recognition of rheumatic complications of hyperlipidemia.
24-hour uric acid excretion	Differentiation of overproduction versus underexcretion as basis for hyperuricemia.
24-hour urine protein Creatinine clearance	Indicators of activity and severity of renal disease in patients with SLE, vasculitis, amyloidosis.

RA = rheumatoid arthritis; SLE = systemic lupus erythematosus; CREST = calcinosis, Raynaud's phenomenon, esophageal dysfunction, sclerodactyly, and telangiectasia; HB = hepatitis B; HLA = human leukocyte antigen; CPPD = calcium pyrophosphate deposition disease; PSS = progressive systemic sclerosis.

should be performed in patients with clinical features compatible with the disease who are antinuclear antibody positive. (The same rule applies to serum complement measurement, although hypocomplementemia has a lower order of specificity for systemic lupus erythematosus). Several antinuclear reactivities have been identified by immunologic techniques, but the procedures for their detection are not routine. For example, anti-Sm is relatively specific for systemic lupus erythematosus, and anti-ribonucleoprotein titers are highest in a "mixed connective tissue disease" that most closely resembles progressive systemic sclerosis. The list of autoantibodies reactive with cellular antigens (Ro, La, Jo-1, phospholipids, and so forth) is not complete and none is diagnostic, but there is a high level of research interest in the clinical associations noted. Rheumatoid factors, usually detected by the latex agglutination test, have the highest association with rheumatoid arthritis, but the results of this test rarely alter clinical impressions.

Pathologic Studies

The relevance of histopathology of biopsy specimens to diagnosis is summarized in Table 1-1. The specificity of such analyses is explicit, but multiple clinical syndromes can be associated with synovitis, myositis, necrotizing vasculitis, or glomerulonephritis. The characteristic lesions of temporal (cranial) arteritis have clear diagnostic and therapeutic implications.

Radiographic Studies

Conventional radiographic studies have significant but limited bearing on rheumatologic diagnosis, but the newer angiographic, radionuclide, and arthrographic techniques have high degrees of specificity for certain conditions (see Table 1-1). Magnetic resonance imaging (MRI) has become the most accepted technique for defining neural lesions of the head and spine. It is also useful in demonstrating internal derangement of joints and early signs of avascular osteonecrosis (Table 1-1).

Summary

The classification and differential diagnosis of rheumatic syndromes are based primarily on the recognition of characteristic clinical patterns, with laboratory data more often confirmatory than diagnostic. The medical history and physical examination can dramatically narrow the range of diagnostic possibilities and direct a more focused and economic use of the laboratory.

Bibliography

Cohen, AS, and Bennett, JC. Rheumatology and Immunology, ed 2. New York, Grune and Stratton, 1986

Katz, WA. Diagnosis and Management of Rheumatic Diseases, ed 2. Philadelphia, JB Lippincott, 1988.

Kelley, WN, Harris, ED, Jr, Ruddy, S, and Sledge, CB. Textbook of Rheumatology, ed 3. Philadelphia, WB Saunders, 1989.

Lahita, R. Systemic Lupus Erythematosus. New York, Wiley, 1986.

McCarty, DJ. Arthritis, ed 11. Philadelphia, Lea and Febiger, 1989.

Scott, JT. Copeman's Textbook of the Rheumatic Diseases, ed 6. London, Churchill Livingstone, 1986.

Utsinger, PD, Zvaifler, JN, and Erlich, GE. Rheumatoid Arthritis: Etiology, Diagnosis and Management. Philadelphia, JB Lippincott, 1985.

Chapter 2
Origin and Clinical Relevance of Autoantibodies*

KEITH B. ELKON, M.D.

Autoantibodies

Autoantibodies are immunoglobulins (Fig. 2-1) that bind via their combining sites to antigens originating in the same individuals or species (*autoantigen*). The *specificity* of the antibody is conveyed by the variable regions of the heavy (V_H) and light (V_L) chains, whereas the biologic properties (e.g., complement fixation, binding to Fc receptors) are dictated by the constant region of the heavy chains (C_H). These biologic effects depend on the immunoglobulin isotype (IgM, IgG, IgA, IgD, IgE) and subclass (IgG1–4, IgA1–2).[1] The autoantigen may be a protein, nucleic acid, carbohydrate, lipid, or a multimolecular complex.

Although any self molecule that is bound by an antibody is an antigen, this does not necessarily imply that the antigen is the *immunogen* (the molecule that induced the production of the antibody). The relationship between the antigen and immunogen is one of the central questions in autoimmunity and is discussed later in this chapter. In addition, although any antibody binding to a self antigen becomes by definition an autoantibody, the binding may or may not be relevant to autoimmune diseases (see below). *Natural* antibodies are immunoglobulins that occur in normal individuals of several species and bind to a variety of self proteins.[2] It may be these autoantibodies that serve a beneficial role in helping to clear self molecules from the circulation.[3]

The significance of an autoantibody should therefore be evaluated by considering the antibody, the antigen, and the assay used for detection. Important features of the antibody are its class, valence, titer, clonality, and affinity. IgM antibodies reflect a primary immune response, are pentavalent (hence, much more efficient in hemagglutination assays), and are usually of low affinity (therefore much more likely to bind nonspecifically). In contrast, bivalent IgG antibodies indicate persistent antigen stimulation analogous to secondary immunization. These antibodies are usually of high affinity and, after binding to their cognate antigen, produce precipitin lines in agarose gels (immunodiffusion and counterimmunoelectrophoresis assays). This type of autoantibody is prominent in multisystem and most organ-specific autoimmune diseases.

The immune response to foreign protein antigens is *polyclonal* (derived from many B cells). *Monoclonal* antibodies arise from neoplastic proliferation of a single B cell clone, or are produced by *in vitro* fusions of individual B cells in the laboratory.[4,5] The failure of monoclonal antibodies to form precipitin lines in agarose gels and their frequent cross-reactivity[6] or "polyspecificity"[7] may make the specificity of monoclonal autoantibodies difficult to establish. A large proportion of monoclonal autoantibodies, especially those obtained from humans, have the properties of natural autoantibodies (namely IgM), low affinity and polyspecificity.[8,9] Solid-phase immunoassays (hemagglutination, enzyme-linked immunoadsorbent assay [ELISA], radioimmunoassay) are influenced by total immunoglobulin levels and readily detect low affinity antibodies.[10] Consequently, these assays are more likely to give false-positive results for autoantibodies than agarose gels,

---
*Supported by grant AR 38915 and a Research Career Development Award from the National Institutes of Health.

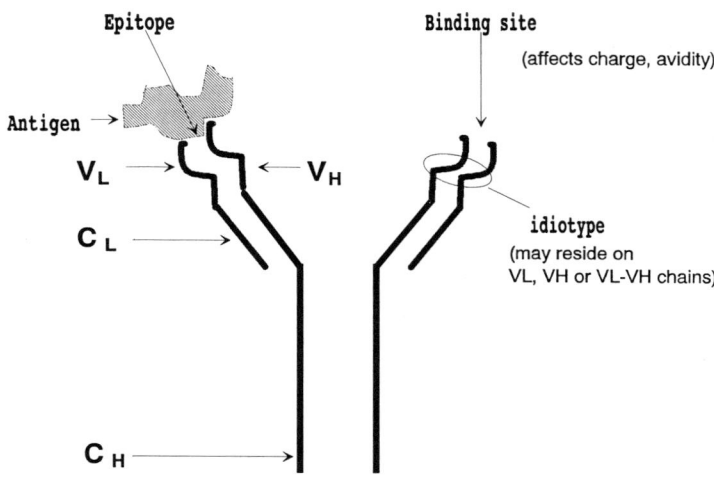

Figure 2-1. Schematic diagram of an IgG immunoglobulin showing the variable (V) and constant (C) regions of the heavy (H) and light (L) chains. The site(s) of the antigen (Ag) recognized by the antibody is called an epitope.

immunoprecipitation, or Western blotting. Finally, the nature of the antigen should be considered. Highly charged moleucles, such as DNA, histones, and IgG itself, may be bound by antibodies with oppositely charged clusters of amino acids. Haptens, by virtue of their small size and rigidity, have less contact with the antibody binding site than do large complex antigens.[11,12] With both these groups of antigens, antibody binding is likely to be less discriminating than for the complex tertiary structures of most protein antigens.

Autoimmune Diseases

Autoimmune diseases are chronic inflammatory disorders in which no obvious etiologic agents are detected, but in which autoantibodies are present in the serum. The autoimmune disease may be restricted to a single cell type or organ system or may involve multiple organ systems throughout the body. In general, the diversity of autoantibodies and immunologic abnormalities parallels the extent of the disease. For example, in one type of hemolytic anemia (paroxysmal cold hemoglobinuria) monoclonal antibodies directed against the I antigen on the red cell surface are the only autoantibodies present. In Hashimoto's thyroiditis, serum antibodies bind to thyroglobulin and thyroid peroxidase. In contrast, multisystem diseases, such as systemic lupus erythematosus (SLE) characteristically show numerous populations of autoantibodies that bind to cell surface membranes as well as to intracellular proteins and nucleic acids. The relationship between autoantibodies and disease is considered in detail later in this chapter.

Significance of Autoantibodies

In the 1960s and 1970s, a considerable volume of research in multisystem autoimmune diseases focused on anti-DNA and anti-IgG (rheumatoid factor) autoantibodies. This was as much due to their clinical diagnostic value (anti-DNA for SLE, and anti-IgG for rheumatoid arthritis) as to the relative ease with which these antigens could be isolated and used for measuring antibody levels. Although a vast amount of information was produced, much of it relevant to disease, the limitations of these studies also became apparent. In general, anti-DNA antibodies show little specificity for either the sequence or source of DNA.[13] Similarly, most rheumatoid factors react with IgG from a variety of species[14] and are induced by many inflammatory stimuli (see below). These autoantibodies, therefore, have not been informative about potential immunogens. (It remains to be seen whether the most recent studies of bacterial DNA and anti-DNA antibodies,[15] and rheumatoid factors arising as anti-idiotypic antibodies in response to Fc binding proteins on bacteria[16] provide important insight into the origins of these autoantibodies.) Additional limitations of nucleic acid and lipid antigens are that very little is known about the normal processing and cellular control of the immune response to these molecules and that the purified antigens may no longer retain the structure of the immunogen.

Proteins have a complex tertiary structure with multiple potential antigenic sites (epitopes, Fig. 2-1). Antibody specificity is, therefore, relatively easy to establish. In a few instances, antigen/antibody complexes have even been crystallized allowing amino acid contact residues to be identified.[17] Not only is the humoral immune response to foreign protein antigens well understood,[18] but the roles of the macrophage in antigen processing and presentation[19] and of T cells in regulating the response[20,21] are now known. Technologic advances of autoantibody precipitation of antigens from radiolabeled cell extracts[22] and Western blotting[23] have led to rapid characterization of protein antigens in autoimmune diseases. Molecular cloning techniques have enabled intracellular protein antigens to be synthesized in large quantities and to be used to develop sensitive immunoassays. For all these reasons much of this chapter focuses on autoantibodies to protein antigens.

The remainder of this chapter presents discussions of four important aspects of autoantibodies:

1. Their diagnostic value.
2. Their ability to cause tissue injury.
3. Their presence as a clue to basic abnormalities in autoimmune diseases.
4. A clinical approach to autoantibody screening.

Diagnostic Value and Clinical Utility of Autoantibodies

Diagnosis

Some autoantibodies, for example, rheumatoid factors, anti–single-stranded DNA and anti-cardiolipin,[24] are produced in infections as well as in a variety of autoimmune disorders, and are therefore of little help in the differential diagnosis of disease. In contrast, most of the autoantibodies found in SLE are not detected in chronic infections.[25] A partial list of autoantibodies that have diagnostic value is shown in Table 2-1. Although the clinical utility of each autoantibody depends on its disease specificity and sensitivity and therefore is different for each autoantibody certain general considerations are relevant. Few, if any, autoantibodies can be used alone to diagnose an autoimmune disease. This is because autoantibodies may be detected in individuals, particularly relatives of patients with autoimmune diseases[26] without overt clinical disease. Also, some autoantibodies, although highly specific, are present in a minority of patients. For example, anti-Sm occurs in only 20 to 30 percent of patients with SLE. For these reasons detection of autoantibodies is usually used to *confirm* a clinical diagnosis.

Table 2-1. Partial Listing of Autoantibodies That Have a High Degree of Diagnostic Specificity

Autoantigen	Disease	Ref.
Single organ/cell		
Acetylcholine receptor	Myasthenia gravis	28
Mitochondrial M2 protein complex	primary biliary cirrhosis	98
Thyroglobulin	Hashimoto's thyroiditis	99
LATS	Grave's disease	43
I	Cold hemolytic anemia	73
130 kd and 85 kd glycopeptide	Pemphigus vulgaris	100
Desmoglein	Pemphigus foliaceus	100, 101
Hemidesmosome 230 kd	Bullous pemphigoid	102
Glomerular basement membrane	Goodpasture's syndrome	103
Multisystem		
Sm	SLE	105
dsDNA	SLE	13
Ribosome P	SLE	106, 107
Ro/La	SLE, SS	108, 109
Topoisomerase, (Scl-70)	Scleroderma	33
Centromere	CREST	33
t RNA synthetases	Polymyositis	110
U1 RNP	MCTD	110, 111
Neutrophil myeloperoxidase	Wegener's granulomatosis	104

Prognosis

For the majority of autoantibodies it is uncertain whether variations in circulating antibody levels have any prognostic significance. This has been due in part to the absence of sensitive and quantitative immunoassays to measure antibody levels. However, even when these requirements have been met (e.g., for anti-DNA or anti-acetylcholine receptor antibodies), it has become apparent that antibody levels rarely show a simple correlation with disease activity and that many biologic variables influence pathogenicity. These variables include the class and subclass of the antibody,[27] epitope specificity of the antibody,[28] and the ability of the host to handle antigen-antibody complexes.[29] Despite current limitations, some autoantibodies clearly have important prognostic implications. The presence of anti-Ro (SS-A), anti-La (SS-B) antibodies in pregnant women with or without a full-blown autoimmune disease conveys a significantly increased risk of the neonatal lupus syndrome.[30] Similarly, prospective studies of anticardiolipin antibodies in pregnant women have shown a significantly elevated frequency of midtrimester fetal loss in women with high levels of such antibodies.[31,32] Certain autoantibodies are also helpful in developing subsets of patients within a disease category. For example, patients with scleroderma and an autoantibody to centromeric proteins almost always have a more benign form of the disease called the CREST syndrome.[33] Patients with SLE and anti-La antibodies are reported to have a lower incidence of renal disease.[34] It is hoped that quantitative immunoassays utilizing the newer synthetic[35] and recombinant[36-38] antigens will allow the predictive value of changes in antibody levels to be established. Initial studies measuring antiribosomal P protein antibodies against a synthetic peptide antigen have suggested that antibody levels parallel the clinical activity of certain neuropsychiatric manifestations in SLE (Fig. 2-2).[39]

Autoantibodies and Tissue Injury

Autoantibodies can be produced in response to tissue breakdown induced by trauma or infection,[40,41] but these antibodies are usually short-lived. Although certain autoantibodies in autoimmune disease may also be produced as a response to tissue injury by some other factor, there are many clear-cut examples of autoantibodies causing disease. The different mechanisms, both established and proposed, for autoantibody-mediated disease are discussed below and illustrated in Figure 2-3.

A direct role for autoantibody-mediated injury is particularly obvious for antibodies directed against cell surface membranes, for example, anti-acetylcholine receptor antibodies in myasthenia gravis,[28] lymphocytotoxic antibodies in SLE,[42] and long-acting thyroid stimulating (LATS) antibodies in thyrotoxicosis.[43] Autoantibodies that bind to surface membranes destroy the cells either by complement-mediated lysis (see Fig. 2-3A,a) or by enhancing phagocytosis by the reticuloendothelial system. Anti-acetylcholine receptor antibodies impair neuromuscular function by markedly enhancing modulation of the receptor from the cell surface (see Fig. 2-3A,b), although some degree of complement-mediated injury also occurs.[44] The LATS autoantibodies cause thyrotoxicosis by activating the thyroid stimulating hormone (TSH) receptor on thyrocytes (see Fig. 2-3A,c).[43,45] Direct autoantibody-mediated injury has also been demonstrated for the three blistering skin conditions (see Table 2-1). In these cases autoantibodies bind to specific components of the desmosomes (epithelial cell adhesion organelles) causing acantholysis and possible complement-mediated damage.[46,47]

Another well-described mechanism of tissue injury in autoimmune diseases is deposition of antigen-antibody complexes (see Fig. 2-3A,d).

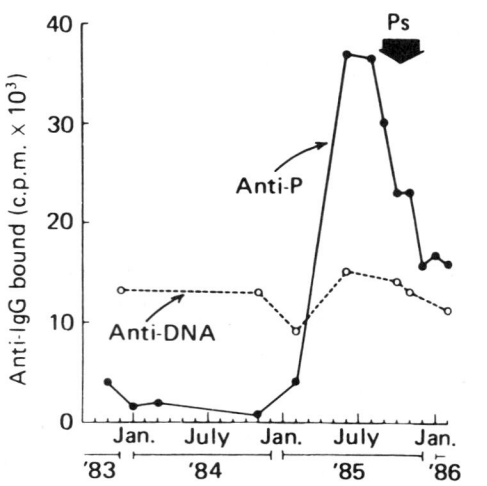
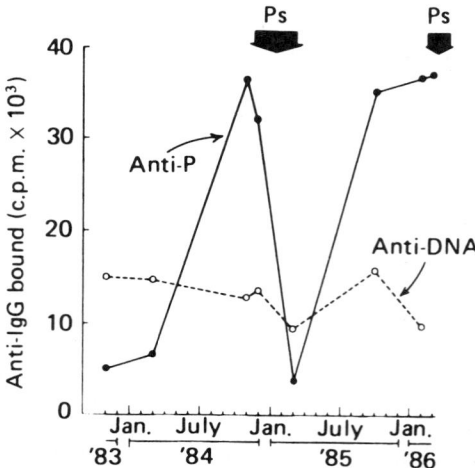

Figure 2-2. Longitudinal studies of antiribosomal P protein levels in two patients with lupus psychosis (PS) using a synthetic peptide as antigen. (Modified from Bonfa et al.[39])

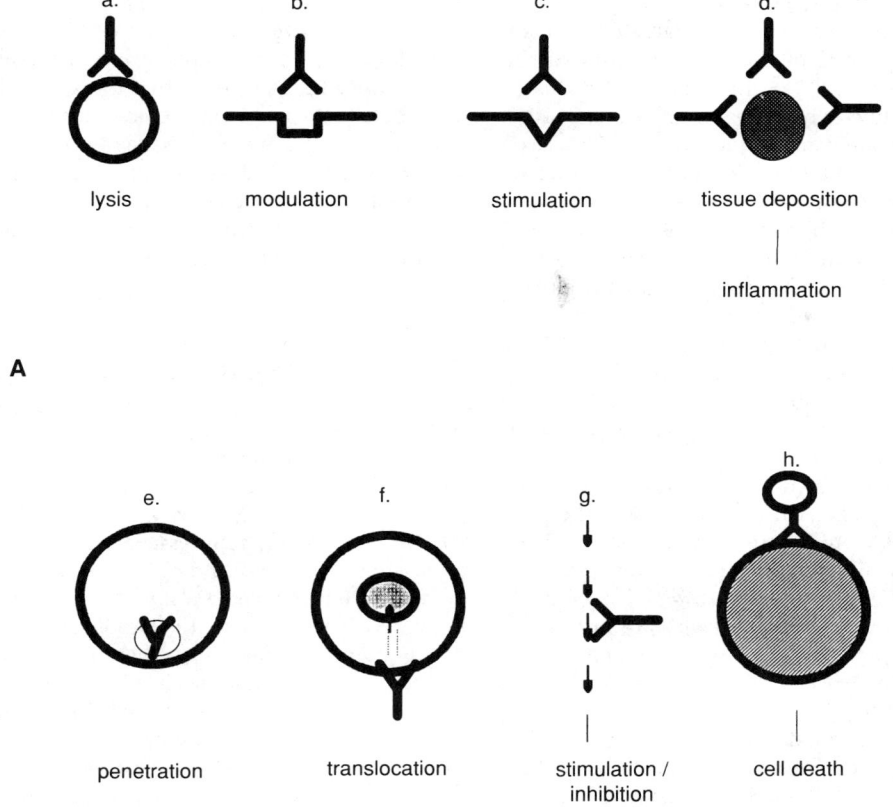

Figure 2-3. Mechanisms of autoantibody-mediated injury. Established (A) and speculative (B) mechanisms of damage. See text for details and examples.

Autoantibodies directed against intracellular proteins and nucleic acids bind to antigens released from dead cells within the circulation and deposit in vessels (causing vasculitis) or in the kidneys (causing glomerulonephritis). Although this model has been very well studied in experimental animals[48] and is at least in part responsible for nephritis in SLE,[48,49] more recent studies have questioned whether autoantibody-containing immune complexes are the major cause of tissue injury in multisystem autoimmune disorders.[50–52] Other possible mechanisms include binding of cationic autoantibodies to antigens in situ,[51] deposition of virus–anti-virus immune complexes,[53] and cell-mediated immunity.[54]

More controversial mechanisms of autoantibody-mediated injury are penetration into living cells (see Fig. 2-3B,e), translocation of intracellular antigens to the cell surface membrane (see Fig. 2-3B,f), interference with complex extracellular cascades (see Fig. 2-3B,g), and antibody-dependent cellular cytotoxicity (ADCC) (see, Fig. 2-3B,h). The evidence for antibody penetration into living cells consists of detection of IgG *within* epidermal cells on skin biopsies of some patients with SLE[55] and of IgG within a subpopulation of T lymphocytes in patients with high titer anti-RNP antibodies.[56] While it has been argued that intracellular IgG is an artefact that occurs at the time of biopsy,[57] in vitro experiments on the effect of temperature suggest that this mechanism cannot be entirely ruled out.[58] Similarly, although it seems highly unlikely that penetration occurs to any significant extent in the majority of cell types, the possibility that cells such as neurons can pinocytose IgG requires formal testing.[59] Further experiments to determine the functional effect of autoantibodies after intracellular uptake are also necessary.

Several recent studies have suggested that autoantibodies to intracellular proteins bind to cell surface membranes.[60-62] In some cases this is thought to be due to cross-reactions (e.g., anti-DNA and the LAMP antigen[60]), whereas in other cases it has been explained by translocation of the intracellular antigen following injury to the cell.[61] While the latter mechanism of tissue damage is of interest, cell surface binding could be influenced by other factors. For example, intracellular particles may be released from dead cells and adhere to the surfaces of live cells in vitro. Also, most studies are performed with polyclonal patients sera, allowing for the possibility that binding to cell surface membranes is due to antibodies primarily directed against uncharacterized membrane antigens.

While it is clear from in vitro studies with monoclonal antiphospholipid antibodies[7] and the association between prolonged clotting times and antiphospholipid antibodies[24] that autoantibodies can interfere with intravascular cascades, it remains to be shown that these autoantibodies are directly responsible for producing the clinical complications associated with their presence. Immunoconglutinins (antibodies to complement components) are another example of autoantibodies to components of an intravascular cascade. The pathogenic effects of these autoantibodies are uncertain. The mechanism shown in Figure 2-3B,h, antibody-dependent cellular cytotoxicity (ADCC), could potentially cause cell injury in vivo. Whether natural killer (NK) cells amplify the cytotoxic potential of autoantibodies directed against the cell surface is not known.

Pathogenic roles for many other autoantibodies not discussed here have been suggested (e.g., antineuronal antibodies and cerebral SLE[63]). For these antibodies, as well as for many of the antibodies mentioned above, a direct pathogenic effect and the mechanism whereby it causes disease remain to be proved. The most clear-cut way to establish a cause-effect relationship is to administer passively the antibody in question to an experimental animal and test for the effect. Such an approach has shown that anti-acetylcholine receptor antibodies are sufficient to induce myasthenia[64] and that IgG fractions from patients with pemphigus and pemphigoid induce damage to keratinocytes in vitro and in vivo.[46,47] This mode of experimental verification is more difficult in multisystem autoimmune diseases, since each patient's serum usually contains multiple autoantibodies. In addition, the possibility that human antibodies have different phlogistic properties in an experimental animal and the difficulties in maintaining high levels of antibody (and possibly of antigen) in the animal are further experimental problems.

In diseases such as scleroderma and polymyositis there is very little evidence that the autoantibodies contribute to the pathology. It seems more likely that mononuclear cells mediate tissue injury and that the autoantibodies reflect an immune response to selected self antigens (see below).

Readers interested in the structure and function of the autoantigens are referred to several reviews.[65-68]

Clues to the Origins of Autoimmunity

Autoimmunity represents a failure in the induction or maintenance of tolerance.[69] While autoreactive T cells are largely deleted in the early neonatal period,[70] potentially autoreactive B cells are not deleted but are actively suppressed.[71] It is therefore not surprising that neoplastic proliferation of B cell clones (as in myeloma or Waldenstrom's macroglobulinemia) may result in the production of monoclonal autoantibodies (e.g., rheumatoid factors,[72] anti-I,[73] anti-myelin-associated glycoprotein[74]). Several investigators have reported that autoantibodies are overrepresented among monoclonal B cell tumors.[72,75,76] While some of this increase could be explained by low affinity interactions between immunoglobulins and charged molecules such as DNA, an increase in the frequency of antibodies to selected protein antigens[76] is more difficult to explain. Whether the proposed increase reflects intrinsic properties of autoreactive B cells, a higher number of autoreactive B cell precursors, or is simply a bias of the assays remains to be determined.

In most autoimmune diseases, however, monoclonal bands are not observed, and the available evidence indicates that the autoantibodies are polyclonal. This is more obvious in multisystem autoimmune diseases in which individual patient sera react with multiple nucleic acid and protein antigens[65-67] and therefore must be derived from different clonal precursors. Moreover, when the humoral immune response to individual protein antigens has been analyzed in detail,[36-38] most sera have been found to contain antibodies to several epitopes (antigenic sites) on each protein. Autoantibody production cannot therefore be explained by an intrinsic B cell abnormality leading to unregulated proliferation of random B cells. Rather, this evidence suggested that autoantibodies are produced as a focused *immune response*. Additional evidence in favor of this theory is: (1) relative to the total number of cellular proteins, only a small number are recognized as antigens in each serum[77,78]; (2) patient sera do not show increased reactivity to the universe of protein antigens[77]; (3) the proteins recognized as antigens are often structurally or functionally related (e.g., the Sm/RNP group of proteins[65]); (4) the antibodies have the characteristics of a secondary immune response (high titer antibodies of the IgG isotype[79]); (5) analysis of the genes encoding some autoantibodies in lupus mice have shown extensive somatic mutation characteristic of an antigen-driven immune response[80]; (6) analysis of the idiotypes of anti-DNA antibodies in lupus-prone mice reveals a marked restriction[81]; and (7) as mentioned previously, antibodies considered specific for diseases, such as SLE (see Table 2-1) are not detected in chronic infectious diseases with polyclonal B cell activation.[25] A more detailed discussion of other possible mechanisms of autoantibody production, such as molecular mimicry, is presented elsewhere.[82]

While a global defect of B (e.g., intrinsic hyperactivity[83]) or T (e.g., defective suppressor function[84,85]) lymphocytes therefore seems an unlikely explanation of autoantibody production, abnormalities of either of these cell populations cannot be excluded. For example, in one model of autoimmunity, graft-versus-host disease, in which donor T helper cells stimulate host B cells, autoantibodies with some specificities similar to SLE may be observed.[86] Another important functional component of the immune system is the idiotype/anti-idiotype network[87] Although it has been shown experimentally that autoantibodies to cell surface receptors may be induced by anti-idiotypic antibodies[88] and it has been suggested that autoantibodies may arise as anti-idiotypes to anti-virus antibodies,[89] the role of the network in autoimmune disease is controversial. Nevertheless, detection of cross-reactive (public) idiotypes among certain[90] but not all[91] autoantibodies, and the identification of apparently pathogenic subsets of idiotypes[92] indicate an important role for structurally related autoantibodies.

The reasons why patients should mount an immune response to acetylcholine receptors in myasthenia gravis or to topoisomerase in scleroderma are still unknown. In theory there could be intrinsic abnormalities of any component of an immune response—the antigen, the macrophage, the B lymphocyte, or the T lymphocyte. Alternatively, it may be the interaction between an environmental factor and certain polymorphic variants in the immune system that result in a response against certain cell components. It is clear from drug-induced syndromes that environmental factors can produce autoantibodies and autoimmune diseases, although these syndromes are reversible upon withdrawal of the drugs. Since susceptibility to drug-induced[93] as well as idiopathic autoimmune diseases is influenced by age, sex, race, and major histocompatibility (MHC) type, it has frequently been proposed that idiopathic autoimmune diseases arise from an environmental agent (such as a virus) in genetically predisposed hosts. Such an agent could induce autoantibodies by modifying host (self) antigens directly, by associating with self MHC determinants, by inducing aberrant MHC class II expression and presentation of self antigens,[94] or by interfering with more complex mechanisms of lymphocyte function. Both human infectious retroviruses discovered recently, human T-cell lymphoma virus (HTLV) and human immunodeficiency virus (HIV), are lymphotropic and produce major abnormalities of T cell function. Moreover, HIV infection is associated with autoantibodies reactive with platelets, lymphocytes, and phospholipids.[95-97]

Autoantibodies in Clinical Practice

Organ-specific Autoimmune Diseases

Since most patients usually have only one organ system involved, detection of the appropriate autoantibody (see Table 2-1) in the serum is most useful to confirm the autoimmune nature of the disease. While autoantibodies are occasionally produced in infections (as discussed previously), persistently elevated titers of antibodies directed against the diseased organ indicate an autoimmune process. For the most part organ-specific autoantibodies are identified by specific patterns of staining of the appropriate cell by indirect immunofluorescence (e.g., linear staining of the glomerular basement membrane in Goodpasture's disease or staining in pemphigus). Consequently, the clinician should request the specific diagnostic test from the clinical laboratory rather than broad screening tests such as the antinuclear antibody assay (also see discussion of multisystem autoimmune diseases, below). While autoantibody levels may broadly parallel the extent of organ inflammation, therapy is dictated more by organ function than by autoantibody titers.

Multisystem Autoimmune Diseases

Autoimmune diseases are frequently considered in the differential diagnosis of skin, kidney, joint, lung, and other disorders. The simplest screening test and practical starting point is the antinuclear antibody (ANA) assay. The ANA assay is a test for any autoantibody that binds to non-tissue-specific antigens within a cell. Currently, the test is performed by indirect immunofluorescence using an epithelial cell line, Hep 2, as a substrate. This substrate is far better than mouse kidney or liver in terms of sensitivity and ability to distinguish staining patterns of autoantibodies. A negative test makes the diagnosis of a systemic autoimmune disease highly unlikely, whereas a positive test, especially at a titer ≥ 1/80, strongly supports the diagnosis. Exceptions to this rule are polyarteritis nodosa and Wegener's granulomatosis in which the ANA assay is positive in only about one third of cases. Anticytoplasmic autoantibodies are, however, more frequently detected in these diseases when neutrophils are used as a cell substrate.[104] Although the exclusive presence of anti-Ro antibodies was at one time thought to be associated with "ANA negative lupus,"[112] most patients with anti-Ro have positive ANA assays on Hep 2 cells, due possibly to the presence of the associated anti-La antibodies. Some SLE sera with exclusive antiribosomal activity are truly antinuclear antibody negative, but show strong cytoplasmic staining on Hep 2 cells.[113]

Once a positive ANA assay is obtained, identification of the actual autoantibody specificity frequently provides additional useful information. As mentioned above, certain autoantibodies have diagnostic specificity (see Table 2-1), and others help to divide patients into clinical subsets (e.g., antitopoisomerase and anti-centromere in scleroderma). Most autoantibody specificities are identified by double immunodiffusion or counterimmunoelectrophoresis, simple techniques that are available in the clinical laboratory. Autoantibodies in multisystem autoimmune disease of clinical interest are describe in Table 2-2.

Since most autoantigens are now cloned, it is highly likely that sensitive ELISAs utilizing recombinant or chemically synthesized antigens will soon replace immunodiffusion as the method of choice for detecting specific autoantibodies. The frequencies of detection and clinical applications of autoantibodies to intracellular proteins are therefore likely to change in the near future.

Table 2-2. Multisystem Autoimmune Diseases with Positive Immunofluorescence (ANA) on Hep 2 Cells

Disease	ANA Positive (%)	ANA Pattern*	Antibody Specificity	Frequency (%)	Clinical association
SLE	95	H, N	dsDNA	70	General activity, renal disease
			Ro	3	Subacute cutaneous lupus, neonatal lupus
		Fine S, N	La	15	? Less renal disease
		Coarse S, N No unstained	Sm	15–30	SLE
			RNP	50	MCTD†
		C	ribosomal P proteins	12	Psychosis
Drug-induced lupus	90	H, N	Histones	90	
Sicca syndrome	85	fine, S, N	Ro, La	70	
Myositis	50	S, N + C	Jo-1	30	
Scleroderma	80	H, N	Topoisomerase	25	Diffuse disease
		discreet S, N	Centromere	80	CREST variant
		No	RNA polymerase	10	

*H = homogeneous, S = speckled, N = nuclear, No = nucleolar, C = cytoplasmic
†Anti-RNP without anti-Sm occurs in SLE/myositis/scleroderma overlap called mixed connective tissue disease (MCTD).

Summary

Autoantibodies are heterogeneous. Some low-affinity autoantibodies may be present at low concentrations in normal sera, some are readily induced by inflammatory stimuli but decline following resolution of inflammation, and others are high affinity, persistent, and show strong associations with individual autoimmune diseases. Among the last group of autoantibodies are those that clearly cause disease (by a variety of different mechanisms) and others that more likely reflect tissue injury.

During the last 10 years there have been major advances in identifying the structure and function of intracellular protein antigens. Large-scale production of these antigens by molecular cloning and chemical synthesis (synthetic peptides) has provided essential reagents to test the role of the autoantibodies in clinical diseases. Major improvements in methods of detection of antiphospholipid antibodies have already been made and have been used to confirm the association between these antibodies and certain clinical complications.

Most autoantibodies arise from the expansion of multiple B cell clones. These antibodies have the properties of a secondary immune response. This response is highly focused on a relatively limited number of antigens that are often related in structure or function. These findings indicate that the autoantigen is itself playing an important role in induction or maintenance of autoantibody production. Exactly where the breakdown in self tolerance occurs—at the level of the antigen, the macrophage, or the lymphocyte—is still not clear, nor is it known whether exogenous agents are necessary for the breakdown to occur. Despite these uncertainties, recent insights into the genetic susceptibility to autoimmune diseases as well as intensive research in tolerance induction in the thymus and the periphery should provide important groundwork for understanding autoimmunity.

References

1. Goodman, JW: Immunoglobulins I: Structure and function. In Stites, DP et al (eds): Basic and Clinical Immunology, ed. 5. Los Angeles, Lange, 1984, p 30.
2. Guilbert, B, Dighiers, G, and Avrameas, S: Naturally occurring antibodies against nine common antigens in normal human sera. I. Detection, isolation, and characterization. J Immunol 128:2779, 1982.
3. Grabar, P: Autoantibodies and immunological theories: An analytical review. Clin Immunol Immunopathol 4:453, 1975.
4. Kohler, G, and Milstein C: Continuous cultures of fused cells secreting antibody of predefined specificity. Nature 256:495, 1975.
5. Steinitz, M et al: EB-induced B lymphocyte cell lines producing specific antibody. Nature 269:420, 1977.
6. Dales, S, Fujinami, RS, and Oldstone, MBA: Infection with vaccinia favors the selection of hybridomas synthesizing autoantibodies against intermediate filaments, one of them cross-reacting with the virus hemagglutinin. J Immunol 131:1546, 1983.
7. Lafer, EM et al: Polyspecific monoclonal lupus autoantibodies reactive with both polynucleotides and phospholipids. J Exp Med 153:897, 1981.
8. Garzelli, C et al: Epstein-Barr virus transformed lymphocytes produce monoclonal autoantibodies that react with antigens in multiple organs. J Virol 52:722, 1984.
9. Seigneurin, JM et al: Polyspecific natural antibodies and autoantibodies secreted by human lymphocytes immortalized with Epstein-Barr virus. Blood 71:581, 1988.
10. Jemmerson, R: Antigenicity and native structure of globular proteins: Low frequency of peptide reactive antibodies. Proc Natl Acad Sci USA 84:9180, 1987.
11. Padlan, EA et al: Model building studies of antigen binding sites: The hapten binding site of MOPC—315. Cold Spring Harbor Symp Quant Biol 41:627, 1976.
12. Padlan, EA et al: Structural basis for the specificity of phosphorylcholine-binding immunoglobulins. Immonochem 13:945, 1976.
13. Stage, DE, and Mannik, M: Rheumatoid factors in rheumatoid arthritis. Bull Rheum Dis 23:720, 1973.
14. Zouali, M, Stollar, BD, and Schwartz, RS: Origin and diversification of anti-DNA antibodies. Immunol Rev 105:137, 1988.
15. Karounos, DG, Grudier, JP, and Pisetsky, DS: Spontaneous expression of antibodies to DNA of various species origin in sera of normal subjects and patients with systemic lupus erythematosus. J Immunol 140:451, 1988.
16. Oppliger, IR, et al: Human rheumatoid factors bear the internal image of the Fc binding region of staphylococcal protein A. J Exp Med 166:702, 1987.
17. Amit, AG et al: Three-dimensional structure of an antigen-antibody complex at 2.8 A resolution. Science 233:747, 1986.
18. Berzofsky, J: Intrinsic and extrinsic factors in protein antigenic structure. Science 229:932, 1989.
19. Unanue, ER: Antigen presenting function of the macrophage. Ann Rev Immunol 2:395, 1984.
20. Howard, JC: Immunological help at last. Nature 314:494, 1985.
21. Kronenberg, M et al: The molecular genetics of the T cell antigen receptor and T cell antigen recognition. Ann Rev Immunol 4:529, 1986.
22. Lerner, MR, and Steitz, JA: Antibodies to small nuclear RNAs complexed with proteins are produced by

patients with systemic lupus erythematosus. Proc Natl Acad Sci USA 76:5495, 1979.
23. Towbin, HT, Staehelin, T, and Gordon, J: Electrophoretic transfer of proteins from polyacrylamide gels to nitrocellulose sheets: Procedure and some applications. Proc Natl Acad Sci USA 76:4350, 1979.
24. Harris, EN et al: Anticardiolipin antibodies: Detection by radioimmunoassay and association with thrombosis in systemic lupus erythematosus. Lancet ii:1211, 1983.
25. Bonfa, E et al: Comparison between autoantibodies in malaria and leprosy with lupus. Clin Exp Immunol 70:529, 1987.
26. Cleland, LG et al: Familial lupus: Family studies in HLA and serologic findings. Arthritis Rheum 21:183, 1978.
27. Schur, PH: IgG subclasses: A review. Ann Allergy 58:89, 1987.
28. Tzartos, SJ, Seybold, MF, and Lindstrom, JM: Specificities of antibodies to acetylcholine receptor in sera from myasthenia gravis patients measured by monoclonal antibodies. Proc Natl Acad Sci USA 79:188, 1982.
29. Haakenstad, AO, and Mannik, M: Saturation of the reticuloendothelial system with soluble immune complexes. J Immunol 112:1939, 1974.
30. Lockshin, MD et al: Neonatal lupus risk to newborns of mothers with systemic lupus erythematosus. Arthritis Rheum 31:697, 1988.
31. Derue, GJ et al: Fetal loss in systemic lupus: Association with anticardiolipin antibodies. J Obstet Gynol Neonatal Nurs 5:207, 1985.
32. Lockshin, MD et al: Antibody to cardiolipin predicts fetal distress or death in pregnant patients with systemic lupus erythematosus. N Engl J Med 313:152, 1985.
33. Tan, EM et al: Diversity of antinuclear antibodies in progressive systemic sclerosis. Arthritis Rheum 23:617, 1980.
34. Wasicek, CA, and Reichlin, M: Clinical and serological differences between systemic lupus erythematosus patients with antibodies to Ro versus patients with antibodies to Ro and La. J Clin Invest 69:835, 1982.
35. Elkon, KB et al: The identification and synthesis of a ribosomal protein antigenic determinant in systemic lupus erythematosus. Proc Natl Acad Sci USA 83:7419, 1986.
36. Earnshaw, WC et al: Analysis of anticentromere autoantibodies using cloned autoantigen CENP-B. Proc Natl Acad Sci USA 84:4979 1987.
37. St. Clair, EW et al: Quantitative immunoassays of anti-La antibodies using purified recombinant La antigen. Arthritis Rheum 31:506, 1988.
38. Netter, HJ et al: A recombinant autoantigen derived from the human (U1) small nuclear RNP-specific 68 Kd protein. Arthritis Rheum 31:616, 1988,
39. Bonfa, E et al: Association between lupus psychosis and antiribosomal P protein antibodies: Measurement of antibody using a synthetic peptide antigen. N Engl J Med 317:265, 1987.
40. Tardiou, M et al: Autoimmunity following viral infection. Eur J Immunol 14:561, 1984.
41. Bacon, PA, Davidson, C, and Smith, C: Antibodies to Candida and autoantibodies in subacute bacterial endocarditis Q J Med 43:537, 1974.
42. Terasaki, PI, Motticoni, VD, and Barnet, EV: Cytotoxins in disease: Autocytotoxins in lupus. N Engl J Med 283:724, 1970.
43. Adams DD, and Kennedy, TH: Occurrence in thyrotoxicosis of a gamma globulin which protects LATS from neutralization by an extract of thyroid gland. J Clin Endocrin Metab 27:113, 1967.
44. Drachman, DB et al: Humoral pathogenesis of myasthenia gravis. Ann NY Acad Sci 505:90, 1987.
45. Kohn, LD et al: Monoclonal antibody studies defining the origin and properties of autoantibodies in Graves' disease. Ann NY Acad Sci 475:157, 1986.
46. Schiltz, JR, and Michel, B: Production of epidermal acantholysis in normal human skin in vitro by the IgG fraction from pemphigus serum. J Invest Dermatol 67:254, 1976.
47. Anhalt, GJ et al: Induction of pemphigus in neonatal mice by passive transfer of IgG from patients with the disease. N Engl J Med 306:1189, 1982.
48. Cochrane, CG, and Koffler, D: Immune complex disease in experimental animals and man. Adv Immunol 18:67, 1974.
49. Krishnan, C, and Kaplan, MH: Immunopathologic studies of systemic lupus erythematosus. II. Antinuclear reaction of gammaglobulin eluted from homogenates and isolated glomeruli of kidneys from patients with lupus nephritis. J Clin Invest 46:569, 1967.
50. Izui, S, Lambert, DH, and Miescher, PA: Failure to detect circulating DNA–anti-DNA complexes by four radioimmunological methods in patients with systemic lupus erythematosus. Clin Exp Immunol 30:384, 1977.
51. Vogt, A: New aspects of the pathogenesis of immune complex glomerulonephritis: Formation of subepithelial deposits. Clin Nephrol 21:15, 1984
52. Tanaka, A et al: Etiopathogenesis of rheumatoid arthritis-like disease in MRL/lpr mice. II. Ultrastructural basis of joint destruction. J Rheumatol 15:6, 1988.
53. Yoshiki, T et al: The viral envelope glycoprotein of murine leukemia virus and the pathogenesis of immune complex glomerulonephritis of New Zealand mice. J Exp Med 140:1011, 1974.
54. Zamvil, S et al: T cell clones specific for myelin basic protein in induce chronic relapsing paralysis and demyelination. Nature 317:355, 1985.
55. Tan, EM, and Kunkel, HG: An immunofluorescent study of the skin lesions in systemic lupus eyrthematosus. Arthritis Rheum 9:37, 1966.
56. Alarcon-Segovia, D, Ruiz-Arguelles, A, and Fishbein, E: Antibody to nuclear ribonucleoprotein penetrates

live human mononuclear cells through Fc receptors. Nature 271:67, 1978.
57. Gilliam, JN: The significance of cutaneous immunoglobulin deposits in lupus erythematosus and NZB/NZW F1 hybrid mice. J Invest Dermatol 65:154, 1976.
58. Galoppin, L, and Saurat, JH: In vitro study of the binding of antiribonucleoprotein antibodies to the nucleus of isolated living keratinocytes. J Invest Dermatol 76:264, 1981.
59. Graus, F et al: Sensory neuropathy and small cell lung cancer: An antineuronal antibody that also reacts with the tumor. Am J Med 80:45, 1986.
60. Jacob, L et al: Presence of antibodies against a cell surface protein, cross-reactive with DNA in systemic lupus erythematosus: A marker of the disease. Proc Natl Acad Sci USA 84:2956, 1987.
61. Lefeber, WP: Ultraviolet light induces binding of antibodies to selected nuclear antigens, on cultured human keratinocytes. J Clin Invest 74:1545, 1984.
62. Holers, VM, and Kotzin, BL: Human peripheral blood monocytes display surface antigens recognized by monoclonal antinuclear antibodies. J Clin Invest 76:991, 1985.
63. Zvaifler, NJ, and Bluestein, HG: The pathogenesis of central nervous system manifestations of systemic lupus erythematosus. Arthritis Rheum 25:862, 1982.
64. Tokya, KSV et al: Myasthenia gravis: Passive transfer from man to mouse. Science 397, 1975.
65. Steitz, JA et al: Small ribonucleoproteins from eukaryotes: Structure and roles in RNA biogenesis. Cold Spring Harbor Symp Quant Biol 47:893, 1983.
66. Christian, CL, and Elkon, KB: Autoantibodies to intracellular proteins: Clinical and biological implications. Am J Med 80:53, 1986.
67. Tan, EM: Antinuclear antibodies: Diagnostic markers for autoimmune diseases and probes for cell biology. Adv Immunol 44:93, 1989.
68. Chan, EKL, and Tan, EM: Human autoantibody reactive epitopes on SS-B/La are highly conserved in comparison with epitopes recognized by murine monoclonal antibodies. J Exp Med 166:1627, 1987.
69. Nossal, GJV: Cellular mechanisms of immunological tolerance. Ann Rev Immunol 1:33, 1983.
70. Kappler, JW, Roehm, N, and Marrack, P: T cell tolerance by clonal elimination in the thymus. Cell 49:273, 1987.
71. Goodnow, CC et al: Altered immunoglobulin expression and functional silencing of self reactive B lymphocytes in transgenic mice. Nature 334:676, 1988.
72. Seligman, M, and Brouet, JC: Antibody activity of human myeloma globulins. Semin Hematol 10:163, 1973.
73. Cooper, AG: Purification of cold agglutinins from patients with chronic cold haemagglutinin disease. Clin Exp Immunol 3:691, 1968.
74. Ilyas, AA et al: Polyneuropathy with monoclonal gammopathy: Glycolipids are frequently antigens for IgM paraproteins. Proc Natl Acad Sci USA 82:6697, 1985.
75. Livneh, A et al: Preferential expression of the systemic lupus erythematosus-associated idiotype 8.12 in sera containing monoclonal immunoglobulins. J Immunol 139:3730, 1987.
76. Sestak, AL: Lupus/Sjögren's autoantibody specificities in sera with paraproteins. J Clin Invest 80:138, 1987.
77. Gharavi, AE, Chu, JL, and Elkon, KB: Autoantibodies in systemic lupus erythematosus are not due to random polyclonal B cell activation. Arthritis Rheum 31:1337, 1988.
78. Hardin, JA et al: Antibodies from patients with connective tissue diseases bind specific subsets of cellular RNA protein particles. J Clin Invest 70: 141, 1982.
79. Maddison, PJ, and Reichlin, M: Quantitation of precipitating antibodies to certain soluble nuclear antigens in SLE: Their contribution to hypergammaglobulinemia. Arthritis Rheum 20:819, 1977.
80. Shlomchik, MJ et al: The role of clonal selection and somatic mutation in autoimmunity. Nature 328:805, 1900.
81. Hahn, B, and Ebling, FM: Idiotype restrictions in murine lupus: High frequency of three public idiotypes on serum IgG in nephritic NZB/NZW F1 mice. J Immunol 138:2110, 1987.
82. Elkon, KB: Epitope mapping of autoantigens using recombinant proteins and synthetic peptides. Clin Exp Rheumatol, in press.
83. Theofilopoulos AN, and Dixon, FJ: Etiopathogenesis of murine systemic lupus erythematosus. Immunol Rev 55:179, 1981.
84. Abdou, NI et al: Suppressor T cell abnormality in idiopathic systemic lupus erythematosus. Clin Immunol Immunopathol 6:192, 1976.
85. Bresnihan, B, and Jasin, JE: Suppressor function of peripheral blood mononuclear cells in normal individuals and in patients with systemic lupus erythematosus. J Clin Invest 59:106, 1977.
86. Gleichmann, E, Van Elven, EH, and van der Veen, JPW: A systemic lupus erythematosus (SLE)-like disease in mice induced by T-B cell cooperation. Preferential formation of autoantibodies characteristic of SLE. Eur J Immunol 12:152, 1982.
87. Jerne, NK: Towards a network theory of the immune system. Ann Immunol (Inst. Pasteur) 125C:373, 1974.
88. Erlanger, BF et al: The auto-anti-idiotypic route to antireceptor antibodies. Ann NY Acad Sci 475:219, 1986.
89. Plotz, PH: Autoantibodies are anti-idiotype antibodies to antiviral antibodies. Lancet ii, 824, 1983.
90. Fong, S et al: Structural similarities in the kappa light chains of human rheumatoid factor: Paraproteins and serum immunoglobulins bearing a cross-reactive idiotype. J Immunol 135:1955, 1985.
91. Horsfall, AC et al: Idiotypes on antibodies to the La (SS-B) antigen are restricted and associated with the antigen binding site. Clin Exp Immunol 63:395, 1986.
92. Kaine, J, and Hahn, BH: Idiotypic characteristics of immunoglobulins associated with systemic lupus

erythematosus: Studies of antibodies deposited in glomeruli of humans. Arthritis Rheum 32:513, 1989.
93. Batchelor, JR, Welsh, KL, and Tinoco, RM: Hydralazine-induced systemic lupus erythematosus: Influence of HLA-DR and sex on susceptibility. Lancet i, 1107, 1980.
94. Londei, M et al: Epithelial cells expressing aberrant MHG class II determinants can present antigen to cloned human T cells. Nature 312:639, 1984.
95. Stricker, RB et al: Target platelet antigen in homosexual men with immune thrombocytopenia. N Engl J Med 313:1375, 1985.
96. Pruzanski, W, Jacobs, H, and Laing, LP: Lymphocytotoxic antibodies against peripheral blood B and T lymphocytes in homosexuals with AIDS and ARC. AIDS Res 3:211, 1984.
97. Gold, JE, Haubenstock, A, and Zalusky, R: Lupus anticoagulant and AIDS. N Engl J Med 314:1252, 1986.
98. Berg, PA et al: ATPase associated antigen (M2): Marker antigen for serological diagnosis of primary biliary cirrhosis. Lancet ii, 1423, 1982.
99. Roitt, IM et al: The cytoplasmic autoantigen of the human thyroid: Immunological and biochemical characteristics. Immunology 7:375, 1964.
100. Stanley, JR, and Koulu-Thioviolet, C: Distinction between epidermal antigens binding pemphigus vulgaris and pemphigus foliaceus autoantibodies. J Clin Invest 74:313, 1984.
101. Jones, JCR, Yokoo, KM, and Goldman, RD: Further analysis of pemphigus autoantibodies and their use in studies on the heterogeneity, structure, and function of desmosomes. J Cell Biol 102:1109, 1986.
102. Mueller, S, Klaus-Koutun, V, and Stanley, JR: A. 230 kD basic protein is the major bullous pemphigoid antigen. J Invest Dermatol 92:33, 1989.
103. Saus, J et al: Identification of the Goodpasture antigen as the alpha 3 (IV) chain of collagen IV. J Biol Chem 263:1337, 1988.
104. Falk, RJ, and Jenette, JC: Antineutrophil cytoplasmic autoantibodies with specificity for myeloperoxidase in patients with systemic vasculitis and idiopathic necrotizing and crescentic glomerulonephritis. N Engl J Med 318:1651, 1988.
105. Notman, DD, Kurata, N, and Tan, EM: Profiles of antinuclear antibodies in systemic rheumatic diseases. Ann Intern Med 8:464, 1975.
106. Elkon, KB, Parnassa, AP, and Foster, CL: Lupus autoantibodies target ribosomal P proteins. J Exp Med 162:459, 1985.
107. Francoeur, AM et al: Identification of ribosomal protein autoantigens. J Immunol 135:2378, 1985.
108. Clark, G, Reichlin, M, and Tomasi, TB: Characterization of a soluble cytoplasmic antigen reactive with sera from patients with systemic lupus erythematosus. J Immunol 102:117, 1969.
109. Alspaugh, MA, Talal, N, and Tan, EM: Differentiation and characterization of autoantibodies and their antigens in Sjögren's syndrome. Arthritis Rheum 19:216, 1976.
110. Nishikai, M, and Reichlin, M: Heterogeneity of precipitating antibodies in polymyositis and dermatomyositis: Characterization of the Jo-1 antibody system. Arthritis Rheum 23:881, 1980.
111. Matthews, MB et al: Anti-threonyl-tRNA synthetase, a second myositis-related autoantibody. J Exp Med 160:420, 1984.
112. Provost TT: Subsets in systemic lupus erythematosus. J Inv Dermatol 72:110, 1979.
113. Bonfa, E, and Elkon, KB: Clinical and serological associations of the antiribosomal P protein antibody. Arthritis Rheum 29, 1986.

Chapter 3
Rheumatoid Arthritis

NINA BHARDWAJ, M.D., PH.D.
STEPHEN A. PAGET, M.D.

Rheumatoid arthritis (RA) is a chronic, systemic, inflammatory disease manifested by a symmetric polyarthritis, constitutional features and, at times, significant visceral involvement. The disease has a broad range of clinical manifestations and presentations. The inflammatory joint disease may vary from mild arthralgias to destructive, erosive disease involving all joints of the upper and lower extremities. Rarely, patients may develop a polyarteritis nodosa–like disorder manifested by major visceral disease due to an inflammatory, occlusive vasculopathy.[1] There are both clinically and serologically defined subsets of RA stimulating the concept that what we call RA may not be a single disease. Instead it could represent a collection of several diseases with similar features.[2] The truth may be defined by further investigation of the etiology and pathogenesis of this inflammatory polyarthritis. It is now believed that RA probably results from complex interactions and sequences of events related to the host's genetic makeup, environment, and inciting agents.[3] For over 50 years, an infectious etiology for RA has been sought. The characterization of a Borrelia spirochete as the cause of Lyme disease, a disorder with many RA-like clinical phenomena, has further supported an initial infectious stimulus for RA. Despite an extensive array of techniques to isolate microorganisms or identify microbial particles, a microbial cause for RA has not been defined.[4,5] Although the inciting agents of RA have not been identified, it is clear that humoral and cell-mediated immunologic abnormalities do exist in patients with RA and clearly contribute to the prominent inflammatory and destructive processes occurring in joints and other tissues. It is believed that after an initial trigger, a genetically predisposed host develops a self-perpetuating inflammatory and immunologic disorder leading to enzymatic breakdown of joints and other organ systems. Normally protective immunologic and proteolytic mechanisms "turn against themselves" and lead to the characteristic clinical and histologic picture of RA.[6]

Because of our ignorance of the basic pathogenesis of RA, our therapeutic armamentarium remains nonspecific. Anti-inflammatory drugs such as nonsteroidal anti-inflammatory drugs and corticosteroids may have profound effects on the inflammatory process but do not have an ameliorative action on the natural history of the disease.[7] That the disease process can persist despite strong suppressive effects on the state of inflammation supports the concept that the entire story about the inflammatory state and its role in the progression of RA has not been written. Gold salts and antimalarial drugs have been called "remittive drugs" but it is clear that only a portion of patients respond to these agents. Further, while some patients do respond with varying control of the disease state, in many the drugs are discontinued because of eventual lack of efficacy.[8] Immunosuppressive drugs such as azathioprine and methotrexate have been borrowed from oncologists in an attempt to "reset" the aberrant immunologic state found in RA patients. While these drugs are efficacious, many patients do not respond or break through their effectiveness.[9] Plasmapheresis, lymphophoresis, thoracic duct drainage, and total nodal irradiation have been more important in their ability to define immune cell types involved in the pathogenesis of RA than in their efficacy as generally used, practical therapeutic modalities.[10]

Epidemiology

The prevalence (i.e., the frequency of a disease in a defined population) of clinically recognizable RA as defined by the American Rheumatology Association criteria is consistently between 1 and 2 percent of the adult population in every part of the world. The prevalence of RA clearly increases with age in both males and females, exceeding 10 percent in persons age 65 and older. The incidence (i.e., the number of *new* cases of a disease that appear in a defined population within a defined period) of RA varies from a high of 2.9 to a low of 0.097 per 1000 population with an increase with each decade of life. Most population surveys agree that there is a female to male predominance with an overall ratio of 2.5 females to each male. This female predominance may become less prominent in patients over age 65. In one study, women had a mean age of onset of 40.8 years compared with 44.6 years in men. All races have equal susceptibility to RA.[2]

Epidemiologic studies have suggested that certain socioeconomic factors are related to RA. In men, there is a distinct trend toward decreasing prevalence of RA with higher education. Among men, the prevalence of RA in the lowest income bracket was twice that expected. There also appears to be a worse overall prognosis and functional outcome in poorer and less educated patients.[11,12]

Regarding disease outcome, the following statements can be made: (1) A poorer prognosis, erosive radiologic joint changes, and the presence of extra-articular disease manifestations are associated with rheumatoid factor positivity; (2) A poorer prognosis and greater disability is associated with radiographic evidence of erosions; (3) Advanced age at study entry was the most powerful predictor of eventual functional disability. Functional incapacitation was related not only to overall frailty but also to the superimposition of comorbid disorders such as cardiovascular disease; (4) Women tend to have more chronic and disabling disease than men; and (5) Insidious onset, delay in treatment, and poor initial response to treatment have been cited as pointing to poor outcome. A *more favorable outcome* may be associated with the following: disease of short duration, less swollen upper extremity joints in the early course of the disease, initial asymmetric joint involvement, acute onset under age 30, favorable initial response to treatment, male sex, and black race. A followup evaluation of a population study was interesting in that there were a significant number of patients who were initially thought to have probable or definite RA but who, on followup, had no evidence of disease or whose illness was downgraded in disease severity. These findings suggest that RA may exist frequently as a benign, self-limited, nondeforming condition.[2]

Data from the US National Health Examination Survey indicated that one third of 3.6 million adult patients with RA in the United States between ages 35 and 50 in the period 1960 to 1962 were disabled. The impact of RA can be defined not only in terms of physical disability but also in significant financial, social, and psychologic costs.

Recent studies examining survivorship in RA clearly demonstrate that the disease is associated with premature death. It was found that in patients over age 55, the survivorship of men with RA was 6 years less than that in the general population, and, in women, the reduction of life expectancy was 12 years. Age is the most strongly correlated variable and disability the second. Shorter survivorship is thought to reflect functional incapacitation, prolonged immobility, general debility from a chronic wasting disease, increased risk of infection due to a disease-induced immunodepressed state, organ dysfunction from extra-articular disease manifestations, and complications from medications (including infections, peptic ulcer disease, bone marrow suppression, and long-term side effects from corticosteroids).[2,13-16]

Etiology and Pathogenesis

Although the clinical features of RA and its treatment and therapy are now better defined, much still remains to be learned regarding its pathogenesis. The discovery of rheumatoid factor (RF) almost 50 years ago and the detection of other autoantibodies (e.g., antinuclear antibodies, anticollagen antibodies) led to the concept that RA was an autoimmune disorder. It is now clear that immunologic mechanisms are of crucial importance in the development of this chronic disabling disease and it has become apparent that both the cellular and humoral arms are intimately involved. In order to understand and appreciate this statement, it is necessary to review the pathology of the rheumatoid joint during the disease process.

Pathology of the Rheumatoid Joint

Articular Lesions

The early changes accompanying the onset of RA occur in the synovium and blood vessels underlying this tissue. Initially there is exudation with congestion and edema of the synovial lining, followed by effusion into the joint space. Polymorphonuclear cells (PMNs) emigrate into the synovial lining and space and are soon followed by lymphocytic infiltrates.[17] Over the next 3 to 6 months chronic features resulting in the histopathologic changes characteristic of RA appear. These include hyperplasia and thickening of the synovial lining, proliferation of blood vessels, and infiltration of the synovial lining with immunocompetent cells. T cells invade the thickened synovium presumably through high endothelial venules, and form aggregates and even lymphoid follicles resembling germinal centers suggesting that controlled mechanisms govern the development of this "pannus" of granulation tissue (Fig. 3-1).[17] T cells are abundant in the rheumatoid pannus. They consist of CD4+ T cells, the helper subpopulation, and CD8+ T cells, which are the suppressor or cytotoxic T-cell group. An interesting pattern has emerged from the study of the location of these T-cell subsets. The CD4+ cells appear to be closely apposed to dendritic cells near the high endothelial cell bearing venules.[18] Dendritic cells are important stimulator cells for several T-cell dependent responses.[19] The consistent appearance of these aggregates suggests that dendritic cells may be presenting antigen to the T cells in situ. In contrast, the CD8+ cells are less localized and lie between these aggregates adjacent to macrophages.[18] Plasma cells also invade the synovium. These can be found in the germinal centers synthesizing immunoglobulin and even RF.[20] Eventually, the granulation tissue that forms expands and grows over the adjacent articular lining and cartilage damage ensues (see Fig. 3-1). Subchondral bone lesions also develop and there is osteolysis, cyst formation, and bony erosions in regions not covered by articular cartilage.[20] The mechanisms affecting these changes have not been defined.

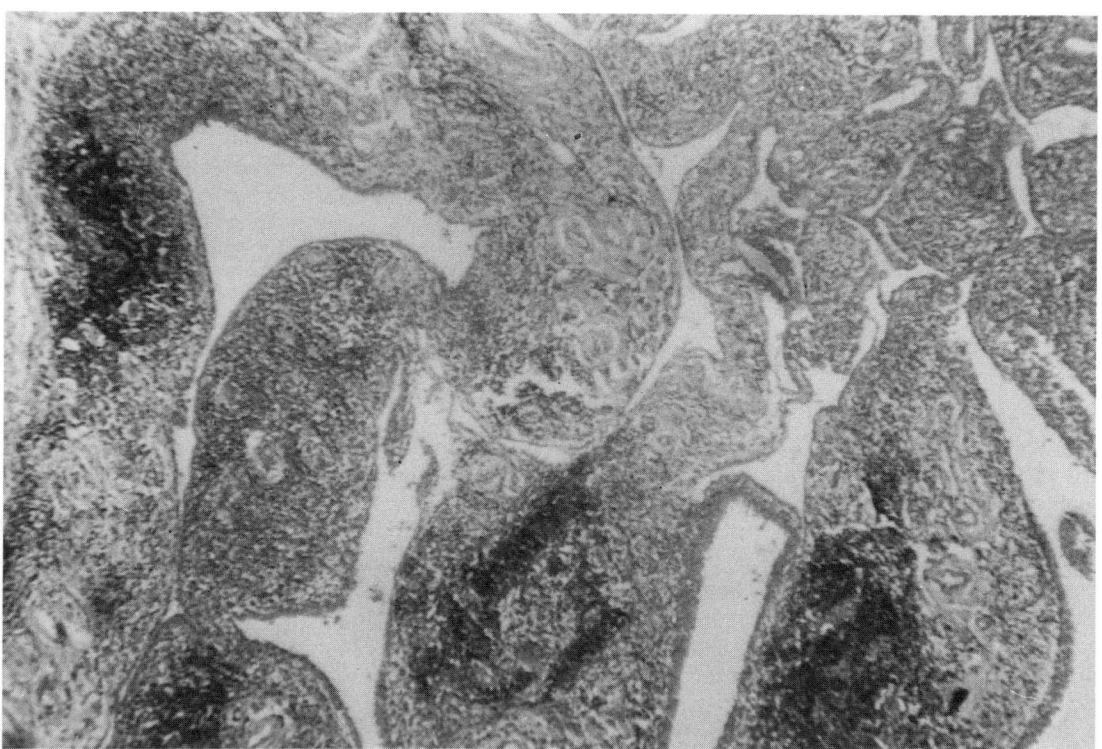

Figure 3-1. Synovial histology in rheumatoid arthritis showing exuberant granulation tissue in proliferating villi and the deeper layers (H and E, × 200). (Courtesy of Gower Medical Publishing Ltd, London, UK. Slide Atlas of Rheumatology. Introduction to Rheumatoid Arthritis, 1983).

Synovial Effusions

Accumulation of exudative fluid in the joint cavity is a counterpart of the pathologic processes that occur within the rheumatoid joint. Most intriguingly, many types of immunocompetent cells localize within this space. The most common cell is the PMN, which may comprise 90 percent or more of the cellular population.[18] The remaining cells consist of monocytes (20 to 40%), T cells (up to 75%), B cells (5%), and dendritic cells (1 to 10% of the mononuclear population).[21] The T-cell CD4/CD8 (helper/cytotoxic) ratio is decreased (1:2) compared with that seen in peripheral blood (2:1), and the T cells bear markers of activation, notably acquisition of surface Ia antigen, Tac antigen (interleukin-2 receptor), and VLA-1 (very late antigen-1), suggesting they have undergone stimulation at some point.[18,22,23] The B cells synthesize RF in vitro also indicating prior activation. Recent studies have identified an important leukocyte known as the dendritic cell in synovial effusions. These cells are distinguishable from monocytes by their dendritic appearance, lack of classic monocyte markers, and inability to phagocytose.[24] Their most important functional characteristic is the ability to present several types of antigen to T cells,[19] and their presence in joint effusions in amounts tenfold to a hundredfold greater than blood suggests that they are involved in the immunopathology of rheumatoid joint disease.[21]

Synovial effusions also contain many soluble biologic mediators including cytokines, proteins that are synthesized by lymphocytes (lymphokines), and monocytes (monokines) usually following activation. These mediators have profound effects on other cellular constituents including synovial cells, chondrocytes, and mononuclear cells of the immune system. For example, interleukin-6 (IL-6), found in large quantities in rheumatoid effusions,[25,26] is a T-cell growth factor and promotes immunoglobulin production by B cells and the release of acute phase reactants by hepatocyte lines.[27] In addition to the ability of these cytokines to modulate the function of immunoreactive cells, they can regulate several properties of connective tissue elements. Interleukin-1 (IL-1) and tumor necrosis factor (TNF) both promote the release of prostaglandin E_2 (PGE_2), plasminogen activator, and collagenase.[28,29] These factors augment tissue destruction in the joint and have adverse vascular effects such as increasing vessel permeability. More recently, interleukin-8 (IL-8) has been shown to be present at high levels in synovial effusions. This cytokine, which has multiple effects on leukocytes, also causes the activation and migration of PMNs.[30] These properties may account for several of the phenomena observed in the joint lining as described above. A listing of the cytokines identified thus far in rheumatoid effusions is presented in Table 3-1.

Other important agents that may mediate connective tissue destruction of the joint in RA are the neutral proteinases stromelysin and collagenase. Messenger ribonucleic acid (mRNA) for both these products has recently been identified in the synovial lining layer[31,33] and these proteins have been described in the joint fluid.[34]

Eicosanoids are also important inflammatory mediators that contribute to the inflammatory process in RA.[37] These products of the cyclo-oxygenase and lipo-oxygenase pathways are central in the goals of antirheumatic therapy, for their inhibition or antagonism of their synthesis can result in improvement of clinical manifestations. Their production in the joint can be activated by several factors including IL-1, TNF, platelet-derived growth factor (PDGF), and epidermal growth factor.[37] Recent studies have suggested that at least in some cases, joint disease and/or autoimmune manifestations may be reduced by the ingestion of marine lipids, which alter the ability of tissues to generate cyclo-oxygenase and lipo-oxygenase byproducts. Some reduction in inflammatory activity in RA has been reported in patients taking large amounts of marine oils.[38] However, more intensive studies will need to be undertaken to determine the efficacy of this therapy in RA.

Table 3-1. Cytokines in Rheumatoid Arthritis Synovial Fluid*

Cytokine	Cellular source
Interleukin-1†	Macrophage
Interleukin-6	Fibroblasts, macrophages
Tumor necrosis factor	Macrophage, ? T cells
Granulocyte-monocyte colony stimulating factor	Macrophage, T cells
Mast cell growth factor	? Macrophages
Transforming growth factor-beta	Macrophage, T cells
Colony stimulating factor	Fibroblasts
Interleukin-8	Monocytes, fibroblasts

*Modified from Firestein and Zvaifler.[35]
†controversial since some studies have detected little IL-1 in synovial fluid.[36]

Humoral and Cellular Immunity in Rheumatoid Arthritis

The histopathologic findings in the rheumatoid synovium and the characteristics of the cellular infiltrate in synovial fluid suggest that both cellular and humoral mechanisms are influential in initiating and perpetuating joint disease. It has been proposed that the initiating event occurs in the joint itself. A potential antigen, either foreign or self, is deposited or exposed in the synovium. Here it is degraded and processed by cells such as macrophages or dendritic cells. The antigenic components are then presented on their surfaces complexed with class II major histocompatibility complex molecules (Ia antigens). T cells then recognize and interact with this complex, and this results in T-cell proliferation along with release of several cytokines that amplify the immune response (e.g., factors that activate B cells to synthesize immunoglobulin and RF factor or T cells to develop cytotoxic activity). The inflammatory response that ensues results in the destruction of joint tissue (Fig. 3-2). In RA the antigens leading to this type of response have yet to be identified, but several have been proposed and will be discussed subsequently.

Major Histocompatibility Complex

The major histocompatibility complex (MHC) consists of several loci encoding groups of polymorphic antigens on chromosome 6 of the human genome. They play an important role in regulating several aspects of the immune response including organ transplantation and recognition of foreign antigen by T cells. Several rheumatic diseases are now known to be associated with certain loci of the MHC complex suggesting that these genes contribute to disease susceptibility or are directly involved in disease expression. The class I and class II MHC molecules are the receptors for antigen on the surfaces of antigen presenting cells such as macrophages and dendritic

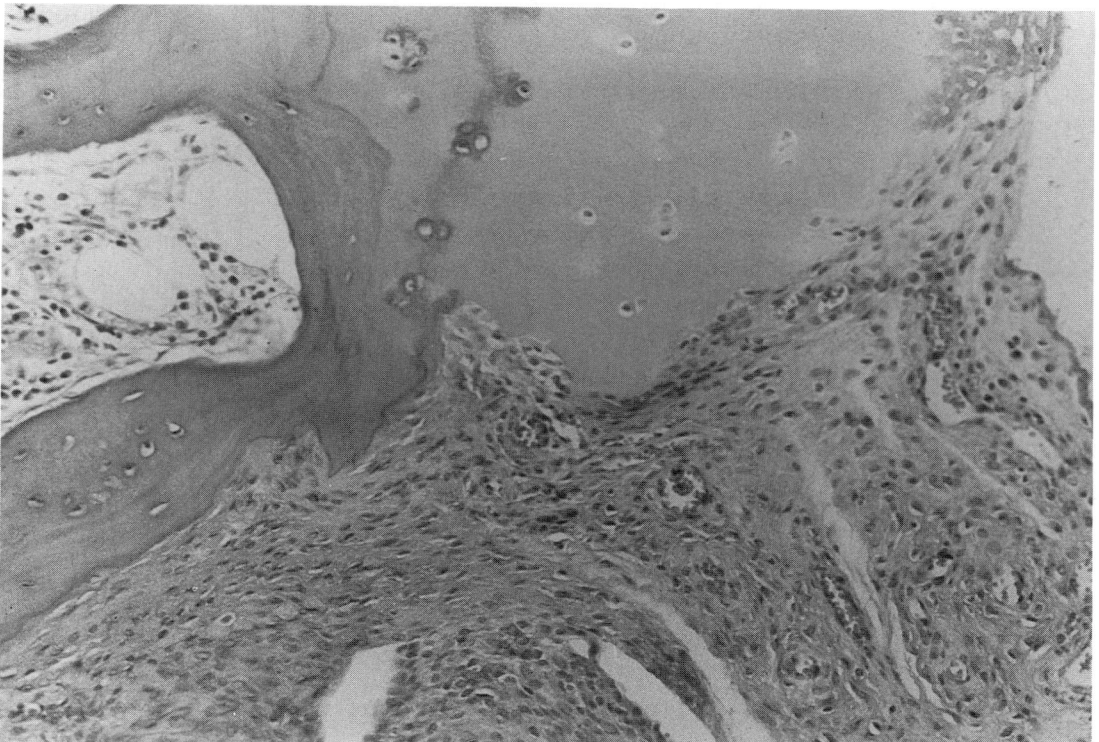

Figure 3-2. This microscopic photograph reveals typical pannus formation. Fibrovascular tissue protrudes from the inflamed synovium into the articular cartilage of an ankle. A portion of the fibrous tissue extends over the surface of the cartilage, which shows death of chondrocytes and loss of basophilia of the matrix. Note the inflammatory exudate in the subchondral bone (H and E, medium power). (Courtesy of the American College of Rheumatology. Clinical Slide Collection on the Rheumatic Diseases, 1989 Supplement).

cells. The class I molecules in association with foreign antigen are recognized by cytotoxic T cells which can then kill cells bearing these complexes. The class II molecules present processed antigen to helper T cells as in delayed-type hypersensitivity reactions. Once helper T cells are sensitized in this fashion, they will recognize the same antigen only in the context of the same MHC molecules to which they were initially exposed.

In RA the primary susceptibility appears to be with certain loci of the class II MHC.[39] The class II MHC consists of several genes that are located in three major subregions, DR, DQ, or DP (Fig. 3-3A). Each subregion has a pair of functional genes, A and B, that encode alpha and beta polypeptides, respectively, as well as some nonfunctional genes or pseudogenes. In general, the products of these two genes form a noncovalently linked heterodimer that is expressed on the surface membrane of certain cell types including dendritic cells, macrophages, and activated T cells (Fig. 3-3B). The DR subregion contains functional A1, B1, and B3,4 genes. The B1 and B3,4 genes express proteins that associate with the gene product of the A gene. The DR B1 gene encodes the DR 1 to 14 specificities while the DR B3,4 gene encodes the specificities DRw52 and DRw53. Both the DR B1 and B3,4 genes are highly polymorphic, while the DR A gene is relatively nonpolymorphic.[39] The functional A and B genes of the DQ subregion are both polymorphic and closely linked to the DR subregion; thus they are usually inherited as a unit, forming distinct haplotypes in individual populations.[39] Both the alpha and beta molecules of the A and B genes resemble immunoglobulins in their structure in that they have variable and constant regions referred to as the alpha 1, beta 1 or alpha 2, beta 2 domains respectively. Because of their homology to these molecules they are part of the immunoglobulin supergene family.[40]

In RA, the primary association appears to be with the DR4 locus, at least in certain populations.[40] The association is not exact since RA can also be associated with DR1 alleles, or non-DR4 haplotypes in some ethnic groups. Seventy percent of white patients with RA will have the DR4 haplotype while less than 30 percent of the normal white population carry this allele.[41] In contrast, 46 percent of black individuals with RA have DR4 in their genome compared with 14 percent of the black normal population.[41] In addition, the DR4 haplotype is associated with other diseases including juvenile rheumatoid arthritis (JRA) and pemphigus vulgaris.[42,43] The DR4 locus can be broken down into various subtypes, and some of these have been associated with RA, including Dw4, Dw14, and Dw15. The last is associated with RA in the Japanese population.[39] The Dw10 subtype is not associated with RA. It is the major subtype, however, in the DR4+ Israeli population where there is a *lack* of association between DR4 and RA.[44]

Recent advances in molecular biology technology have permitted sequencing of DR4 molecules and have provided a rationale for the close association of this haplotype and certain of its subtypes with RA in a particular population. Gregersen and his colleagues[39] have found that it is only the DR B1 gene that has significant differences between the subtypes of DR4 that are or are not associated with RA. They were able to localize these differences to the first domain of the molecule around position 70 (Table 3-2). The Dw10 subtype shows amino acid substitutions in its allele at positions 70 and 71 that lead to major charge differences at these sites. The Dw4, Dw14, and Dw15 subtypes are relatively similar. These findings suggest that a group of epitopes that are similar in primary structure may confer disease susceptibility while those that are dramatically different may confer resistance. To support this argument other investigators have shown that the DR1 haplotype, which is also associated with RA, has sequences in the DR β1 hypervariable region that are identical to the Dw14 subtype of DR4.[45] More recently, Willkins and associates[46] have shown that the DR6, Dw16 allele is associated with RA in the

Table 3-2. Major Differences in Amino Acid Composition in the First Domain of DR Beta 1 Chains Sequenced from Various DR4 Subtypes*

| | \multicolumn{7}{c}{Position of Amino Acid} |
	57	67	69	70	71	74	86
Dw4	Asp	Leu	Glu	Gln	Lys	Ala	Gly
Dw10	—	Ile	—	Asp	Glu	—	Val
Dw13	—	—	—	—	Arg	Glu	Val
Dw14	—	—	—	—	Arg	—	Val
Dw15	Ser	—	—	—	Arg	—	—

Modified from Gregersen et al.[39]
The dashes indicate identity with the amino acid of the Dw4 allele.

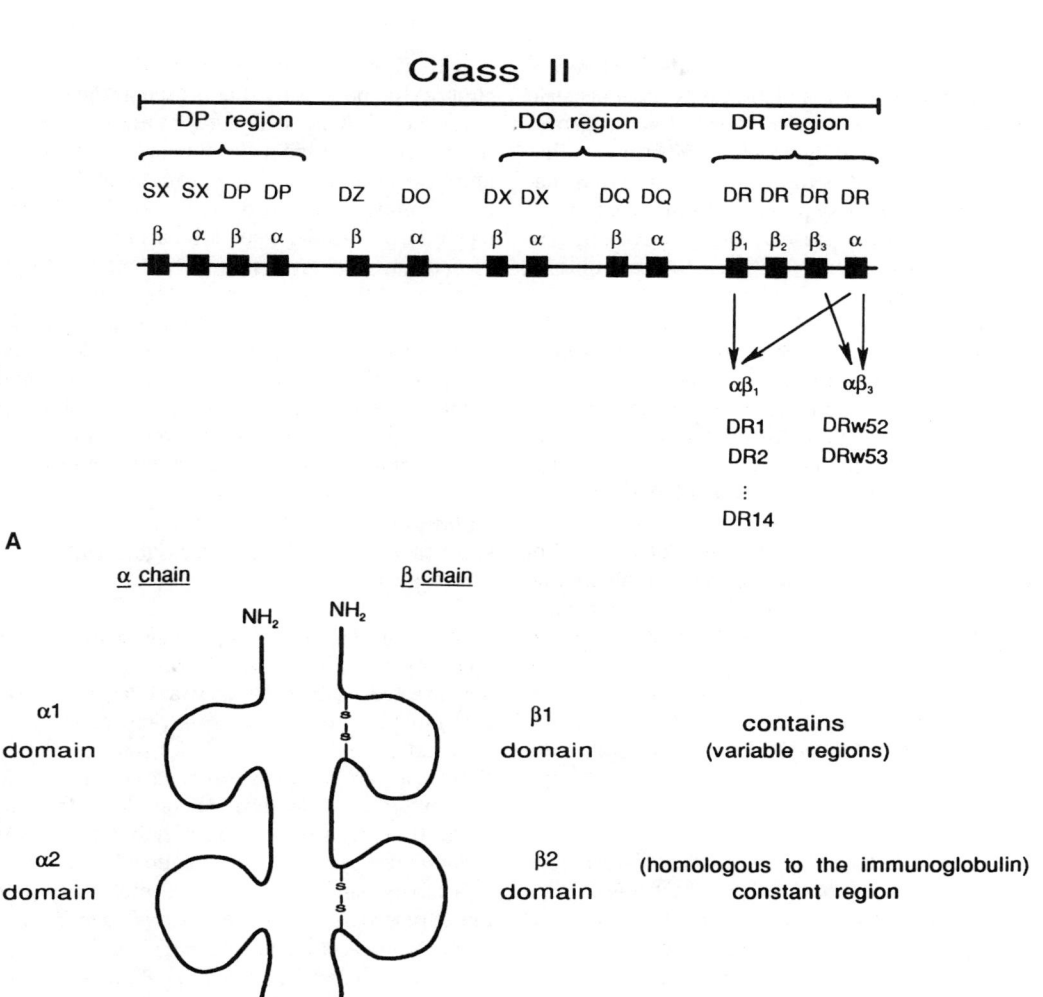

Figure 3-3. *A*, Schematic diagram of the class II MHC genes. The HLA, DR, DP, and DQ loci determine the class II molecules. The function of the remaining genes is not known at this time. Each of these subclasses of class II molecules contains at least one functional heterodimer composed of an alpha and beta chain. The DR subclass expresses two heterodimers of which alpha beta 1 is the most polymorphic. *B*, Schematic diagram of class II MHC molecule. This consists of two noncovalently linked alpha and beta molecules. The alpha chain in the DR molecule is not polymorphic, while the beta chain is highly polymorphic. Both molecules are divided into two domains. The beta 1 domain is the most variable of all the domains and is the most responsible for interacting with antigen and possibly T cells. This region is subdivided further into three hypervariable regions of which the third has been implicated in determining disease susceptibility to RA (see text).

Yakima Indian population. The DR B1 gene encoding this allele has sequence identity with DR4/Dw14 in the region encompassing amino acids 67 to 74.[46] Further studies on genes in multiple populations that have RA and are DR4− will be necessary to determine whether similarities in the hypervariable regional of the DR beta 1 region are all-important in conferring disease susceptibility. Based on these findings, Gregersen and associates[39] have proposed that these shared epitopes affect the way class II molecules interact with antigen and the T-cell receptor. Thus the disease association may arise because these molecules can present a potential antigen to the T cell thus triggering an immune response that could be detrimental to the host. DR4 subtypes that differ in amino acid sequence around position 70 would be unable to present the putative antigen. Alternatively, the shared epitope may resemble or mimic the antigen at the molecular level.

Firestein and Zvaifler[35] have proposed that RA actually results after the development of an abnormal and persistent autologous mixed leukocyte reaction. In this model stimulator cells such as macrophages and dendritic cells which bear Ia antigen on their cell surface interact with T cells in the synovium and promote T-cell activation through interaction of the self Ia molecules and the T-cell receptor. The subsequent release of cytokines and of other mediators of inflammation leads to the chronic inflammatory response characteristic of RA synovitis. The model would require that stimulator cells chronically express Ia antigen and/or that abnormal immunoregulation of T cells occurs. The initial event could be a response to an etiologic agent as suggested earlier followed by a persistent autologous response.

T-Cell Receptor Studies

Little is known about the contribution of specific T cells and their receptors to the pathogenesis of or susceptibility to RA. The T-cell receptor consists of two glycosylated chains, T alpha and T beta, each having a constant and variable region, much like the immunoglobulin and the MHC molecules described earlier. The specificity of the T-cell receptor is determined by several genes that encode the alpha and beta chains. Recently, it has been shown that the T-cell response to certain microbial antigens, termed superantigens, is specified by families of variable region beta genes.[47] These antigens are produced by a number of organisms, including those causing staphylococcal, streptococcal, and mycoplasma arthritides.[47] They are called superantigens since T cells bearing particular V beta chains will proliferate when cultured with these proteins. Streptococcal proteins have been implicated in the pathogenesis of rheumatic fever, while mycoplasma arthritidis is known to cause arthritis in rodents.[48] It has been speculated that a similar agent may be involved in the pathogenesis of RA. In fact, investigators have found that the frequency of T cells bearing the V beta 14 receptor was significantly greater in joint effusions than in the blood of RA patients.[49] In some cases, no V beta 14+ cells could be seen in the blood. Analysis of the T-cell beta chains indicated that they were largely oligoclonal. These findings support the possibility that a superantigen might be involved in RA since changes in numbers of T cells were observed only for the V beta 14+ T-cell population. These studies were supported by those of Howell and his colleagues who found limited heterogeneity of T-cell receptor beta chains in T cells taken from the synovium of patients with RA.[50] They found that three gene families, V beta 3, 14, and 17, predominated in most of the samples studied. Furthermore, these three receptor genes are closely related in an area where superantigens are believed to bind the T-cell receptor. It is likely that more revelations regarding the role of these unusual proteins in the pathogenesis of autoimmune disease will emerge soon.

Rheumatoid Factor, Immune Complexes, and the Immunoglobulin Supergene Family

Rheumatoid factors (RFs) are classically seen in the majority of patients with RA. RFs are antibodies that are directed against the constant region of the IgG molecule (Fc portion, Fig. 3-4) and exist in blood, synovial fluid, and tissue.[51] In synovial fluid and tissue they are found as aggregates of IgG and RF. It is known that these immune complexes fix complement; thus, they may be important contributors to inflammatory joint disease. While a hallmark of RA, RFs have been identified in several other autoimmune disorders including Sjögren's syndrome, systemic lupus erythematosus (SLE), as well as in infectious disorders like hepatitis. Thus the presence of RF is not specific for RA.

Rheumatoid factors can be found among the IgM, IgG, IgA, and IgE classes of immunoglobulin.[51] They are generally polyclonal in rheumatoid patients and can be heterogeneous in their binding specificities. For example, RFs may bind to the Fab region of immunoglobulin, deoxyribonucleic acid (DNA), histone, and nuclear antigens.[51,52] Furthermore, RFs can be related to one another by the presence of shared idiotypes. Idiotypes are the unique antigenic determinants of the variable region of the immunoglobulin (see Fig. 3-4). While originally thought to be unique to individual antibodies, it is now clear that RFs share "families" of idiotypes and are thus related to one another.[52,53] Human RFs utilize a wide range of variable region genes, at least four heavy and light region genes, indicating that there has been significant somatic diversification in terms of variable region usage.[51] The affinity of RFs for IgG molecules is close to, but less than that seen with, conventional antigen-antibody interactions.[51,54] Together these findings support the concept that the formation of

RFs may be an antigen driven phenomenon, and that these antibodies arise secondary to the introduction of antigen into the system.

The agents responsible for RF production in RA have yet to be determined. Stimuli that can elicit RFs from B cells include immune complexes, and polyclonal B-cell activators such as Epstein-Barr virus (EBV) and lipopolysaccharide (LPS).[55] It has been speculated that abnormal activation of B cells plus persistent antigen driven processes lead to chronic production of RFs and this has a pathologic role in RA. The evidence that B cells are abnormally activated has come from a series of studies on the types of B cells that are involved in RF production. Maini and colleagues[56] found that almost 50 percent of the circulating Ig+ B-cell population in RA patients bore the CD5 antigen, an antigen also found on B cells from patients with chronic leukemia.[57] In contrast, only few (up to 20 percent) CD5+ B cells are found in normal blood. The antigen is normally found on T cells and may be involved in the activation of T cells.[58] An intriguing observation is that human cord blood also contains as many as 50 percent CD5+ B cells.[59] It has been suggested that these cells are a distinct population of B cells present in lymphoid cells early in ontogeny but their numbers fall so that at birth significant levels are seen only in cord blood.[56] Subsequently, numbers decline in the peripheral blood except in autoimmune disorders where extrinsic factors such as viral activation or abnormal immunoregulatory T-cell function results in their expansion. Analysis of the function of CD5+ B cells has shown that they are probably the source of polyclonal RFs and other autoantibodies in RA and SLE.[56,60] Further study of these cells and factors controlling their expression and function will be necessary to elucidate the precise role they play in the pathogenesis of RA.

Infectious Agents

Thus far this chapter has eluded to the possibility that RA could develop as a response to either foreign or autologous stimuli. This section summarizes recent evidence in support of infectious agents as etiologic pathogens of this disease. It is important that we continue to evaluate RA for potential infectious agents that cause the disease, especially in light of the recent recognition that Lyme disease is caused by a spirochete. Many of the patients who subsequently were found to have Lyme disease had previously been diagnosed as having JRA.[61] Thus it is reasonable to propose that other agents may well be involved in the development of RA.

Lentiviruses

Lentiviruses are causative agents of polyarticular arthritis in sheep and goats. These are retroviruses that infect monocytes and macrophages and result in a chronic synovitis that involves primarily the carpal joints.[62] Eventually there is cartilage and bone involvement and destruction of the joint. Studies of the replication cycle of this virus have shown that the host is incapable of eliminating the virus. As monocytes mature, the virus, which is otherwise latent in these cells, undergoes replication. Expression of viral antigens on the cell surface of the monocyte leads to T-cell activation and forms the initial stimulus

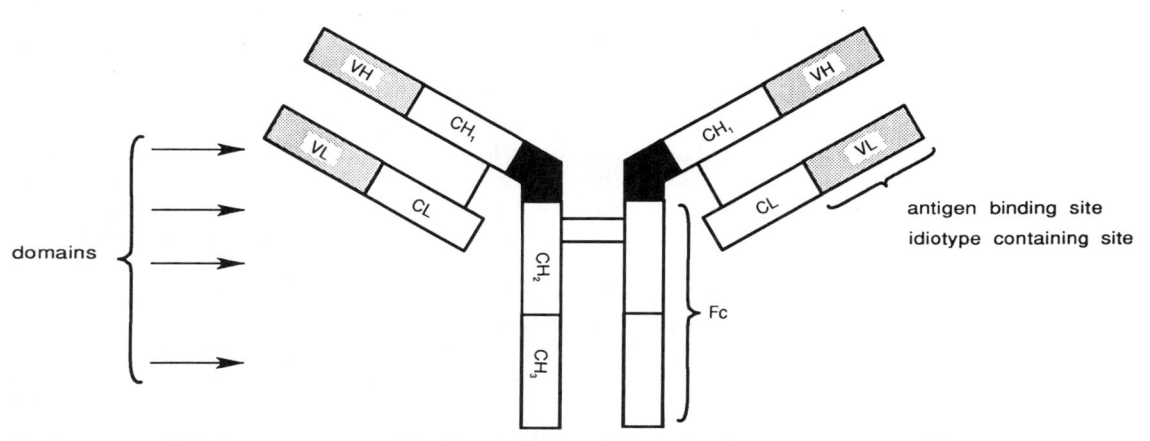

Figure 3-4. A schematic representation of the human immunoglobin molecule. Its major structural features are constant (C) and variable (V) regions of the heavy and light chains, respectively. The constant region of the heavy chain is divided into three subregions, CH1, CH2, and CH3. The V regions of both the heavy and light chains form the antigen binding site and therefore contain unique protein structures. These structures are known as idiotypes. The Fc portion of the molecule is indicated on the diagram and is the binding site on IgG for RFs.

that results in chronic inflammation.[63] Because of the similarities between this model of virus induced arthritis and RA there has been speculation that lentiviruses may also be involved in the latter. To date, however, there has been no convincing evidence to support this possibility.

Studies of patients infected with one retrovirus, the human immunodeficiency virus (HIV-1), have yielded some interesting observations. A number of these patients develop autoimmune-like diseases that resemble psoriatic arthritis, Sjögren's syndrome, SLE, and Reiter's syndrome.[64] Furthermore, it is known that infection with the human T-cell leukemia virus (HTLV-1) causes an oligoarticular arthritis with marked synovial proliferation that is thought to be manifested by products of the tax gene product.[65] With newer molecular biology techniques we now have the technology to determine whether retroviruses and their gene products play a role in the pathogenesis of RA.

Parvoviruses

Parvoviruses are single-stranded DNA viruses that have been shown to cause arthritis in humans.[66,67] One example, parvovirus B19, infects many humans but the illness is usually mild and not noticed.[66] In some cases it causes a rash, "erythema infectiosum," and even an acute or persistent arthritis.[68] The arthritis may present more commonly in women than men,[69,70] and is usually a symmetric arthropathy characterized by swelling and morning stiffness. Small joints of the hand and the knees are commonly involved. The arthritis may persist for over 5 years; it has been linked to an increased prevalence to DR4, and evidence of serologic infection has been noted in small numbers of RA patients.[71] However, RFs are not a feature of this viral infection and their role in the pathology of RA remains undefined at this time.

The parvovirus RA-1 has been isolated from rheumatoid synovial cells maintained in culture.[72] However, further studies are necessary to determine whether it is a common isolate of rheumatoid synovium. With probes prepared from the cloned genome of this family of viruses it will soon be possible to determine whether these agents are actual pathogens in RA.

Rubella Virus

Rubella viruses are ribonucleic acid (RNA) viruses belonging to the togavirus family that cause German measles in humans, usually in childhood.[73] The virus is usually acquired by the respiratory route and multiplies in the respiratory tract. Clinically, there is a prodrome of mild constitutional symptoms, following the incubation period of 2 to 3 weeks, and the appearance of a macular rash usually over the face and trunk. A low-grade fever, pharyngitis, and conjunctivitis may also be present.[73,74] Articular manifestations of this infection occur about 7 days after the appearance of the rash and are most commonly seen in young women. It has been estimated that up to 60 percent of women with natural infection develop arthralgias and arthritis, while about 15 percent may manifest similar symptoms following vaccination.[75] The most commonly involved joints are the hand joints, knees, and wrists followed by the ankles, hips, and joints of the foot. The arthritis is in most cases self-resolving but in a minority, a chronic picture becomes prevalent. Little is known about the characteristics of the inflammatory response in the synovium, and it is unclear whether antinuclear antibodies or RFs are commonly detected in this syndrome.[76] The organism can be isolated from the synovial fluid, and rubella antigens have also been detected.[77] Patients with RA and JRA have been found to have elevated titers of antibody to rubella virus.[78] In one study investigators found that synovial fluid cells from one of ten RA patients and one of eight patients with undiagnosed arthritis of the knee proliferated in vitro to rubella viral antigens.[79] More recently, investigators have shown that the virus can be recovered from the peripheral blood or synovial fluid of several patients with JRA (seven of 19) but not from normal persons or patients with joint effusions secondary to trauma.[80] While many of these patients had previously been immunized to rubella, the onset of their joint disease could not be temporally related to this or known rubella infection. These findings raise the strong possibility that some cases of chronic arthritis diagnosed as RA may in fact be due to persistent rubella virus infection. Rubella virus apparently infects lymphocytes, where it replicates, and may even infect chondrocytes.[73,81] It is likely that the expression of viral antigens in these host cells leads to an immune response on the part of the T cells and eventually results in the onset of inflammatory responses. Why the arthritis persists or appears only in some persons with rubella infection remains a mystery at this time. With the availability of newer recombinant techniques it should be possible to ascertain whether rubella virus or antigen is demonstrable in RA synovial tissue, synovial fluid cells, and peripheral blood mononuclear cells.

Epstein-Barr Virus

Epstein-Barr virus (EBV) belongs to the herpes family of DNA viruses and causes infectious mononucleosis, Burkitt's lymphoma, and nasopharyngeal carcinoma in humans. The virus infects B cells, which have receptors for the agent, and during initial infection there is significant polyclonal B-cell activation.[82] The activation is normally suppressed by the appearance of suppressor T cells. There has been much speculation regarding the role of EBV in the pathogenesis of RA. Several findings implicate this virus: (1) the observation that affected patients have elevated titers of antibody to EBV (EB nuclear antigen, viral capsid antigen) in their serum and synovial fluid[83]; (2) the virus is an activator of RF production[84]; and (3) blood mononuclear cells from rheumatoid patients spontaneously become transformed by EBV in the absence of exogenous infection when cultured long term.[84] It has been suggested that T cells from RA patients are defective in suppressing this transformation[85] and further studies have found that the number of B cells infected in vivo are increased compared with normals.[86-88]

Recently, sequence homologies have been discovered between EB nuclear antigens and host proteins. A major epitope of the nuclear antigen appears to have homology to cytokeratin and collagen.[89] Other investigators[90] have described another interesting homology: part of the EBV viral capsid antigen includes the amino acid sequence that is shared by the RA-associated haplotypes DR1, Dw4, Dw14, and Dw15 on positions 70 to 74 of the DR beta chain (see Table 3-2). It remains to be determined how these homologies between EBV proteins and host proteins relate to the pathogenesis of RA. As with other viral agents, the final determination of whether RA arises from an infection of this nature will come from studies employing tools of immunology and recombinant DNA technology.

Microbial Products

Microorganisms not only directly cause septic arthritis but can also induce the development of chronic inflammatory joint disease by the deposition of nonviable microbial products within the synovial lining. In addition, certain bacteria are known to induce a reactive arthritis following infection of the gastrointestinal or genitourinary tract, for example, Shigella and Salmonella. The mechanisms underlying the development of joint disease in these cases could be due to the presence of microbial antigens within the joint space, antigenic cross-reactivity between bacterial antigens and articular antigens, or both. Animal models have been developed to study the relationship between microorganisms and microbial products as inducers of arthritis. We will review these models and compare their clinical presentation as well as their immunologic associations with RA.

Bacterial Cell Wall Components

Peptidoglycans are polymers of muramic acid and N-acetyl glucosamine that are present in all bacterial cell walls.[91] These molecules are known to directly activate macrophages[92] and induce B cells to synthesize RFs.[93] If administered intravenously to rats, in the form of muramyl dipeptide, there is rapid onset of an acute polyarthritis that lasts about 4 days.[94] Chronic arthritis can be induced by repeated injections of the antigen but usually subsides with termination of injections. Some investigators have found that patients with RA have elevated levels of serum antibody to peptidoglycan.[95] Since these products are active inducers of RFs it has been speculated that these agents may be involved in the pathogenesis of RA; however, little evidence has accumulated thus far to support this.

Bacterial cell walls of gram-positive organisms consist of peptidoglycan linked to polysaccharide units. In organisms such as the group A streptococci and Lactobacillus casei, these structures are poorly degraded and can remain in tissues for long periods.[96] Rats given a suspension of these complexes develop a chronic arthritis that resembles RA histologically.[91] The induction of disease in rats is dependent on the strain and sex employed and the bacterial class. Female rats tend to develop more severe disease. Thus, in many respects, this disease resembles RA and it remains to be seen whether subtypes of RA will have etiologies ascribed to bacterial cell wall fragments.

Adjuvant Arthritis

Adjuvant arthritis results when an intradermal injection of Mycobacterium tuberculosis is given to rats or mice in an oil-water emulsion. A polyarticular arthritis develops in the distal extremities about 7 to 14 days following injection and this lasts several days. The pathology of the synovium is characterized by hypertrophy, and infiltration of the lining with T cells and macrophages.[91] T cells appear to play an important role in the pathogenesis of this disease. T-cell clones reactive with M. tuberculosis have been raised from animals with adjuvant arthritis and they are capable of transferring disease to irradiated recipients. The clone A2b recognizes an M. tuberculosis antigen as well as a component of cartilage proteoglycan.[97] In contrast, another T-cell clone (A2c) functions as a suppressor-inducer population by suppressing the induction of arthritis if given prior to an intradermal injection of emulsified mycobacteria. Van Eden and associates[97] have used these clones to identify particular mycobacterial antigens that stimulate the proliferation of these clones. Both clones responded to whole preparations of M. tuberculosis as well as to a 65-kd fraction of bacille Calmette-Guérin (BCG) derived protein. Fragments of 65-kd protein were obtained by creating mutants of the gene for the protein and it was determined that the critical epitope for both clones resided in the 180 to 188 amino acid sequence of the protein. Four of the nine amino acids were identical to the link protein of rat proteoglycan.[98] The administration of the 65-kd protein emulsified in oil did not result in arthritis in susceptible rats but the treated animals resisted subsequent attempts to induce disease by immunization with M. tuberculosis in oil-water emulsion. It has been speculated that the 65-kd protein induces the emergence of suppressor T cell populations that resemble clone A2c in function and they abort or block the appearance of T cells that would normally mediate the arthritogenic response. Analysis of the 65-kd protein has shown that it is a heat shock protein[97] with homology to related proteins in bacteria as well as eukaryotes. These proteins are normally produced under conditions of stress (e.g., heat shock) but may also be involved in the translocation of secreted organelle proteins from the ribosome to the appropriate membrane surface.[99] Heat shock proteins may also protect the conformational state of proteins,[100] and possibly play a role in antigen presentation.[101]

Mycobacterial and related antigens have been implicated in autoimmunity and specifically in connective tissue disorders based on the above observations and the following findings: (1) recent studies have found that a significant proportion of patients with SLE have antibodies to the human heat shock protein, HSP70[102]; (2) blood T lymphocytes from RA patients show augmented reactivity to acetone-precipitable fractions of M. tuberculosis[103]; (3) synovial fluid cells from patients with RA also proliferate to the 65-kd heat shock protein[104]; (4) the isolation of mycobacteria-reactive T-cell clones from RA synovial fluid[105]; and (5) the gene for human HSP-70 has been localized to the class II region of the MHC and these genes influence many human diseases, including RA.[101]

During infection with mycobacteria it has been postulated that the major antigenic proteins presented to T cells are the heat shock proteins of microbial agents.[106] If the antigens are presented in excessive amounts or at a chronic rate, there may be a breakdown of tolerance to self heat shock proteins and the result is the development of an autoimmune reaction to structures containing cross-reactive epitopes, for example, proteoglycan components (see earlier discussion). Now that the gene for HSP70 has been located on chromosome 6 in the class II MHC,[101] it will be of interest to examine whether it has allelic polymorphisms and how these relate to diseases such as RA which are known to have MHC associations.

Other Animal Models: Collagen Type II Arthritis

This form of arthritis is induced in susceptible strains of rats and mice with native type II collagen emulsified in complete Freund's adjuvant. The arthritis is first evident about 2 weeks following injection of the antigen and usually follows a chronic destructive course.[107] As in RA, there is synovial hypertrophy, pannus formation, marginal erosions of subchondral bone, and development of antibody to collagen.[88] In the animal model antibodies are directed to both native and denatured collagen, while in RA most of the anticollagen antibodies are toward the latter,[108] suggesting that this is a secondary response to degraded material. Recent studies have shown that collagen type II arthritis is dependent on factors like MHC background, class of antibody formed to collagen, complement activity, and particular variable region beta gene usage of the T-cell receptor.[109-111] Further analysis of this model will show the exact mechanisms involved in the manifestation of disease. It is unlikely that a humoral response to collagen is a major mechanism in the pathogenesis of RA but it is possible that it leads to the exacerbation of inflammatory responses that have already been initiated.

Summary

This section reviewed some of the current concepts regarding the etiology and pathogenesis of RA. Several points emerged from the studies described. First, RA is clearly associated with the genes of the MHC complex and DNA sequencing has identified important areas within the DR molecule that could be involved. Second, it is evident that more than one factor is involved in the pathogenesis of RA. Other genes involved in susceptibility to RA should soon be identified by means of restriction fragment length polymorphisms (RFLPs), making it easier to predict susceptibility with accuracy. The target antigen in RA has yet to be defined. However, new information regarding the potential antigens involved, in particular, microbial antigens, has been forthcoming. T-cell receptor studies may lead to clues regarding the nature of the antigen. With the advancement of recombinant technology, identification of the alleles involved and the inciting antigens should lead to better strategies of treatment.

Diagnostic and Clinical Aspects

RA has an impressively broad spectrum of clinical presentations. The characteristic patient is a woman between the ages of 20 and 50 with a symmetric polyarthritis including involvement of the small joints of the hands and feet, fatigue, morning stiffness, an elevated erythrocyte sedimentation rate (ESR), anemia, and a positive rheumatoid factor test. However, there are many other ways in which this disease presents.

Early Symptoms and Joint Involvement

Early in the course, the patient may present with only *prodromal features* such as fatigue, weight loss, sweating, myalgias, arthralgias, and morning stiffness. The *onset of joint disease* varies. Approximately 10 to 15 percent of patients demonstrate an *acute* onset. The suddenness of onset brings to mind the possibility of an infectious origin. This type of onset is more common in the elderly. Between 15 and 20 percent of patients have an *intermediate* onset occurring over a few days or weeks. The most common type of onset, the *insidious* type, takes place over weeks or months and occurs in 60 to 70 percent of patients. Aside from a symmetric polyarthritis affecting the small joint of the hands and feet, patients may have constitutional features, including low-grade fevers, anorexia, and weight loss.[106]

During the *early stages of joint involvement*, when changes are confined to the synovial membrane, capsule, and tendon sheaths, the patient complains of pain, swelling, tenderness, and stiffness of a number of joints. Even when the large joints are affected first, those of the hands and feet are usually involved early in the course of the disease. Swelling of the proximal interphalangeal joints gives rise to fusiform changes, which are characteristic of this disease (Fig. 3-5). The wrists, elbows, shoulders, knees, and feet may all be affected at this stage. Effusions are common, especially in the knees. Swelling of the bursae and tendons, especially related to the wrists and dorsa of the hands and feet, are relatively common. Morning stiffness is prominent, even at an early stage of disease. Morning stiffness remains a prominent symptom throughout the disorder, and can be used as a guide to the activity of the disease and response to therapy. Joint deformities are not usually present and radiologic examination shows only soft tissue swelling and juxta-articular osteoporosis, without erosions. Mild anemia may be present, and the ESR is usually elevated. The rheumatoid factor test may or may not be positive at this stage.

In a *later stage of joint involvement*, destruction of cartilage, necrosis and fibrosis of the synovial membrane, contracture of the joint capsule, and invasion of tendons and their sheaths by granulation tissue lead to increasing and irreversible impairment of function. In the hands, progression of the disease in the metacarpophalangeal joints leads to subluxation and ulnar deviation of the fingers (Figs. 3-6 and 3-7). Muscle wasting becomes more marked and other joints of the upper and lower extremities become progressively involved, including the shoulders, elbows, knees, hips, and feet. Weight loss and fatigue become prominent, and stiffness may persist throughout the day. ESR remains elevated and anemia worsens. Nodules may develop or increase in number (Fig 3-8), and rheumatoid factor is present in a majority of patients.[107]

In about 10 to 25 percent of patients, sustained disease activity leads to severe destruction of many articular surfaces. Severe deformities may develop and the functional status worsens (Fig. 3-9). RA may involve all of the joints of the upper and lower extremities and the cervical spine. Although radiologic and pathologic evidence of RA-related lumbar spine involvement exists, rarely do RA patients present with or develop clinically significant low back syndromes. The presence of significant low back or buttock pain should stimulate the physician's consideration of alternative disorders, such as a septic process or one of the spondyloarthropathies.[108]

Unusual Presentations

Palindromic Rheumatism

This is a clinical syndrome characterized by episodes of arthritis and periarthritis recurring at variable intervals, lasting for a few hours or days, and

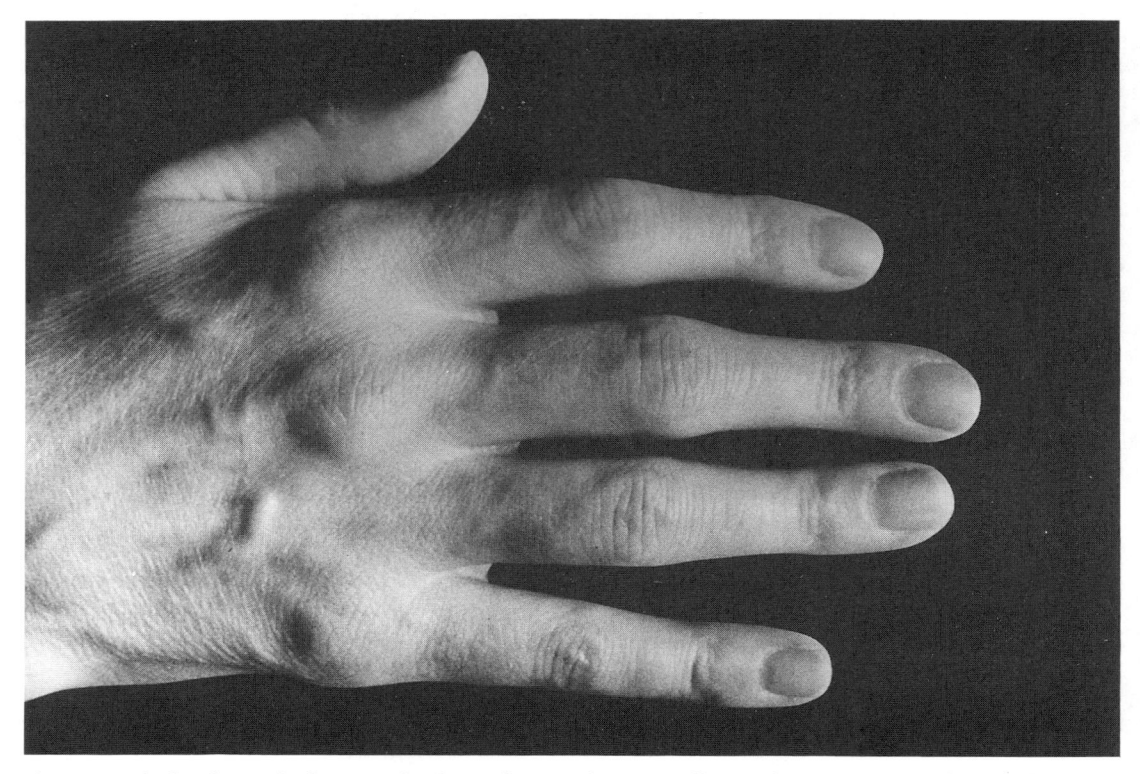

Figure 3-5. The hand in early rheumatoid arthritis showing obvious swelling at the proximal interphalangeal joints together with involvement of the metacarpophalangeal joints. (Courtesy of the Gower Medical Publishing Ltd, London, UK. Slide Atlas of Rheumatology. Introduction to Rheumatoid Arthritis, 1983.).

subsiding completely between attacks. The fingers, wrists, shoulders, and knees are most commonly involved, and laboratory and radiologic tests are usually normal. Approximately 50 percent of patients with this diagnosis go on to develop RA, at times as long as 20 years after the onset of the first attack. Rarely, patients presenting in this fashion go on to develop other systemic disorders, such as systemic lupus erythematosus or systemic vasculitides.[109]

Polymyalgia Rheumatica-type Presentation

It is, at times, difficult to differentiate between polymyalgia rheumatica (PMR) and this uncommon presentation of RA. This is particularly true in the elderly patient who has a negative test for rheumatoid factor. If the patient is young, seropositive and has obvious symmetric inflammatory peripheral joint disease, RA is more likely despite the predominance of proximal soreness and stiffness. Clinical points supporting the diagnosis of PMR are the development of the disease at age 65 or older, onset of less than 2 weeks' duration, bilateral shoulder pain or stiffness, an initial ESR greater than 40 mm per hour, and temporal arteritis-type symptoms. A symmetric synovitis is consistent with both disorders. A trial of low-dose corticosteroids may be needed. A rapid response is said to favor PMR as a diagnosis. However, both diseases may respond quickly to a dose of 10 to 15 mg of prednisone per day.[110]

Adult Still's Disease

This rare presentation of RA occurs primarily in the third and fourth decades. The presentation is usually with a fever of unknown origin, frequently associated with lymphadenopathy, pharyngitis, splenomegaly, and an evanescent, erythematous, maculopapular rash. Involvement of the lung, liver, and pericardium occurs in 30 percent of patients. Arthritis often involves proximal joints, but may also present in a typical rheumatoid pattern or as an ankylosing disorder in the wrists and cervical spine. The diagnosis can be a difficult one, especially if the

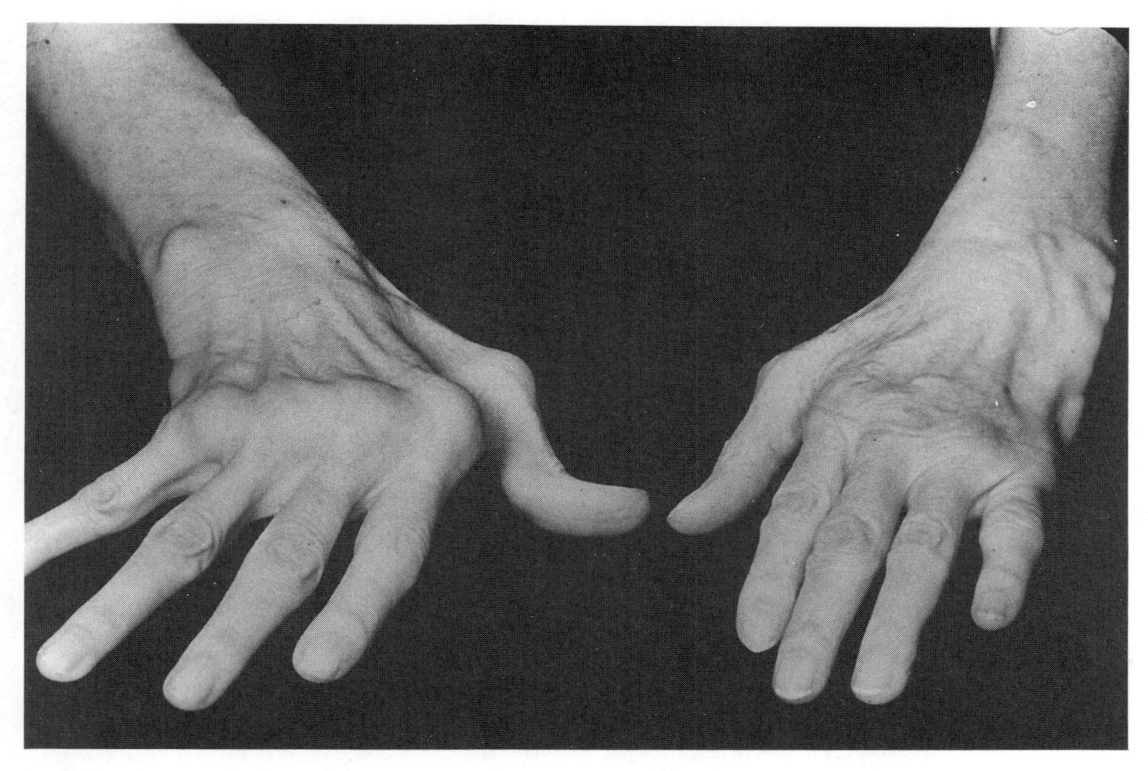

Figure 3-6. Ulnar deviation and subluxation of metacarpophalangeal joints have occurred in this rheumatoid patient's right hand. These joints appear swollen. Muscle atrophy has developed in the dorsal musculature of both hands. (Courtesy of the American College of Rheumatology. Clinical Slide Collection of the Rheumatic Diseases, 1989 Supplement.)

joint disease has not yet developed or become a prominent part of the clinical picture.[111]

Monoarticular Onset

While RA may present with inflammatory joint disease in a single joint, the definitive diagnosis of RA is usually made only with the benefit of time. One must always consider the possibility of a joint infection (e.g., bacterial infection, Lyme disease, tuberculosis) in a patient with monoarticular synovitis. Other considerations include the seronegative spondyloarthropathies (e.g., reactive arthritis/Reiter's syndrome, psoriatic arthritis, colitic arthropathy), crystal induced disease, or traumatic arthritis/mechanical derangement. Arthroscopy with synovial biopsy is appropriate in a patient with a persistent monoarticular synovitis of unknown cause. This is performed mainly to rule out infection but the histologic changes on synovial biopsy may be supportive of a diagnosis of RA or other types of inflammatory arthropathy.[108,112]

Tenosynovitis and Carpal Tunnel Syndrome

The initial presentation of RA may be in the form of either tenosynovitis of the joints of the hands or feet, and/or a median nerve entrapment syndrome. In the hands, patients may present with dorsal tendon inflammation or prominent palmar tenosynovitis, with or without triggering phenomena. When there is substantial volar wrist tenosynovial involvement, the median nerve may become entrapped under the volar carpal ligament and patients may develop the characteristic carpal tunnel syndrome. This includes numbness, tingling and pain of the first three and one half fingers of one or both hands (most prominent at night or elicited by the Phalen's and Tinel's signs), and signs of muscle weakness (early signs may include weakness of the opponens pollicis or the abductor pollicis brevis; late findings may include thenar atrophy). Eventually the patient will develop characteristic involvement of the small joints of the hands and feet, making the diagnosis of RA more obvious.[106]

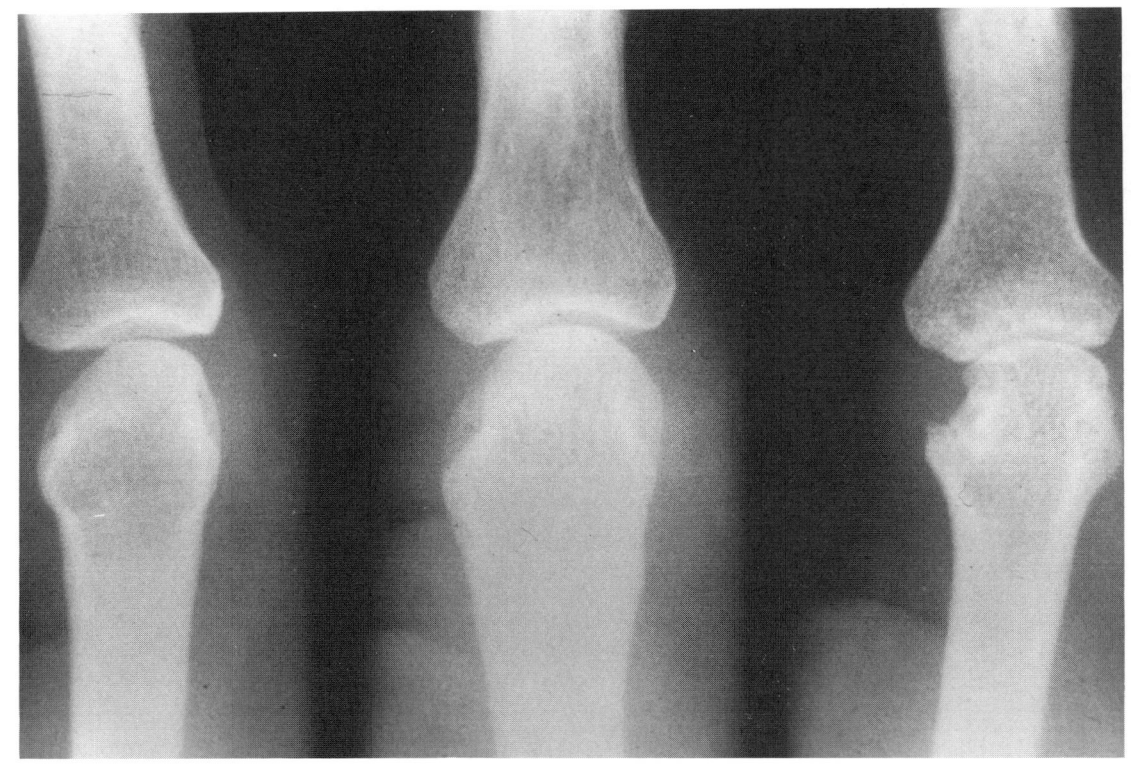

Figure 3-7. Progressive changes can be seen in this metacarpophalangeal joint beginning with (A) soft tissue swelling, but with intact underlying cortex and no erosions. This is followed by (B) thinning of the radial side of the cortex with minimal disturbance of underlying trabeculae and minimal joint space narrowing. Then (C) marginal erosion changes appear involving the radial aspect of the metacarpal head. There is a loss of bone substance and joint space narrowing. (Courtesy of the American College of Rheumatology. Clinical Slide Collection of the Rheumatic Diseases, 1989 Supplement.)

Extra-articular Manifestations

While the inflammatory joint disease of RA maintains center stage, extra-articular manifestations may be quite prominent and, at times, may dominate the clinical picture (Fig. 3-10). These abnormalities occur in a small subset (10 to 20 percent) of rheumatoid patients (men more often than women) but they are clearly associated with more severe, erosive joint disease, worse functional outcome, increased incidence of constitutional features, and an overall more aggressive inflammatory state. When such disorders occur *prior to* the development of the characteristic RA joint involvement (as with pleural effusions), difficult differential diagnostic problems exist. Some of these manifestations are related to an underlying small vessel vasculitis (e.g., nail infarcts, neuropathy, rheumatoid nodules, palpable purpura due to leukocytoclastic angiitis), but the incidence of a full-blown, true polyarteritis-like disorder is, fortunately, quite low.[113-115]

Fever

Fever may be a manifestation of disease activity in some patients with RA. These patients present with one or more episodes of a "pseudoseptic" picture with a high, spiking fever, chills, and a severe flare of inflammatory joint disease. If the joint disease is asymmetrical the possibility of a septic joint should be entertained. Despite the existence of the subset of patients who present in this fashion, fever should *not* be considered a common manifestation of active RA and should alert the physician to rule out infection carefully.

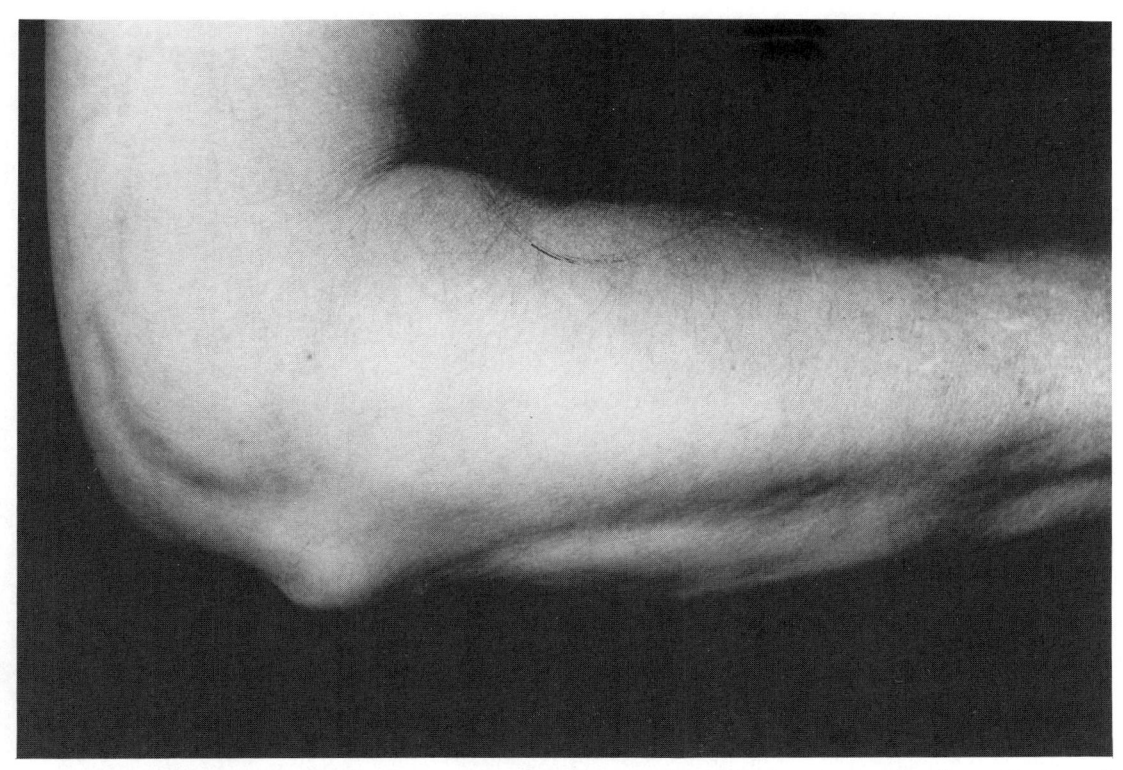

Figure 3-8. A large subcutaneous nodule is located on the extensor surface of the forearm near the elbow. (Courtesy of the American College of Rheumatology. Clinical Slide Collection of Rheumatic Diseases, 1989 Supplement.)

Weight Loss

Weight loss may be prominent, especially in those patients with severe, active disease and extra-articular manifestations of RA. This "malignoid" presentation is characteristic of many severe, chronic medical disorders. Weight loss however, should always alert the physician to the possibility of a superimposed malignant or infectious process, and appropriate testing and surveillance should be carried out when appropriate (e.g., stool guaiacs, mammograms, chest roentgenograms, gastrointestinal series, prostate evaluations). *Nutritional factors* must also be taken into consideration because patients with RA, especially those with major upper or lower extremity joint deformity or dysfunction, may not be able to shop for food, prepare nutritious meals, or physically deliver food to their mouths.

Rheumatoid Nodules

Rheumatoid nodules occur in approximately 20 percent of patients with RA and are considered to be associated with a poor prognosis and the presence of other extra-articular disease manifestations. They are most prominent on the extensor surfaces of the forearms, but they may also exist in other body areas subjected to trauma or pressure (e.g., buttocks) (see Fig. 3-8). Other sites include tendons, bones, lungs, heart, and dura. Rarely, such nodules may lead to organ dysfunction (e.g., cardiac arrhythmia or valvular dysfunction). Nodules may ulcerate and become infected, an important potential source of infection in patients with prosthetic joints in place.

Pulmonary Lesions

Pulmonary lesions include pleural involvement with or without effusion, rheumatoid pneumoconiosis, pulmonary nodules, interstitial pulmonary fibrosis, obliterative bronchiolitis, and pulmonary hypertension. Of note is the fact that pleural effusions and interstitial pneumonitis may *predate* the onset of arthritis by years.

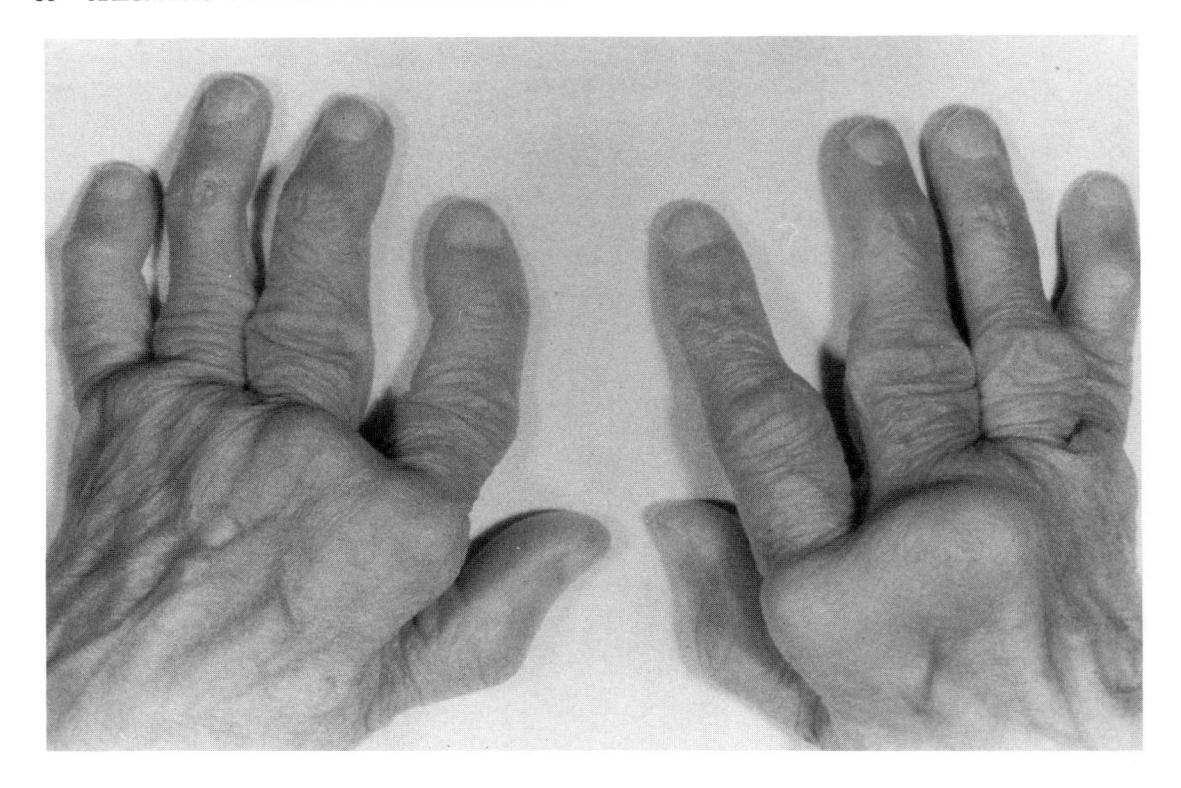

Figure 3-9. Rheumatoid "arthritis mutilans" showing subluxation of the metacarpophalangeal joints and foreshortening of the fingers due to bone erosion and resorption. All the fingers are involved. (Courtesy of Gower Medical Publishing Ltd, London, UK. Slide Atlas of Rheumatology. Rheumatoid Arthritis of the Hands and Feet.)

Sensory and Motor Neuropathies

Sensory and motor neuropathies may occur either as a manifestation of the inflammatory state or due to compression phenomena (e.g., carpal tunnel syndrome, tarsal tunnel syndrome). A mononeuritis multiplex pattern of nerve involvement is usually a manifestation of an underlying vasculitis. *Myelopathy* may occur in patients with atlantoaxial or subaxial cervical spine dislocation. The physician must have a high index of suspicion for the development of myelopathic symptoms, such as new onset of weakness, progressive alteration in the gait pattern, severe cervical spine pain, or a clunking feeling in the neck.

Ocular Disease

Ocular disease may present as keratoconjunctivitis sicca (Sjögren's syndrome), episcleritis, scleritis, scleromalacia perforans, or drug-induced injuries (e.g., corticosteroids leading to cataracts, antimalarials to retinal disease).

Cardiac Disease

Cardiac involvement may take the form of pericarditis (rarely with tamponade or constriction), myocarditis, valvular disease and conduction abnormalities due to rheumatoid nodules, or coronary vasculitis as part of a systemic vasculitis.

Felty's Syndrome

This syndrome occurs in 1 percent of RA patients, usually those with severe, active disease. It is diagnosed when patients with RA present with splenomegaly and severe leukopenia. Although the occurrence of infection leads to both morbidity and mortality in patients with this disorder, in approximately one third of patients persistent or recurrent infections are not observed. The cause of the tuberculosis, and aplastic anemia. A drug-induced neutropenia must always be considered.[116]

Sjögren's Syndrome

Sjögren's syndrome is a systemic connective tissue disorder manifested by salivary, lacrimal and other exocrine gland infiltration by mononuclear cell infiltration, leading to the "sicca complex" (dry eyes and dry mouth), salivary gland enlargement, and dryness of other mucosal surfaces. While the most prominent manifestations are related to dry mucosal membranes, other visceral disease may occur, including interstitial nephritis, adenopathy, pancreatitis, neurologic disorders, and an increased incidence of neoplasia (e.g., pseudolymphoma, lymphoma, Waldenstrom's macroglobulinemia, skin tumors). Thirty percent of RA patients develop SS, and 50 percent of patients with SS have RA. In general, those patients with coexistence of RA and SS have a worse prognosis.

Rheumatoid Vasculitis

Rheumatoid vasculitis (also called malignant rheumatoid arthritis) is an immune complex-mediated systemic vasculitis with a clinical presentation similar to that of polyarteritis nodosa. The small subset of RA patients with advanced, erosive disease who develop this disorder present with fever, leg ulcers, mononeuritis multiplex, and significant visceral disease (e.g., mesenteric infarction and coronary vasculitis). Fortunately, this disease presentation is very rare.[117,118]

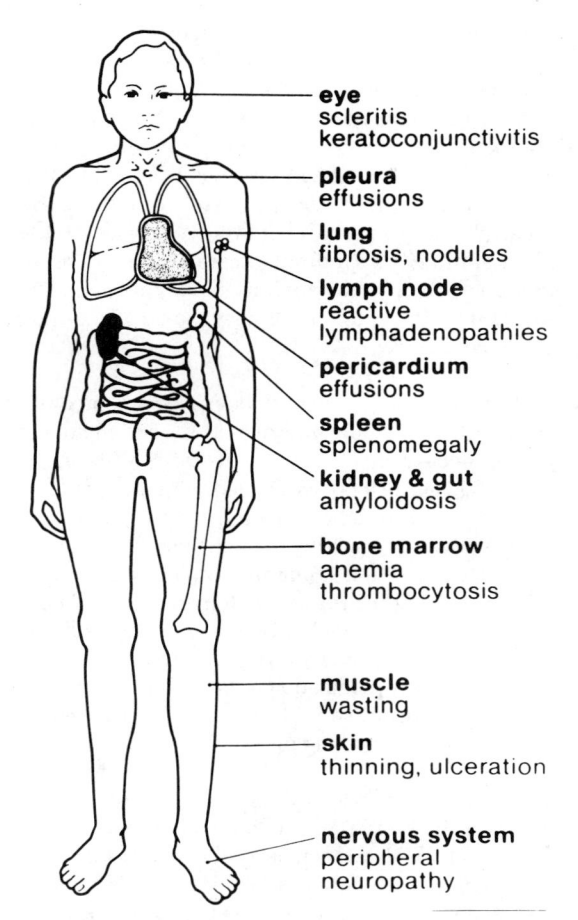

Figure 3-10. Other organs commonly involved in rheumatoid disease. (Courtesy of the Gower Medical Publishing Ltd, London, UK. Slide Atlas of Rheumatology. Introduction to Rheumatoid Arthritis, 1983).

leukopenia is thought to be multifactorial and includes sequestration due to splenomegaly, PMN-specific antibodies and PMN-associated immune complexes leading to PMN dysfunction and destruction, and serum factors suppressing bone marrow colony stimulating activity. There is not a good correlation between the tendency to infection and the absolute neutrophil count. The diagnosis of Felty's syndrome is dependent upon the criterion used for leukopenia (strict criteria are less than 2000 WBC or PMN less than 1000); in most patients the WBC count is between 1000 and 2500 per mm^3. The differential diagnosis of splenomegaly and neutropenia in RA patients includes viral infection, amyloidosis, preleukemia, myeloproliferative or lymphoproliferative disorders, systemic lupus erythematosus,

Amyloidosis

Amyloidosis, usually of the SSA or secondary type, occurs in a small subset of RA patients with long-standing disease (e.g., 20 years of severe, erosive disease). While there may be widespread deposits in the spleen, kidneys, liver, gastrointestinal tract, and blood vessels, renal disease (with nephrotic syndrome) is the usual problem demanding clinical attention and has been the leading cause of death in every series. Renal and rectal biopsies have the highest diagnostic yields, but gingival and anterior abdominal wall fat biopsies have a low frequency of complications and reasonable diagnostic sensitivity. For some unknown reason, amyloidosis complicating RA is much more common in European RA patients.[119]

Laboratory and Radiologic Manifestations

As with many connective tissue disorders, the diagnosis of RA is usually based upon clinical examination, with support from laboratory and radiologic tests. Such supporting information, however, is quite helpful in guiding therapy and in defining the response or lack of response to therapy. In addition, in certain difficult-to-diagnose inflammatory joint disorders such tests may increase the database to the point at which a diagnosis of RA will become more likely.

Hematologic and Serologic Abnormalities[120]

Anemia. Normochromic, normocytic, or hypochromic anemia may accompany *active* RA. A *low* serum iron, total iron binding capacity (TIBC), and mean corpuscular volume (MCV) are characteristic of the anemia of chronic disease seen in RA. The extent of anemia usually correlates with the RA disease activity and improves when the clinical picture improves. Examination of the bone marrow most commonly demonstrates hypercellularity with normal or increased iron stores. The physician must be alert to the possibility that the anemia of a patient with RA could be due to NSAID- or steroid-induced gastritis or peptic ulceration or gastrointestinal (GI) tumor-related blood loss from the GI tract. Close monitoring of stool guaiacs is indicated to rule out this possibility. While RA patients are not particularly prone to develop GI tumors, neither are they immune from them. RA patients do appear to have an increased incidence of peptic ulcer disease, with or without NSAIDs or steroids. Because pernicious anemia is more common in patients with other "autoimmune" disorders such as RA, the possibility of a superimposed megaloblastic anemia should be considered, especially in those patients with pancytopenia, hypersegmented polymorphonuclear leukocytes on the peripheral smear, and an elevated MCV. Other possible causes include glucose 6-phosphate dehydrogenase deficiency-related anemia triggered by NSAIDs, antimalarial drugs, or azulifidine; megaloblastic anemia due to azulfidine or methotrexate; anemia due to bone marrow suppression secondary to drugs such as gold, penicillamine, azathioprine, or cyclophosphamide. Thus, while it is true that anemia may be a manifestation of active RA, the physician must rule out drug-related anemia or anemia due to other, superimposed diseases.

Leukocytosis or Leukopenia. Leukocytosis may be seen in RA patients and usually reflects active, inflammatory disease. This is especially true in patients with rheumatoid vasculitis. Leukopenia may be seen in patients with Felty's syndrome (see above), or may be related to drugs (e.g., gold salts, penicillamine, immunosuppressive drugs, azulfidine, NSAIDs) employed in the treatment of the disease. In Felty's syndrome, there appears to be an immune and/or sequestration etiology for leukopenia. Drugs appear to have a direct toxic effect upon the bone marrow.

Platelet Disorders. Thrombocytosis accompanies active RA and usually improves as the activity of the disease decreases. This so-called "reactive thrombocytosis" is not usually associated with a hypercoagulable state. Thrombocytopenia may occur in patients with Felty's syndrome and is usually due both to sequestration and immune mechanisms. A drug-related etiology for thrombocytopenia must always be strongly considered. Gold salts, penicillamine, and immunosuppressive drugs are the most likely culprits, but any medication must be suspect, and all nonessential drugs should be stopped in the setting of a significant lowering of the platelet count.

Elevated Erythrocyte Sedimentation Rate. An elevation of the Westergren sedimentation rate is common in active RA and can be a good guide to the state of the inflammatory process. An increase in the ESR represents the nonspecific elevation of the level of acute phase reactants, specifically various types of proteins, in the setting of inflammation. These proteins allow red blood cells in a tube to fall faster, in a more linear pattern (rouleaux formation). It is important to note that an elevated ESR is quite a *nonspecific* finding and may reflect not only inflammation due to active RA, but also infections and neoplasms. In addition, the ESR may be minimally elevated or normal in overtly inflammatory clinical situations. The physician should be guided more by the patient than the result of a laboratory test. An elevated ESR may fall slowly and lag behind the clinical improvement. This differs from the *C-reactive protein*, another acute phase reactant, which correlates better with the status of inflammation.

Hyperglobulinemia, Polyclonal Gammopathy. The inflammatory state of RA leads to a polyclonal immunologic response. Thus, many RA patients have elevated serum globulins, and quantitative immunoelectrophoresis demonstrates a polyclonal elevation of IgG, IgM, and IgA. Uncommonly, patients with RA have a monoclonal gammopathy, but this is usually benign and is very rarely associated with typical myeloma-associated bone marrow abnormalities.[121]

Elevated Alkaline Phosphatase. Patients with more advanced, active RA may have an elevated serum alkaline phosphate (AP), gamma-glutamyl transpeptidase (GGTP) and 5′-nucleotidase. These elevations may represent RA-related liver inflammation, but are not usually associated with clinically significant liver or biliary tract dysfunction. Recent evidence supports the likelihood that AP elevations represent an acute phase protein reflecting the liver response to circulating mediators such as interleukin-1 and that the origin of elevated 5′-nucleotidase levels may be the joint, not the liver.[122] Rarely, RA patients (especially those with Sjögren's syndrome) may have coexistent hepatobiliary disorders such as primary biliary cirrhosis, chronic active hepatitis, or sclerosing cholangitis. If a patient develops jaundice or biliary symptoms, ultrasonography, computerized transaxial tomography, or more invasive techniques (e.g., endoscopic retrograde cholangiopancreatography, percutaneous cholangiography) may be necessary to rule out a superimposed malignancy or stone.

Rheumatoid Factor. A rheumatoid factor is an immunoglobulin (IgM, IgG, or IgA) that has immunologic reactivity with the second and third constant region domains of an IgG molecule. The actual role of RFs in the causation of disease remains unknown. The most common assay for serum IgM RF is the latex fixation test in which IgG molecules are attached to latex particles and then mixed with test serum. If patients have RFs in their serum, the latex particles become cross-linked and agglutination can be viewed under the microscope. Doubling dilutions are then carried out to arrive at the final RF titer. The finding of such immunoglobulins is nonspecific, since they are found in many disease states, such as rheumatoid arthritis, sarcoidosis, bacterial endocarditis, and tuberculosis. Seventy to eight percent of rheumatoid patients have rheumatoid factors in their serum and many have them in synovial fluid. In practice, it is *not* helpful to do serial evaluations of rheumatoid factor, since a change in the titer does not correlate with changes in disease activity. Low RF titers (1:40, 1:80, and 1:160) are thought to be nonspecific and may be seen in diseases other than RA. While low titers may be seen in early RA, the more common RF titers are 1:320 or greater. The absence of serum RF (so-called seronegativity) does not rule out the possibility of rheumatoid arthritis, but in this circumstance other causes of inflammatory joint disease (e.g., psoriatic arthritis, Reiter's syndrome, crystal-induced disease) should be reconsidered.[108,112]

Antinuclear Antibody Test. A subset of rheumatoid arthritis patients have a positive antinuclear antibody (ANA) test, usually of the homogeneous (nonspecific) pattern. Some patients have a positive ANA and a negative rheumatoid factor test. In general, this group of patients presents with typical rheumatoid arthritis and no systemic features of systemic lupus erythematosus. Most of these patients maintain the RA-type illness despite the fact that they maintain ANA positivity and rheumatoid factor negativity. Rarely, patients in this group develop typical SLE.[123]

Synovial Fluid Analysis. Synovial fluid analysis is useful for the diagnosis of RA and coexistent arthritis of other causes. It gives a rough estimate of the degree of inflammation present, helps the physician to determine the pace at which diagnostic and therapeutic intervention must proceed, and is the only means by which complicating infectious or crystal-induced arthritis can be definitively excluded. Aside from evaluation for crystals and culture of the synovial fluid, the synovial fluid cell count remains the most important piece of information to be obtained from arthrocentesis. By convention, a synovial fluid white blood cell count of 2,000 per mm^3 is the cutoff to differentiate between noninflammatory and inflammatory synovial fluids. The usual rheumatoid fluid has a WBC between 10,000 to 30,000 per mm.^{3} If the WBC count goes beyond 50,000 per mm^3, RA may still be the appropriate diagnosis, but infection must be appropriately ruled out with a culture. The predominant cell found is the neutrophil, usually constituting 70 percent or more of the total leukocytes. Synovial fluid differential counts in early or mild RA may demonstrate a mononuclear predominance.[112]

Synovial Tissue Evaluation. Because the diagnosis of RA is almost invariably made on the basis of the clinical presentation, rarely does the physician need to obtain synovial tissue for histologic confirmation. The inflammatory/infiltrative histologic synovial changes of RA (see Fig. 3-1) have *no* diagnostic specificity. The pathologist, even armed with well-documented clinical information and ample tissue, will most commonly make a nonspecific, anatomic diagnosis of "chronic arthritis, rheumatoid type." A synovial biopsy finds its greatest usefulness in distinguishing RA from infectious (e.g., tuberculosis), crystal-induced, and neoplastic disorders. In general, synovial biopsy is rarely needed for the diagnosis of inflammatory joint disease in the everyday practice of rheumatology.

Radiologic Abnormalities

While juxta-articular bony erosions are characteristic of the rheumatoid inflammatory process, it may take up to 6 months for such changes to become obvious on serial joint x-rays, if they are to occur at all. Plain x-rays usually suffice in determining the presence or extent of joint involvement. Ultrasonography can be used to demonstrate noninvasively the presence of popliteal (Baker's) cysts of the knee joint. At times, more sophisticated radiologic techniques, such as magnetic resonance imaging (MRI) and computerized transaxial tomography (CTT) are indicated for better definition of the anatomy, especially in the setting of cervical spine disease. Bone scanning can be used to define the symmetric pattern of joint inflammation in cases in which such information is not readily available on the physical examination. One or more of the following roentgenographic changes may be seen in a patient with RA and may also develop over time:

Soft Tissue Swelling. Such swelling about the typical joints involved in RA (e.g., proximal interphalangeal and metacarpophalangeal joints) is a typical soft tissue change.

Juxta-articular Osteoporosis. This finding is a characteristic early x-ray abnormality.

Juxta-articular Erosions. These erosions reflect the destructive changes of the rheumatoid process. In the hand, they are usually located radially. Some drug trials employing cyclophosphamide and gold salts have demonstrated a decrease in the size of such erosions. Figure 3-1 demonstrated the characteristic erosive changes seen in RA patients with progressive disease over a 5-year period.

Joint Space Narrowing. Joint space narrowing may be seen in more advanced RA and reflects major changes in the anatomy of the joint.

Ankylosis. Ankylosis of joints may be seen in some patients with severe RA and also in patients with JRA.

Atlantoaxial and/or Subaxial Cervical Spine Abnormalities. These abnormalities may exist in patients with severe RA. They can lead to significant neurologic dysfunction, and thus optimal definition of the anatomy often necessitates MRI or CTT scanning.

Differential Diagnostic Considerations[108,112]

Systemic Lupus Erythematosus

Patients with SLE often present with, or eventually develop, an RA-like *symmetric* joint disorder involving many joints of the upper and lower extremities, especially the small joints of the hands and feet. Given the fact that SLE and RA occur in the same patient population (i.e., young women), the physician must always consider SLE in the differential diagnosis of an RA-like polyarthritis. While this type of inflammatory joint involvement may be the sole clinical manifestation of SLE, most patients will eventually develop, or already have, some other signs or symptoms of this systemic disease. These include fever, skin rash, alopecia, mouth or nasal ulcers, serositis, cytopenias (e.g., leukopenia, thrombocytopenia, and hemolytic anemia), renal involvement, or nervous system disorders. Most patients with SLE have a positive serum test for ANA, but some may also have a positive serum test for RF. In general, it is the *clinical presentation*, not the serologies, that helps to define the diagnosis. In the subgroup of RA patients who have positive ANA tests and negative RF tests, the joint presentation remains RA-like for long periods and the patient never develops any SLE-associated disease manifestations. Thus, the patient is thought to have RA and is treated as such. Nevertheless, given the reported instances in which some of these patients do eventually develop SLE, physicians would be wise to observe the clinical status of this subgroup of patients closely for SLE manifestations. Further, they should consider starting with an antimalarial drug as a first step in disease modifying therapy because both mild RA and SLE-related joint inflammation respond to this therapy.

Seronegative Spondyloarthropathies

Psoriatic Arthritis. Patients with psoriatic arthritis may present with a symmetric polyarthritis indistinguishable from RA. Some physicians feel that this presentation represents the coexistence of two common disorders, RA and psoriasis. Most rheumatologists see this as one of the presentations of psoriatic arthritis. A more common pattern of psoriatic arthritis presents as an asymmetric, large-joint, lower-extremity synovitis, at times associated with sacroiliitis and spondylitis. Patients with psoriatic arthritis often have nail pitting and dactylitis (so-called sausage-shaped digits because the global inflammation of the tendons, soft tissues, and joints of the toes make them appear like little sausages). These patients are generally seronegative, that is, they have negative tests for RF.

Reiter's Syndrome. Patients with Reiter's syndrome rarely present with symmetric polyarthritis. Their joint inflammation is characteristically asymmetric and involves the large joints of the lower extremities. They, too, may have sacroiliitis and spondylitis and may also present with toe dactylitis. Their psoriasiform rashes (keratodermia blennorhagica and circinate balanitis), urethritis, and eye inflammation (conjunctivitis and uveitis) are helpful clinical guides to the diagnosis.

Ankylosing Spondylitis. This disorder mainly involves the spine and sacroiliac joints. Thirty percent of patients, however, will develop peripheral joint inflammation, most commonly in an asymmetric fashion involving the hips and shoulders.

Colitic Arthropathy. This condition most often presents as an asymmetric, lower extremity, large-joint synovitis, at times with associated spine and sacroiliac involvement. Rarely, joint inflammation may predate the inflammatory bowel disease, making the differential diagnosis difficult.

Crystal-induced Joint Disorders

Gouty Arthritis. This disorder presents as a polyarticular synovitis in one third of patients. At times, patients with gout have initially been diagnosed as having RA because of the multiplicity of joint involvement and the presence of subcutaneous nodules (which were actually gouty tophi). Patients with gout commonly have an elevated serum uric acid level (although uric acid level may be normal during an acute attack of gout), a monoarticular presentation (with podagra eventually developing in 90 percent of patients), and negatively birefringent needle-shaped crystals in the polymorphonuclear leukocytes of joint fluid. A personal or family history of gout or urate kidney stones may be helpful in supporting the diagnosis of gout. Probably for genetic reasons, the coexistence of gouty arthritis and RA is very rare!

Pseudogout or Calcium Pyrophosphate Deposition Disease (CPPD). CPPD may present in a polyarticular fashion, but the more common presentation is monoarticular. Weakly-positively-birefringent rhomboid crystals are commonly seen within synovial fluid polymorphonuclear leukocytes. At times the crystals are so small that the diagnosis of CPPD is missed. Radiographs demonstrating chondrocalcinosis (especially in the knee cartilage or menisci, symphysis pubis, and triangular cartilage of the wrist) are helpful in supporting this diagnosis.

Calcium Hydroxyapatite. Calcium hydroxyapatite crystals do not cause polyarthritis of the RA-type. The characteristic presentation is that of a shoulder disorder manifested by osteoarthritis, rotator cuff tears due to tendon erosion and bony and cartilage destruction (the so-called Milwaukee shoulder).

Osteoarthritis

While osteoarthritis (OA) may present in a polyarticular fashion, the joint involvement is usually noninflammatory and involves the distal interphalangeal (DIP) and proximal interphalangeal (PIP) joints of the hands with the characteristic Heberden's (DIP) and Bouchard's (PIP) nodes. OA, however, may coexist with CPPD and calcium hydroxyapatite crystals and may lead to an inflammatory and destructive pattern of joint disease. OA generally presents in an asymmetric fashion and involves not only the hand and foot joints but also large joints such as the knee and hip. OA patients do *not* have a systemic disease, thus distinguishing them from patients with RA.

Infectious Arthritis

Monoarticular Synovitis. There is rarely a diagnostic problem in patients who present with monoarticular synovitis, fever and chills, an elevated peripheral leukocyte count, and a high synovial fluid white blood cell count with positive synovial fluid cultures for gram-positive or -negative bacteria. Patients with any preexisting arthritis (RA, seronegative spondyloarthropathies, osteoarthritis, and crystal-induced disorders) are predisposed, however, to developing superimposed septic arthritis. RA patients have a particularly high incidence of Staphylococcus aureus infections. Thus, the physician must have a high index of suspicion for infection when such patients have a monoarticular flare.

Gonococcal Arthritis. Gonococcal arthritis may present in a polyarticular fashion, at times with a migratory pattern. The sexual history, migratory joint and tenosynovial involvement, and the presence of a pustular, vesicular, or necrotic rash help to define the correct diagnosis.

Viral Polyarthritis. This disease may mimic RA and some patients who develop a "self-limited" RA disorder may have had a virally-induced disorder.[44]

Hepatitis B. This infection may lead to a serum sickness-like illness, and these patients may develop a self-limited RA-like polyarthritis associated with a rash (urticaria, purpura) and liver function test abnormalities.[45]

Rubella. Whether acquired via infection or immunization, rubella may lead to a similar rheumatoid-type disorder.[46]

Parvovirus B19. These infections (in the child called erythema infectiosum, or fifth disease) in both children and adults may lead to an acute RA-like polyarthritis. The associated facial (slapped cheek) and leg rash and the epidemic nature of the presentation help to define the etiology. Most such cases of arthralgia or arthritis are self-limited, but long-term followup is indicated because this arthropathy may be characterized by episodic flares separated by symptom-free intervals.

Lyme Disease. While Lyme disease most commonly presents (in late stages) with a monoarticular synovitis of the knee, some patients may present early with arthralgias and myalgias or, in the tertiary, late phase, with an RA-like illness. The early diagnosis of Lyme disease is based on the presence of arthralgias and myalgias in a patient in an endemic area who also has other systemic features, such as fever, malaise, headache, a history of a tick bite, and/or the development of the characteristic erythema chronicum migrans rash. ELISA or indirect immunofluorescence serologic testing is commonly negative within the first 6 weeks after the tick bite. In the tertiary, or late, stages of Lyme disease, patients may develop frank arthritis. The most common presentation is that of a *remitting* synovitis of a knee. At times, the inflammatory knee involvement may become chronic. By this time, most patients will have developed clearly abnormal Lyme serology in the form of IgG antibodies. There is a small subgroup of patients who may have negative serologies in this late phase, but this is uncommon and may reflect early antibiotic treatment leading to ablation of the humoral response to the Borrelia infection. Other associated systemic features may support the Lyme diagnosis, including neurologic disease (e.g., Bell's palsy, meningoencephalitis, peripheral neuropathy) and cardiac dysfunction (including heart block).

Therapy

Basic Concepts

The main thrust of any therapeutic program should be directed at the following manifestations of rheumatoid arthritis[124]:

An aggressive inflammatory/immunologic process within joints and other organs in which the final common pathologic process involves enzymatic destruction of cartilage, bone, tendons, ligaments, and other connective tissue components. The initial stimulus for this self-perpetuating process is unknown, and thus therapeutic modalities have been directed at the inflammatory process rather than the actual cause of the disease. "Chemotherapy" for this disorder has *not* been specially crafted to alter well-defined, basic cellular and humoral abnormalities of RA. Rather, it reflects drugs chosen to nonspecifically treat inflammation (so-called nonsteroidal anti-inflammatory drugs and corticosteroids), drugs chosen by serendipity (e.g., gold salts and antimalarials), and drugs borrowed from oncologists (e.g., immunosuppressive drugs such as azathioprine and methotrexate). Although one of the concepts of the pathogenesis of RA continues to stress the probability of an infectious basis for this chronic inflammatory disorder, to date no infectious agent has been definitively implicated, and antibiotic therapy (e.g., tetracycline) has not been proven to be efficacious.

The tendency of joints to stiffen and fuse. A specific program of anti-inflammatory agents, disease modifying drugs, and physical therapy are employed to counter these processes basic to the rheumatoid syndrome.

The eventual destructive process leading to joint deformity and alteration in joint function. It is here that the impressive advances in orthopedic surgery and prosthetic design in conjunction with physical therapy have helped rheumatoid patients to regain function and resume their desired activities of daily living.

General Concepts Regarding Treatment

Concepts regarding the treatment of RA are rapidly changing. The stimuli for a more aggressive approach include (1) the realization that the erosive, destructive joint process begins within the first 2 years of the onset of disease and our ability to reverse erosions and deformities is limited; (2) the increasing appreciation that RA shortens life; and (3) RA can rapidly lead to profound and progressive alteration in the patient's functional status.

In the past, patients might have been treated with a NSAID until erosions developed, and then a disease-modifying drug (DMARD) would be instituted. If, after 1 to 3 months, there was no obvious clinical improvement or disease progression was found, an alternative DMARD would be instituted. Rheumatologists now feel that once a diagnosis of active disease is made, one or more DMARDs is indicated to attempt altering the natural history of the disease and prevent the development of erosions.

With these thoughts in mind, three different therapeutic approaches have evolved over the past 5 years:

1. *Continuation of the "traditional approach."* This is outlined in Table 3-3, and involves the use of combinations of one NSAID, one DMARD, and possibly short courses of oral or intra-articular steroids for systemic or local disease flares. With this approach, if one NSAID or DMARD either does not improve the disease activity or is associated with unacceptable side effects, an alternative drug is employed. Rheumatologists differ in their initial and subsequent choices of these drugs, and the variation usually depends on their past experience, the drugs used in their training programs, interaction with drug detail personnel, and the impact of published placebo controlled trials and symposia. A common approach would be to begin a NSAID of choice, and one DMARD, usually either hydroxychloroquine sulfate (Plaquenil), sulfasalazine (Azulfidine), or oral or parenteral gold. Lack of clinical improvement in 3 weeks leads to a change of NSAID, and in 1 to 3 months to a change in the DMARD. Over the past few years, the use of methotrexate has gained acceptance, and it is instituted earlier and earlier in the course of RA. Some physicians only institute methotrexate after one or more of the above drugs have failed to improve the patient's status. They note concern about the ill-defined, long-term potential liver and pulmonary toxicity, and question its capacity as a disease-modifying agent. Others begin it as their first DMARD because they feel that it works rapidly, has the best ability to alter the course of the illness, and is well tolerated. They stress the idea that the physician and patient have a narrow window of opportunity in which to alter the destruction process.

2. The use of *combination 2-DMARD therapy* has been fueled by the same concepts noted above, that is, to assume an aggressive approach to the treatment of a severe disease. An additional stimulus to the use of this type of regimen comes from the success of combination chemotherapy in the treatment of malignant disorders. Despite our ignorance of the mechanism of action of any one of the DMARDS, the basic principle here is that if one drug works well two will work better. Studies vary greatly regarding the

Table 3-3. Treatment Approaches to Rheumatoid Arthritis

1. **Traditional approach**
    a. Diagnosis and assessment of clinical activity and extent of disease. The definition of comorbid states may alter the therapeutic regimen. Patient and family education, reassurance, and support. Physical and occupational therapy assessment and treatment plan.
    b. Institution of medications to control the inflammatory state, and limit or reverse the damage to joints and soft tissue.
        (1) Nonsteroidal anti-inflammatory drugs (NSAIDs)—control a component of the inflammatory process but do not have the capacity to alter the natural history of the disease.
        (2) Disease modifying drugs (DMARDs)—all patients with active RA should be treated with a drug in this class. Included in this group of drugs (in order of increasing potential toxicity, not efficacy) are hydroxychloroquine, sulfasalazine, oral gold, parenteral gold, methotrexate, azathioprine.
        (3) Corticosteroids—both systemic and intra-articular.
        (4) Cyclophosphamide—reserved for the treatment of rheumatoid vasculitis.
        (5) D-Penicillamine—reserved for cases in which extra-articular disease manifestations are prominent.
        Note: Rheumatologists vary with regard to which NSAID or DMARD should be used before another. Other modalities can be employed when clinically indicated including analgesics and other forms of pain control, the use of splinting of actively inflamed joints or tendons, and surgical intervention when needed for correction of joint deformities.
2. **Two-DMARD combination therapy.** Employed in an attempt to establish a more aggressive approach to a severe disease. Common combinations include antimalarial drugs with most other DMARDs.
3. **Stepwise multidrug approach.** Employs a cancer chemotherapy–type approach to the treatment of early, active RA. The initial regimen includes hydroxychloroquine + oral gold + methotrexate + azathioprine + oral corticosteroids. As the disease is controlled, drugs are shed until the patient remains solely on hydroxychloroquine. While this is not a commonly used regimen, it does reflect the increasing appreciation and concern about the destructive nature of RA.

efficacy of two-drug combination of DMARDS over the use of single DMARDS, and there may be more side effects when two drugs are combined. There are reports of almost all combinations of DMARDS, but many include the addition of hydroxychloroquine to another DMARD.

3. The use of a *multi-DMARD stepwise approach* is the most aggressive and revolutionary concept in the care of RA patients. The rationale for this approach is borrowed from oncologists and cancer treatment and includes the fact of disease aggressiveness; the successful, multidrug chemotherapy approach to malignancy; and the probability that RA patients may develop a cancerlike resistance to one DMARD, but not multiple ones. Patients are initially treated with a combination of oral steroids, oral gold, hydroxycholoroquine, azathioprine, and methotrexate. Once the disease is brought under control, drugs are discontinued in a stepwise manner until the patient is treated with only one of the most benign DMARDS, hydroxychloroquine. The argument against this approach includes the fact whereas oncologists know how their drugs work, rheumatologists do not. Further, there is debate as to whether any one of the DMARDS actually reverses or arrests the development of erosions, joint and soft tissue damage, and self-perpetuating deformities. The potential additive toxicities are also a concern.

Thus, we are moving from the wait-and-see approach of the past to an activist one in which all RA patients are treated early in the course of their illness with the strongest and most effective drugs available. While not all rheumatologists use multi-DMARD regimens, and all await the definition of the pathogenesis of this disorder and the availability of more effective treatment modalities, the approach to this disease will never be the same.

Every new step should be carefully thought out by the physician and the patient. The risks and benefits of each new modality should be completely understood by *both* the patient and the physician. It must be noted that although drugs such as nonsteroidal anti-inflammatory agents are still employed early in the course of RA and are thought of as having a "low" toxicity profile, as many as 25 percent of patients develop gastritis or gastric ulceration on these medications. This is especially true in the elderly, a subgroup of patients with a generally higher propensity for developing side effects from all categories of medications.[126] Such toxicities have led many rheumatologists to reassess the order in which RA-directed medications are given, and some advocate the use of disease modifying, antirheumatic drugs (DMARDs) earlier in the course of the disease because they may be more effective in controlling the basic disease process before destructive joint changes occur. Also, they may not actually be more toxic, in individual cases, than drugs such as NSAIDs. We still employ NSAIDs early, but are more cognizant of their potential toxicities. We respect the severe potential toxicities of drugs such as gold and immunosuppressive agents, but are tending to use them earlier, before joint erosions develop.

An educated medical consumer is the best patient, and an open-minded, communicative, caring, and thoughtful physician is the best caretaker. This is especially true because the majority of RA patients go on to develop a chronic disease with a constant need for single or combination drug therapy. Fortunately, only a small percentage develop a highly destructive (mutilans) disorder unresponsive to *all* therapies. A respect for this chronicity and the many potential frustrations along the road of therapeutics enables the physician to guide or pace the patient through the vagaries of this unpredictable disease. Although no specific or curative treatment is available, most patients can benefit by a comprehensive approach using medical, rehabilitative, and surgical services.[125]

Therapeutic Goals

The management of RA involves the following goals:

1. Education, motivation, and emotional support.
2. Induction of remission through the suppression of the joint and systemic inflammatory/immunologic process.
3. Maintenance of joint function and prevention of deformities.
4. Repair of joint damage if it will relieve pain, improve range of motion, or facilitate function.

Patient and Family Education

A health education program should take the form of frank discussions between the physician and the patient and the family, supplemented by literature dispensed by the doctor.[127] In addition to familiarizing patients with the concepts of RA and its management, specific points must be stressed regarding individual drug and physical therapies used, nutritional information, quackery, social services available to the patient, sex and vocational counseling, and support groups.[128] The patient should also contact the national or local Arthritis Foundation in order to obtain the available reading material regarding RA.

Systemic and Articular Rest

The patient must strike a balance between resting and exercising joints that fall short of significant pain and fatigue. Systemic rest includes at least 10 hours a day of sleeping or remaining in bed prior to beginning the day's activity. At times a nap or rest period is needed in the middle of the morning and afternoon.[129] Splints provide rest for the inflamed joints or tendons, relieve spasm and prevent deformities. Wrist splints are particularly useful during bouts of acute wrist synovitis and for management of carpal tunnel syndrome. At times, hospitalization is needed to impose a strict balance of rest and activity and also to institute new, anti-inflammatory agents and disease-modifying drugs. A reassessment of the patient's lifestyle is important in order to define those activities clearly associated with exacerbation of disease. Practical changes in those inciting activities at home, at work and at play may markedly alter disease activity. A change in footwear may improve the gait pattern and decrease foot pain and inflammation. Running shoes and shoes with cushioned soles and rocker bottoms with a wide, high toe box can mean the difference between being able to work and having to curtail one's activities (Recommendation: Rockport shoes initially, specially crafted orthopedic shoes in advanced cases).

Hospitalization

Despite the rising costs of in-hospital care and the general trend toward outpatient management of non-emergency medical care, one or two weeks in the hospital can be a valuable adjunct in the management of active inflammatory disease. Specific indications include: (1) active joint and/or systemic disease not responding to, or flaring in spite of, conventional therapy as an outpatient. Removing the patient from the home and work environment, and instituting an appropriate balance of rest and activity are effective means of reducing joint inflammation, fever, and fatigue. Institution of new drugs, physical therapy modalities, patient education, and emotional support are all important goals of hospitalization; (2) treatment of active vasculitis; (3) treatment of rheumatoid emergencies, such as atlantoaxial subluxation, septic arthritis, drug-induced side effects (e.g., gastrointestinal hemorrhage due to NSAIDs, cytopenias related to remittive drugs), and osteoporosis with vertebral compression fractures related to steroid therapy; and (4) the need for surgical treatment. This might involve joint replacement surgery, repair of tendon ruptures, synovectomy, joint fusion, correction of an unstable cervical spine, or surgical care of an infected native or prosthetic joint.[129]

Physical Medicine

This includes: (1) a regular exercise program, with goals being maintenance of maximum range of joint motion and preservation of hip and shoulder girdle muscle tone. Adequate aerobic exercise is also important. Non-weight-bearing exercises are most appropriate and patients should avoid exercises that involve sudden stops, starts, or twisting motions; (2) appropriate use of heat modalities, such as paraffin baths and hot packs; (3) the use of splinting; (4) education in the principles of joint protection; and (5) activities of daily living assessment. These modalities should be guided by a physical therapist and an occupational therapist. It must be stressed that such therapy should be considered as important as drug therapy and should be prescribed *early* in the disease, with reassessments during the course of the disorder.[130,131]

Medications [132]

General Concepts

Prior to starting any drug in the armamentarium directed at RA it is important, both practically and medicolegally, that the patient be educated about the following: (1) why the drug has been recommended and, if appropriate, alternative drugs to use in the clinical situation, (2) what factors may alter their effectiveness (i.e., drug interactions and complicating illnesses), (3) the importance of compliance in drug administration, (4) the exact dosage and schedule of drug administration and relationship of dosing to meals, and (5) how the drug is to be monitored, drug-related side effects, and when and how to contact the physician about potential drug reactions.

The physician should maintain ongoing education about new facts, about old, tried, and tested drugs, and should become familiar with new forms of drug therapies, their potential side effects, and appropriate monitoring schedules. In order to detect early trends in laboratory changes due to medications, flow sheets should be maintained. Physicians should maintain control of medications and prescribe only the amount of drug needed until the next scheduled testing rather than "open-ended" refill orders. In this way, the patient can only receive refills after the physician has carefully reviewed the appropriate laboratory tests and has questioned the patient about possible adverse side effects of the medication.

Nonsteroidal Anti-inflammatory Drugs (NSAIDs)[133,134]

All NSAIDs have anti-inflammatory, analgesic, and antipyretic properties. Although much of the anti-inflammatory effect of this class of drugs has been associated with their effect upon arachidonic acid metabolism (e.g., prostaglandin synthesis inhibition), it is likely that multiple stages of the inflammatory process are affected in individual patients by different NSAIDs. It is clear that although many of these agents are potent inhibitors of inflammation, they do *not* appear to alter the natural history of RA. The disease progresses, in most patients, despite the continued use of these drugs throughout the course of the illness. Appendix 3-1 at the end of this chapter lists the acetylated and nonacetylated salicylates and nonsalicylate NSAIDs, their recommended dosages, average monthly costs, and specific clinical facts. Appendix 3-2 lists the potential side effects of the NSAIDs in general.

The use of NSAIDs as the initial step in the effective management of synovitis in rheumatoid arthritis is well established. In most, additional anti-inflammatory or disease modifying drugs are added because of the progression or persistence of the disease process (as demonstrated by systemic features, joint deformities, and x-ray defined bony erosions).

Despite the introduction of many newer NSAIDs, salicylates remain important agents, not only in the initial phases of treatment but in all stages of RA therapy. The ability to obtain serum salicylate levels, unavailable with other NSAIDs, is helpful in individualizing treatment programs and evaluating compliance. The recent introduction of nonacetylated forms of salicylate has improved their safety, reduced dosage frequency, and improved patient compliance. These nonacetylated salicylates offer decreased GI and renal toxicity, b.i.d. dosing, and decreased bleeding potential. Although all of the newer NSAIDs (i.e., non-ASA drugs) have been associated with gastric and other side effects, these agents are, in general, better tolerated than ASA.

Response Time. Benefits of treatment with NSAIDs may be apparent within the first few days of administration, but it takes approximately two to three weeks for NSAIDs to demonstrate their full clinical effect. Unfortunately, it takes only two to three days for such drugs to lose their efficacy after discontinuation. Thus, RA patients with ongoing joint inflammation and undergoing a switch from one NSAID to another will be without effective anti-inflammatory coverage for a relatively long period of time. The patient should be made aware of such a hiatus and appropriate pain medications should be given to fill the gap.

Choice of NSAID. One cannot predict which NSAID will work in a given patient and thus one employs a largely empiric technique in choosing them. There is great variation in patient response and adverse reactions with all these drugs. Most physicians have a group of NSAIDs with which they are familiar and they use them in a "round robin" manner, starting with their most effective and least toxic drug and then moving to another if a drug proves ineffective after three or four weeks or is associated with an adverse drug reaction. Little evidence to date suggests that one NSAID is more effective than another, or that combinations are more beneficial than single drug therapy.

Unresponsiveness. Although a drug may work initially, patients very often become unresponsive (tachyphylactic) to NSAIDs, and alternative drugs may have to be instituted as time goes on.

Patient Compliance. Whether the drug employed is a salicylate or nonsalicylate NSAID, a single daily or b.i.d. dose schedule will meet with the highest rate of patient compliance.

Adjustment of Dosage. Because individual responses to different NSAIDs vary markedly, adjusting the dosage to the patient's response is essential, especially in the elderly. Using the lowest possible dose initially and then increasing the dosage slowly and carefully is optimal.

NSAIDs in Combination with Disease Modifying Drugs. NSAIDs continue to be used as baseline therapy despite the addition of other forms of medical management. The withdrawal of NSAIDs at the time of institution of the slower acting, disease-modifying drugs may lead to a flare of the inflammatory state.

Cost. Cost is an important consideration in the use of NSAIDs. As noted in Appendix 3-3 at the end of this chapter, many of the newer NSAIDs cost 10 times as much as aspirin. Thus, a clear cost (in both side effects and monetary cost) vs. benefit decision must be made prior to the institution of this class of drugs.

Gastrointestinal Toxicity. Gastrointestinal toxicity, including gastritis and gastric and duodenal ulceration with hemorrhage or perforation, may occur in both the young and old. These potentially fatal disorders may occur in an asymptomatic patient or may be signaled by a prior or recent history of GI disturbance. Unfortunately, the physician cannot distinguish between "benign" GI symptoms and those reflecting gastric or duodenal damage. As many as two thirds of those with GI complaints discontinue their NSAID. Patients reporting symptoms tend to be young, to be female, to have somewhat more severe disease, and to have a history of previous gastric upset and use of gastroprotective therapy. In contrast, those with severe endoscopic lesions, hospitalizations for GI problems, or death were frequently older, with strikingly more severe disease. Multiple therapies, smoking, and, in particular, low-dose prednisone more than doubles the frequency of severe side effects.[126] Attention to these facts is important when physicians are prescribing these medications, especially in the elderly. Although NSAIDs are used as first-line drugs in the treatment of RA, their toxicity profile is higher than previously appreciated and initial risk assessment is indicated prior to the institution of this class of drugs, especially in the elderly. The availability of cytoprotective measures (e.g., misoprostol, Cytotec) enables the physician to protect the stomachs of patients at high risk for GI problems while on NSAIDs. The indications for the use of these medications should be better defined in the near future.

Elderly Patients. Physical and pharmacologic changes associated with aging may increase older patients' sensitivity to both the therapeutic and toxic effects of some drugs. Because of the many alterations that occur in the metabolism of drugs in the elderly, NSAIDs with a shorter half-life (e.g., drugs with t.i.d.–q.i.d. dosing such as ibuprofen) are optimal in an attempt to avoid side effects. Further, one must carefully take into consideration drug interactions in a potentially ill, elderly population. An attempt to avoid "polypharmacy" makes good clinical sense. Great care should be taken when one uses NSAIDs in the elderly because of their increased propensity for side effects, including life-threatening GI and renal toxicity. In general, in the elderly, the concept of hemeostenosis should be considered. This represents the limited ability of the elderly to compensate for pertubations in their own organ systems.

Slow-acting or Disease Modifying Antirheumatic Drugs (DMARDs)[135-138]

Most patients with RA ultimately require these agents. As a general rule, of any 100 patients taking any DMARDS, about 50 percent will have a satisfactory response within 6 months of use. Another 20 percent will stop taking the drug during the first 6 months because of side effects, and about 30 percent will stop treatment after 6 months because of lack of efficacy. Conventional DMARDs include antimalarial drugs and gold salts (parenteral and oral). Azathioprine is an immunosuppressive drug and, while it may lead to a significant improvement in the basic disease state, it is potentially oncogenic. Methotrexate is both well-tolerated and effective. Its long-term hepatic toxicity has not been defined and it differs from other DMARDs in that patients respond quickly to its institution and flare rapidly after its discontinuation. The concept that these drugs are specific antirheumatic agents derives from the observation that they are active in treating RA but have minimal demonstrable nonspecific anti-inflammatory effects. Patients responding to these agents show significant improvement by clinical and laboratory parameters. Although controversy exists with each of these agents, they appear, clinically, to have the potential to modify the natural history of rheumatoid arthritis. Whether or not these drugs actually decrease the rate of progression or accelerate the rate of healing of radiologically defined bone erosions or other characteristic manifestations of joint destruction remains controversial. They are to be differentiated from the various nonspecific anti-inflammatory agents that may effectively control symptoms but have not been demonstrated to modify the course of the disease. The use of DMARDs is based almost entirely on clinical experience rather than the knowledge of their specific drug action. None of these drugs was initially developed to treat rheumatoid arthritis. Many aspects of their use in this disease are based upon accumulated experience and not documented fact. Despite this, there is a broad clinical experience supporting the capacity of these drugs to alter the course of rheumatoid arthritis.

An important characteristic of this group of drugs is their delayed onset of action, thus the name "slow-acting drugs." The suppression of disease is gradual, may not be apparent until weeks or months after the initiation of therapy, and may take from 4 to more than 6 months to reach a maximum. The inflammatory process may remain inactive for weeks or months after the drug is stopped, in contrast to the quicker inflammatory flare after stopping nonsteroidal anti-inflammatory drugs. Methotrexate, however, has a more rapid onset of action, and flares may occur within 2 to 4 weeks after stopping the medication. Physicians and patients must appreciate this fact because the flares can be quite severe.

Although these drugs may cause an improvement in many patients, induction of a total clinical remission remains an *uncommon* event. More commonly, the remission is a temporary reduction in the rate of disease progression.

Indications[138]

1. **Active, systemic, seropositive rheumatoid disease.** Active and progressive disease is defined clinically by joint pain, swelling, stiffness, and deformity, and radiologically by the development of new erosions, joint space narrowing, or other structural joint changes. The presence of an elevated ESR, thrombocytosis, and anemia are further manifestations of active systemic disease. Fatigue is, for most patients, one of the most disturbing features of active disease and is an excellent clinical sign of the systemic activity of the disease.
2. **Inability to continue another DMARD** because of lack of effectiveness and/or toxicity.
3. **The need for a "sparing agent" for corticosteroids.** In those patients already on corticosteroids and with unacceptable side effects, the use of DMARDs may allow for disease control and taper of steroids.

Decision to use DMARDs. The patient and the physician must take the likelihood of success and the potential toxicity into consideration when deciding on these drugs. The patient must balance the potential side effects against potential gains in the quality of life. Antecedent therapy with one disease-modifying agent appears to have little predictable effect on the likelihood of either a therapeutic response or a toxic side effect when taking a second DMARD. It appears that the same percentage of patients will respond to treatment with a DMARD irrespective of antecedent therapy with another DMARD. It is important to note that one cannot predict the likelihood of either a therapeutic response or a toxic side effect in a given patient. As noted above, over time, significant numbers of patients stop taking these drugs, either because of early or late lack of clinical response or toxicity. One would hope that a drug used to modify a chronic, inflammatory disease such as RA could be taken over a long period of time. Recent evidence has demonstrated that at 5 years, only 8 to 20 percent of patients are still taking many of the so-called disease modifying drugs (specifically oral and parenteral gold, sulfasalazine, antimalarial drugs, and D-penicillamine). Most of these drug discontinuations were due to lack of drug efficacy. However, 50 percent of patients on methotrexate remain on it after 5 years, and the primary reason for its discontinuation is side effects. Such data have led to the emergence of methotrexate as a favored drug, one which is instituted earlier and earlier in the treatment protocol of RA.

Choice of DMARD. As is appropriate, the decision regarding the choice of DMARD should be made in close consultation with an informed patient. The patient should be given extensive reading material about these drugs, including information about their positive and negative effects. At times, although a specific drug would be appropriate in the clinical situation, an alternative drug is chosen because of logistical problems, specific patient fears about certain medications, cost factors, and potential problems with patient compliance or reliability.

Rheumatologists vary greatly in their choice and order of use of DMARDs. However, a few general points can be made:

1. Whether one uses DMARDs singly or in combination, there is a consensus to use them *early* in the course of RA to attempt to alter the natural history of the disease. There is still great debate whether any of these drugs have the capacity to modify the RA disease process.
2. While physicians are using methotrexate[139,149-152] (Appendix 3-4 at the end of this chapter) early in the course of disease (at times as their first DMARD), others still use parenteral gold[140] (Appendix 3-5) first because of a long therapeutic experience with it as an effective drug with an acceptable profile of side effects.
3. DMARDs such as sulfasalazine (Appendix 3-6),[144,145] hydroxychloroquine (Appendix 3-7),[142,143] and oral gold (Appendix 3-5) are commonly used in the early phase of RA or in combination with other DMARDs because of patient acceptance, reasonable toxicity profile, and many controlled trials demonstrating their efficacy.

In general, they are considered to have relatively equal efficacy. Our experience with the two former drugs is good, but oral gold appears to be the least effective drug in our armamentarium. We do avoid sulfasalazine and specifically use hydroxychloroquine in those situations in which the patient may have systemic lupus rather than RA.

4. D-Penicillamine, a drug commonly used in the past especially in those patients with prominent extra-articular disease manifestations, has fallen out of favor because of its unacceptably high toxicity profile, and its slow onset of action (Appendix 3-8).[146,147]
5. Methotrexate has a steroidlike, rapid onset of action (in 4 to 6 weeks), and is also the most likely of all DMARDs to be tolerated and/or effective on a long-term basis. However, if methotrexate has to be stopped because of side effects or lack of efficacy, the majority of RA patients will have a disease flare, at times more severe than prior to its institution. Thus, an alternative DMARD should be started immediately after stopping methotrexate, and we tend to use azathioprine or sulfasalazine in this setting. There is still uncertainty about the long-term liver and pulmonary toxicity of methotrexate. Recent studies have demonstrated that severe liver toxicity may develop in one in 1000 methotrexate-treated RA patients, and that an increased frequency of methotrexate-induced pneumonitis has been appreciated. Most rheumatologists recommend a liver biopsy after 1500 to 2000-mg cumulative dose of methotrexate (approximately 3 to 4 years of therapy).
6. Azathioprine has been shown to be effective in the treatment of RA, but its early use has been avoided because of its oncongenicity (Appendix 3-9).[148] Cyclophosphamide is one of the most effective disease modifying drugs (only intramuscular gold and cyclophosphamide have been clearly demonstrated to lead to healing of erosions), but its high profile of significant side effects (e.g., oncogenicity, hemorrhagic cystitis, sterility) has limited its use to those patients with rheumatoid vasculitis.[153] Cyclosporine is also effective in controlling the RA inflammatory state, but it is used mainly in those patients with refractory disease because of its renal toxicity and high cost.

Corticosteroids

Although these drugs are the most potent of the anti-inflammatory agents, systemic corticosteroids have a high incidence of toxicity and do not appear to have an effect upon the underlying disease process.

Indications

Before these drugs are used, the patient and the physician must balance the desired effects against the toxic effects. Further, one must consider the fact that RA patients may need chronic treatment with escalating doses of steroids with all their attendant cumulative side effects. Indications include:

1. Sustained or progressive, severe polyarticular joint disease unresponsive to a regimen of antirheumatic therapy (including antimalarials, azulfidine, gold salts, NSAIDs, and physical therapy).
2. An acute episode of severe arthritis that is predictably (from prior experience with clinical flares) short-lived.
3. The presence of systemic rheumatoid disease manifested by (a) serositis (pleuritis and/or pericarditis), (b) inflammatory pulmonary disease, (c) episcleritis/scleritis (unresponsive to topical treatment), (d) vasculitis of the polyarteritis nodosa type or severe systemic features of disease including fever, anemia, weight loss, or neuropathy.
4. The presence of "social indications" such as a long-awaited vacation trip, honeymoon, or an unexpected, stressful situation. One- or 2-week courses of tapering doses of corticosteroids in these situations can be very valuable and there is little risk of side effects.
5. Patients with severe, active disease despite NSAIDs in whom it will take 1 to 2 months for a DMARD to be effective. In this situation, the patient can remain functional until the DMARD begins to control the disease. The steroids can then be tapered in the setting of the "steroid sparing effect" of DMARDs.
6. Intra-articular or intralesional injection of microcrystalline corticosteroid esters for the treatment of severe, local disease and in order to avoid the need for systemic steroids.[155]

Contraindications and Side Effects. As a result of disease chronicity in the majority of RA patients, many may develop chronic steroid dependency. Such patients, especially when treated with prednisone doses of more than 7.5 mg per day for long periods, are likely to develop one or more side effects. These include osteoporosis, peptic ulcer disease/gastritis, increased propensity for infections, diabetes, cataracts, and hypertension.

Topical Steroids. Topical steroids are used in the treatment of uveitis or scleritis and for cutaneous use in the treatment of drug-related dermatitis (e.g., gold salts, penicillamine).

Intra-articular and Intralesional Steroids. Injectable corticosteroids are used within joints and peri-articular tissues to locally control severe inflammation. *Indications* for local corticosteroids in RA include: (1) recalcitrant synovitis of one or very few joints (inflammation of a single joint should be disproportionate compared with other joints; infection must always be considered in any RA patient with a monoarticular synovitis), (2) palliation of selected joints pending response to DMARDs, (3) limited, mild RA not warranting aggressive systemic therapy, with one or a few joints most severely affected, and (4) nonarticular, soft-tissue "rheumatoid" disease, including entrapment neuropathies (e.g., carpal tunnel syndrome), popliteal and antecubital cysts, tenosynovitis (digital flexor, wrist extensor, rotator cuff, Achilles tendon), and bursitis (olecranon, subacromial, trochanteric, anserine, infrapatellar, retrocalcaneal).

Complications of local corticosteroid injections include (1) postinjection flare (This evanescent inflammatory reaction is due to leukocyte ingestion of corticosteroid microcrystals and occurs within 12 hours of the injection. This possibility should be brought to the patient's attention and, if it occurs, the patient should apply ice and take acetaminophen; the attack should clear within 24 to 48 hours.), (2) possible accelerated joint destruction (limit injections to no more than three times per year) and tendon rupture (especially true when Achilles tendons are injected), (3) septic arthritis usually due to Staphlococcus aureus, develops after approximately one in 14–50,000 injections, (4) skin atrophy and hypopigmentation at injection sites, and (5) hypersensitivity reaction to steroid vehicle and transient facial flushing.

The value of *postinjection rest* has recently been stressed. With a strict regimen of three days of bedrest after knee injection, followed by three weeks of guarded ambulation, there is a significant prolongation of response to intra-articular steroids. Of course, such restrictions are, at times, difficult to impose on a patient who works or runs a household. Enforced rest may also diminish the risk of the articular abuse and damage that may result from steroid-mediated joint analgesia.

In the future, corticosteroid esters may be incorporated into dipalmitoyl phosphatidylcholine liposomes. In experimental situations, liposome-entrapped steroids produced greater and more sustained anti-inflammatory effects than did comparable doses of conventional microcrystalline steroids.[155]

Systemic Corticosteroids. Systemic corticosteroid therapy consists of (1) low-dose oral steroids, (2) high-dose oral steroids, and (3) very-high-dose intravenous steroids.

Of the *low-dose oral steroids*, prednisone is the preferred agent because its cost and mineralocorticoid activities are low. Tablets are available in 1-, 5- and 10-mg tablets. When used to suppress synovitis, the regimen is 5.0 to 7.5 mg prednisone, preferably in a single morning dose, although divided dose schedules may be required. The total dose should be the smallest possible dose needed to ameliorate symptoms. The physician should attempt to decrease steroid requirement by using NSAIDs and/or remittive agents. RA patients tolerate alternate-day administration of corticosteroids poorly because synovitis tends to flare on the "off" day. However, they generally have a lower incidence of side effects and are better than no steroids at all. At times, an acute RA flare may require in-hospital management with the institution of prednisone 20 to 30 mg per day in divided doses for three to five days with tapering, but only if more conservative management has failed.[156]

High-dose oral steroids are used to treat rheumatoid vasculitis, if manifested by mesenteric and other internal organ ischemia or mononeurtis multiplex. Prednisone is administered in doses of 40 to 60 mg per day, in divided doses, because of its malignant, life-threatening nature. Eventual taper by 5 to 10 mg every five to seven days is started after the clinical (organ ischemia, fever, weight loss) and laboratory (hemoglobin, ESR, thrombocytosis) status has improved and remains stable.

For *very-high-dose intravenous steroids*, 1 g of Solu-Medrol is infused over 1 to 2 hours, once a day for three consecutive days, as a current "vogue" in the treatment of many severe, active connective tissue and other inflammatory disorders unresponsive to NSAIDs and/or remittive agents or low-dose oral steroids. Although patients do respond to this very-high-dose regimen, the long-term effectiveness in both controlling active disease and slowing the radiographic progression of the arthritis remains unknown. In the setting of "pulse" therapy for SLR, this type of therapy is not as benign as initially thought, and may lead to infections, osteonecrosis, electrolyte abnormalities, seizures (especially in patients with hypertension), myocardial ischemia due to coronary vasospasm, and sudden death thought to be related to arrhythmia/electrolyte imbalance. This type of therapy remains *experimental*.[157]

Felty's Syndrome

Those patients who have a low neutrophil count without a history of infection should be observed and treatment should be directed at the underlying inflammatory state of the RA. In those patients with a history of infection, the use of lithium carbonate is appropriate in an attempt to increase the white blood cell count by stimulation of colony-stimulating activity. Gold and penicillamine have also been useful in the treatment of the underlying inflammatory and immunologic state of RA and also the leukopenia of Felty's syndrome. If patients continue to develop infections, splenectomy is considered. Splenectomy leads to improvement in the white blood cell count in over 70 percent of Felty's patients, but recurrent or persistent infections occur in as many as 60 percent. Given the increased susceptibility to infection in patients undergoing splenectomy, the benefits of this operation must be weighed against this potential complication. If patients continue to have infections after this splenectomy, accessory splenectomy, lithium carbonate, and gold or penicillamine should be reconsidered. Corticosteroids are usually avoided because they reduce the functional capacity of granulocytes (increasing the risk for infection) and are infrequently effective in the treatment of Felty's syndrome. Immunosuppressive agents cannot be recommended except in rare instances in which the patient has a systemic vasculitis.[158]

Extra-articular Manifestations

Constitutional Features

Fatigue, anemia, weight loss, and low-grade fever are usually managed as part of the overall treatment of RA (after ruling out other causes of these symptoms/signs, such as malignancy, blood loss, infection).

Pulmonary and Cardiac Disease

Patients with pleural effusions/pleurisy or pericardial disease may be treated with NSAIDs, or with corticosteroids if these problems are more severe. Pericardiocentesis or thoracentesis may be needed for diagnostic or therapeutic reasons, depending upon the clinical presentation. Infection with pyogenic bacteria or tuberculosis must always be considered in patients who present with pericardial or pleural effusions, especially if fever is present and if the patient is on steroids. Patients with progressive pulmonary dysfunction due to interstitial pulmonary disease may need to be treated with steroids along with discontinuation of medications potentially contributing to the lung disorder (e.g., methotrexate, penicillamine, gold can lead to interstitial pneumonitis or obliterative bronchiolitis).

Rheumatoid Nodules

Rheumatoid nodules may, at times, ulcerate. This should be treated locally and with antibiotics if infection is present. Rarely, surgical removal is needed. Following surgical removal, the nodules very often return in the same area.

Neuropathy

Usually neuropathy is due to an underlying vasculitis or amyloidosis, and the nerve disorder is treated along with the other disease manifestations. Alternative causes for neuropathy should be sought, including heavy metal poisoning, diabetes, and malignancy.

Cervical Spine Disease

The treatment of cervical spine disease (atlantoaxial and subaxial dislocation) should be guided by the extent of actual or potential neurologic dysfunction and varies from soft to hard to Philadelphia collars, and potentially may involve surgical intervention. If the patient develops progressive weakness or clear neurologic dysfunction, definition of the anatomic distortion of the cervical spine area due to RA may need to be defined by MRI scanning. The upper cervical spine (atlantoaxial) area is more capacious than the lower cervical area and there is a lower potential for cord compression, especially if there is erosion of the odontoid process. Superior migration of the odontoid process can lead to foramen magnum invagination and potential neurologic dysfunction.

Rheumatoid Vasculitis or Malignant Rheumatoid Disease

In patients with significant visceral disease (i.e., major vascular compromise, including mesenteric vasculitis, mononeuritis multiplex, coronary vasculitis), fever, and leukocytosis, one uses 40 to 60 mg of prednisone in three to four divided daily doses initially, with a slow taper of steroids when the inflammatory process is stable. If the disease process advances despite high doses of steroids, or if the side effects from the steroids are intolerable, immunosuppressive agents such as azathioprine or cyclophosphamide are indicated in a dosage of 2 mg per kg per day.

Surgery

Surgical treatment plays a major role in the management and rehabilitation of RA patients with erosive, destructive, and deforming disease. Traditional techniques of joint fusion and synovectomy remain in the orthopedist's armamentarium, while joint arthroplasty (especially total hip and knee replacement) is achieving an even higher level of acceptance and efficacy. Surgical reconstruction in RA patients must be regarded as part of a comprehensive care plan and judiciously balanced with medical management. The pattern of joint involvement and the eventual functional goals of the patient must be considered. The indications, goals, and timing of surgery must be individually tailored to each patient and depend on the course of disease, functional impairment, and rehabilitation potential. The possible benefits of surgery are to prevent further tissue destruction, to relieve pain, and to improve function.

Additional Therapeutic Modalities

Radiation Synovectomy

The local joint installation of various isotopes has been employed over the years in order to obliterate intensely inflamed synovium. Such a procedure, said to have long-term safety in extensive clinical experience in Europe, avoids the morbidity and recuperative period of a surgical synovectomy. The problem with arthroscopic synovectomy is the limited amount of synovial tissue that can be removed through the arthroscope. Dysprosium and newer isotopes with longer half-lives have been effective and practical agents for use in the treatment of persistent joint synovitis. Enthusiastic endorsement of radioisotope synovectomy must await the results of additional cooperative controlled studies. The general public and physicians must also be convinced that such therapy will not lead to late chromosomal damage or neoplasm.

Diet

Physicians and patients have been intrigued for many years with the possibility that arthritis might be the result of hypersensitivity to environmental toxins, specifically to food and food-related products. The Arthritis Foundation, in its informational pamphlets for patients, summarized:

> **The Truth About Diet and Arthritis.**
> The possible relationship between diet and arthritis has been thoroughly and scientifically studied. The simple proven fact is: no food has anything to do with causing arthritis and no food is effective in treating or curing it.

Some observations, however, support the suggestion, but do not prove, that individualized dietary manipulations may be beneficial for selected patients with rheumatic diseases. Controlled, blinded studies are needed to resolve this issue. As a general rule, however, if a patient has found a strong relationship between the eating of a certain type of food and an exacerbation of the arthritis, it is practical to avoid that inciting food. Some authorities think that about 1 in 400 RA patients may have a food allergy which may lead to a flare. Several studies have shown that cow's milk may induce or exacerbate rheumatic symptoms in some patients, and that a controlled fast can help to alleviate such symptoms.[159]

Fish Oil Supplements

New evidence suggests that dietary fish oil supplements may help alleviate symptoms of rheumatoid arthritis. The oil, obtained from cold-water fish, contains omega-3 polyunsaturated acids. These competitively inhibit synthesis of prostaglandins and leukotrienes, both of which may mediate the inflammatory response in patients with RA. Fish oil is known to prolong bleeding time and to inhibit platelet aggregation. These effects could be dangerous in patients taking other anticoagulants, including aspirin. Fish oil capsules, sold in health food stores and pharmacies, are currently touted for the prevention of heart disease with a maximal dose of 6 g per day. In a double-blind, controlled, crossover trial involving 33 patients with RA, 15 g of fish oil appeared to reduce joint inflammation and improve function in some patients with active disease. Until further information on optimum dosage and duration is available, however, such supplementation cannot be generally recommended for the treatment of RA. Patients should be told that if they take fish oil capsules and NSAIDs, an additive anticoagulant effect may occur. Such drugs should be stopped, along with NSAIDs, in the perioperative period in order to decrease the propensity for intraoperative or postoperative bleeding due to drug-induced platelet defects. A preoperative bleeding time will define the effect of these drugs on platelets.[160]

Novel Immunotherapies for the Treatment of Rheumatoid Arthritis

A number of drugs are currently being evaluated in the treatment of refractory disease. These can be divided into three groups. The first are cytokines. An example is interferon-gamma, which can have certain downregulatory effects on synovial cells. However, its full efficacy has yet to be determined and it is not certain whether patients have sustained improvement on this drug.[161] The second group includes inhibitors of cytokines. One such inhibitor is the IL-1 receptor antagonist, which is being evaluated based on its ability to block IL-1 function[162] and the fact that some RA patients develop anti-IL-1 antibodies.[163] Inhibitors for tumor necrosis factor[164] have also been described but they have not been studied in vivo yet. A recent adaptation has been to make use of recombinant fusion proteins conjugated to cytokines themselves. Sewell and Trentham[165] have used IL-2 conjugated to diphtheria toxin that is cytotoxic to cells with high affinity receptor. Preliminary studies in a noncontrolled trial suggest some efficacy; longer term studies are needed. A third group makes use of chimeric monoclonal antibodies that are targeted toward specific cell types. These include anti-CD4, which is on the helper T cell population[166]; and anti-CD5, which is on T cells and a subset of B cells that are thought to be responsible for RF production.[167]

Potentially valuable therapies in the future include anti–T-cell receptor antibodies and newer immunologic agents designed to suppress the immune system, for example, FK506, a cyclosporine relative.

Summary

In general, 70 percent of patients with rheumatoid arthritis experience chronic disability with alternating remission and exacerbation. While 10 to 20 percent have sustained remissions, a similar number develop a severe, crippling disorder. Indicators of a poor prognosis include multiple inflamed joints, subcutaneous nodules, strongly positive rheumatoid factor tests, other serologic abnormalities (antinuclear antibody, circulating immune complexes), bone erosions or cartilage loss on x-ray, and onset at an older age. Although remittive drugs may cause improvement in many patients, induction of total clinical remission as a result of therapy with these agents remains a relatively uncommon event, and the term remission-inducing implies more of a hope than an expectation. More usual is a temporary reduction in the rate of disease progression. While some patients develop long-term improvement on a single remittive agent taken over many years, most will be switched from one NSAID or remittive drug to another either because of initial or eventual lack of clinical improvement and/or an adverse drug reaction. However, an overall program of physical therapy, medications, surgical intervention when indicated, and emotional support, go a long way in improving the overall functional status of the patient. In the long run, a defintion of the etiology and a better understanding of the immunopathogenesis of this chronic, inflammatory disorder will enable physicians to more specifically and effectively target therapies at basic disease processes.[161]

References

1. Harris, E: The clinical features of rheumatoid arthritis. In: Kelley, WN, et al (Eds): Textbook of Rheumatology. Philadelphia, WB Saunders, 1989, p 943.
2. Mitchell, D: Epidemiology of rheumatoid arthritis. In: Utsinger, PD, Zvaifler, NJ, and Ehrligh, GE (Eds): Rheumatoid Arthritis. Philadelphia, JB Lippincott, 1985, p 133.
3. Zvaifler, N: New perspectives on the pathogenesis of rheumatoid arthritis. Am J Med 85 (suppl 4A):12, 1988.
4. Phillips, PE: Infectious agents in chronic rheumatic disease. In: McCarty, DJ (Ed): Arthritis and Allied Conditions. A Textbook of Rheumatology. Philadelphia, Lea and Febiger, 1989, p 482.
5. Steere, AC: Lyme disease. In: Kelley, WN, et al (Eds): Textbook of Rheumatology. Philadelphia, JB Lippincott, 1985, p 71.
6. Silver, RM, and Zvaflier, NJ: Pathogenesis immunological considerations. In: Utsinger, PD, Zvaifler, NJ, and Ehrlich GE (Eds): Rheumatoid Arthritis. Philadelphia, JB Lippincott, 1985, p 71.
7. Schlegel, SI, and Paulus, HE: Update on NSAID use in rheumatic diseases. Bull Rheum Dis 36:1, 1986.
8. Lipsky, PE: Disease modifying drugs in rheumatoid arthritis. In: Utsinger, PD, Zvaifler, NJ, and Ehrlich, GE (Eds): Rheumatoid Arthritis. Philadelphia, JB Lippincott, 1985, p 601.
9. Ward, JR: Role of disease-modifying anti-rheumatic drugs versus cytotoxic agents in the treatment of rheumatoid arthritis. Am J Med 85 (suppl 4A):39, 1988.
10. Gaston, JSH, et al: Dissection of the mechanism of immune injury in rheumatoid arthritis using total lymphoid irradiation. Arth Rheum 31:21, 1988.
11. Pincus, T, and Callahan, LF: Formal education as a marker for increased mortality and morbidity in rheumatoid arthritis. J Chronic Dis 38:973, 1985.
12. Callahan, LF, and Pincus, T: Formal education level as a significant marker of clinical status in rheumatoid arthritis. Arth Rheum 31:1346, 1988.
13. Pincus, T: Is mortality increased in rheumatoid arthritis? J Musculoskel Med 5(6):27, 1988.
14. Pincus, T, and Callahan, LF: Taking mortalilty in rheumatoid arthritis seriously: Predictive markers, socioeconomic status and comorbidity. J Rheumatol 13:841, 1986.

15. Rasker, JJ, and Cosh, JA: Cause and age at death in a prospective study of 100 patients with rheumatoid arthritis. Ann Rheum Dis 40:115, 1981.
16. Mitchell, DM, et al: Predictors of mortality in RA (abstr). Eighth Pan American Congress of Rheumatology, Washington, DC, 1982.
17. Firestein, GS, Tsai, V, and Zvaifler, NJ: Cellular immunity in the joints of patients with rheumatoid arthritis and other forms of chronic arthritis. Rheum Dis Clin North Am 13:191, 1987.
18. Kobayashi I, and Ziff, M: Electron microscopic studies of lymphoid cells in the rheumatoid synovial membrane. Arthritis Rheum 16:471, 1973.
19. Van Voorhis, WC, et al: The relative efficacy of human monocytes and dendritic cells as accessory cells for T cell replication. J Exp Med 158: 174, 1983.
20. Sokoloff, L: Pathology of rheumatoid arthritis and related disorders. In: McCarty, DJ (ed): Arthritis and Allied Conditions, ed 10. Philadelphia, Lea & Febiger, 1985, pp 571–592.
21. Zvaifler, NJ, et al: Dendritic cells in synovial effusions of patients with rheumatoid arthritis. J Clin Invest 76:789, 1985.
22. Burmester, GR, Jahn, B, and Gramatzki, M: Activated T cells in vivo and in vitro: Divergence and expression of Tac and Ia antigens in the nonblastoid small T cells of inflammation and normal T cells activated in vitro. J Immunol 133: 1230, 1984.
23. Hemler, ME, et al: Very late activation antigens on rheumatoid synovial fluid T lymphocytes: Association with stages of T cell activation. J Clin Invest 78: 696, 1986.
24. Van Voorhis, WC, Witmer, M, and Steinman, RM: The phenotype of dendritic cells and macrophages. Fed Proc 42: 114, 1983.
25. Bhardwaj, N, et al: Interleukin-6/interferon beta$_2$ in synovial effusions of patients with rheumatoid arthritis and other arthritides: Identification of several isoforms and studies of cellular sources. J Immunol 143:2153, 1989.
26. Houssiau, FA, et al: Interleukin-6 in synovial fluid and serum of patients with rheumatoid arthritis and other arthritides. Arthritis Rheum 31:784, 1988.
27. Sehgal, PB, et al: Human beta$_2$ interferon and B cell differentiation factor BSF-2 are identical. Science 235:731, 1987.
28. Dayer, JM, et al: Human recombinant interleukin-1 stimulates collagenase and prostaglandin E production by human synovial cells. J Clin Invest 77:645, 1986.
29. Dayer, JM, Beutler, B, and Cerami, A: Cachectin/tumor necrosis factor stimulates collagenase and prostaglandin E$_2$ production by human synovial cells and dermal fibroblasts. J Exp Med 162:2163, 1985.
30. Brennan, FM, et al: Detection of interleukin 8 biological activity in synovial fluids from patients with rheumatoid arthritis and production of interleukin 8 mRNA by isolated synovial cells. Eur J Immunol 20:2141, 1990.
31. Firestein, GS, Paine, MM, and Littman, BH: Gene expression (collagenase, tissue inhibitor of metalloproteinases, complement, and HLA-DR) in rheumatoid arthritis and osteoarthritis synovium. Arthritis Rheum 34:1094, 1991.
32. Gravallese, EM, et al: In situ hybridization studies of stromelysin and collagenase messenger RNA expression in rheumatoid synovium. Arthritis Rheum 34:1076, 1991.
33. Walakovits, LA, et al: Detection of stromelysin and collagenase in synovial fluid from patients with rheumatoid arthritis and post-traumatic knee injury. Arthritis Rheum (in press).
34. Cawston, et al: Metalloproteinases and collagenase inhibitors in rheumatoid synovial fluid. Arthritis Rheum 27:285, 1984.
35. Firestein, GS, and Zvaifler, NJ: The pathogenesis of rheumatoid arthritis. Rheum Dis Clin North Am 13:447, 1987.
36. Bhardwaj, N, et al: Interleukin-1 production by mononuclear cells from rheumatoid synovial effusions. Cell Immunol 114:405, 1988.
37. Robinson, DR: Lipid mediators of inflammation. Rheum Dis Clin North Am 13:385, 1987.
38. Kremer, JM, et al: Effects of dietary supplementation in active rheumatoid arthritis. Ann Intern Med 106:497, 1987.
39. Gregersen, PK, Silver, J, and Winchester, RJ: The shared epitope hypothesis. Arthritis Rheum 30:1205, 1987.
40. Larhammar, D, et al: Complete amino acid sequence of an HLA-DR antigen like beta chain as predicted from the nucleotide sequence: Similarities with immunoglobulins and HLA-A, -B, and -C antigen. Proc Natl Acad Sci USA 79:3687, 1982.
41. Karr, RW, et al: Association of HLA-DRw4 with rheumatoid arthritis in black and white patients. Arthritis Rheum 23:1241, 1980.
42. Nepom, BS, et al: Specific HLA-DR4 associated histocompatibility molecules characterize patients with seropositive juvenile rheumatoid arthritis. J Clin Invest 74:287, 1984.
43. Hochman, PS, and Huber, BT: A class II gene conversion event defines an antigen specific Ir gene epitope. J Exp Med 160:1925, 1984.
44. Amar, A, et al: HLA-D locus in Israel: Characterization of 14 local HTC's and a population study. Tissue Antigens 20: 198, 1982.
45. Bell, JI, et al: DNA sequence and characterization of human class II major histocompatibility complex beta chains from the DR1 haplotype. Proc Natl Acad Sci USA 82:3405, 1985.
46. Willkens, RF, et al: Association of HLA-Dw16 with rheumatoid arthritis in Yakima Indians: Further evidence for the "shared epitope" hypothesis. Arthritis Rheum 34:43, 1991.
47. Kappler, J, et al: V beta-specific stimulation of human T cells by staphylococcal toxins. Science 244:811, 1989.

48. Cole, BC, et al: Mycoplasma induced arthritis. In: Razin, S, and Barile, MF (Eds): The Mycoplasmas, Vol IV. New York, Academic Press, 1985, pp 107–160.
49. Paliard, X, et al: Evidence for the effects of a superantigen in rheumatoid arthritis. Science 253:325, 1991.
50. Howell, MD, et al: Limited T-cell receptor beta-chain heterogeneity among interleukin 2 receptor-positive synovial T cells suggests a role for superantigen in rheumatoid arthritis. Proc Natl Acad Sci USA 88:10921, 1991.
51. Chen, PP, Fong, S, and Carson, DA: Rheumatoid factor. Rheum Dis Clin North Am 13:545, 1987.
52. Agnello, V, et al: Evidence for a subset of rheumatoid factors that cross-react with DNA-histone and have a distinct cross-reactive idiotype. J Exp Med 151:1514, 1987.
53. Kunkel, HG, et al: Cross-idiotypic specificity among monoclonal IgM proteins with anti-gammaglobulin activity. J Exp Med 137:331, 1973.
54. Manser, T, et al: The molecular evolution of the immune response. Immunol Today 6:94, 1985.
55. Carson, DA: Rheumatoid factor. In: Kelley, WJ, Harris, ED, Jr, and Ruddy, S, (Eds): Textbook of Rheumatology. Philadelphia, WB Saunders, 1985, p 664.
56. Maini, RN, Plater-Zyberk, C, and Andrew, E: Autoimmunity in rheumatoid arthritis. Rheum Dis Clin North Am 13:319, 1987.
57. Wang, CY, et al: Identification of a p69, 71 complex expressed on human T cells sharing determinants with B-type chronic lymphatic leukemia cells. J Exp Med 151: 1539, 1980.
58. Thomas, Y, et al: Biologic functions of the OK T-1 T cell surface antigen. 1. The T-1 molecule is involved in helper function. J Immunol 133:724, 1984.
59. Hardy, RR, and Hayakawa, K: Development and physiology of Ly-1 B and its human homolog Leu-1 B. Immunol Rev 93:53, 1986.
60. Burastero, SE, et al: Monoreactive high affinity and polyreactive low affinity rheumatoid factors are produced by CD5+ B cells from patients with rheumatoid arthritis. J Exp Med 168:1979, 1988.
61. Steere, AC, and Malawista, SE: The epidemiology of Lyme disease. In: Lawrence, RC, and Schulman, LE (Eds): Current Topics in Rheumatology: Epidemiology of the Rheumatic Diseases. Proceedings of the Fourth International Conference. New York, Gower Medical Publishing. Lyme arthritis: An epidemic of oligoarticular arthritis in children and adults in three Connecticut communities. Arthritis Rheum 20:7, 1977.
62. Kennedy-Stoskopf, S, et al: Lentivirus-induced arthritis. Rheum Dis Clin North Am 13: 235, 1987.
63. Gendelman, HE, et al: Tropism of sheep lentiviruses for monocytes: Susceptibility to infection and virus gene expression increase during maturation of monocytes and macrophages. J Virol 58:67, 1986.
64. Calabrese, LH: The rheumatic manifestations of infection with human immunodeficiency virus. Semin Arthritis Rheum 18:225, 1989.
65. Nishioka, K, et al: Novel mechanism of synovial proliferation caused by human T leukemia/lymphotropic virus type 1 (HTLV-1) (Abstract No. 3, P.S33). ACR 55th Annual Meeting, 1991.
66. Siegl, G: In: Berns, KI (Ed): The Parvoviruses. New York, Plenum, 1984, p 297.
67. Smith, CA, Woolf, AD, and Lenci, M: Parvoviruses: Infections and arthropathies. Rheum Dis Clin North Am 13:249, 1987.
68. Ager, EA, Poland, TDY, and Poland, JD: Epidemic erythema infectiosum. N Engl J Med 275:1326, 1966.
69. Tuckerman, JG, Brown, T, and Cohen, BJ: Erythema infectiosum in a village primary school: Clinical and virological studies. J R Coll Gen Pract 36:267, 1986.
70. White, DG, et al: Human parvovirus arthropathy. Lancet i:419, 1985.
71. Woolf, AD, et al: An epidemiological study of human parvovirus infection in adults. Br J Rheumatol 25:2, 1986.
72. Simpson, RW, et al: Association of parvoviruses with rheumatoid arthritis of humans. Science 224:1425, 1984.
73. Smith, CA, Petty, RE, and Tingle, AJ: Rubella virus and arthritis. Rheum Dis Clin North Am 13:265, 1987.
74. Horstmann, DM: Rubella. In: Viral Infections of Humans. New York, Plenum, 1982, pp 519–539.
75. Tingle, AJ, et al: Rubella associated arthritis. I. Comparative study of joint manifestations associated with natural rubella infection and RA 27/3 rubella immunization. Ann Rheum Dis 45:110, 1986.
76. Martinis, TW, Bland, JW, and Phillips, CW: Rheumatoid arthritis after rubella. Arthritis Rheum 11:683, 1968.
77. Ogra, PL, et al: Rubella virus infection in juvenile rheumatoid arthritis. Lancet i:24, 1975.
78. Ogra, PL, and Herd, JK: Serologic association of rubella virus infection and juvenile rheumatoid arthritis. Arthritis Rheum 15:121, 1972.
79. Ford, DK, et al: Synovial mononuclear cell responses to rubella antigen in rheumatoid arthritis and unexplained persistent knee arthritis. J Rheumatol 9:420, 1982.
80. Chantler, JK, Tingle, AJ, and Petty, RE: Persistent rubella virus infection associated with chronic arthritis in children. N Engl J Med 313:1117, 1985.
81. London, WT, et al: Concentration of rubella virus antigen in chondrocytes of conjecturally infected rabbits. Nature (London) 226:172, 1970.
82. Tosato, G, et al: Activation of suppressor T cells during Epstein-Barr-virus induced infectious mononucleosis. N Engl J Med 301:1133, 1979.
83. Alspaugh, MA, et al: Elevated levels of antibodies to Epstein-Barr virus antigens in sera and synovial fluids of patients with rheumatoid arthritis. J Clin Invest 67:1134, 1981.

84. Slaughter, L, et al: In vitro effects of Epstein-Barr virus on peripheral blood mononuclear cells from patients with rheumatoid arthritis and normal subjects. J Exp Med 148:1429, 1978.
85. Depper, JM, Bluestein, HG, and Zvaifler, NJ: Impaired regulation of Epstein-Barr-virus-induced lymphocyte proliferation in rheumatoid arthritis is due to a T cell defect. J Immunol 127: 1899, 1981.
86. Tosato, G, Steinberg, AD, and Blaese, RM: Defective EBV-specific suppressor T-cell function in rheumatoid arthritis. N Engl J Med 305:1238, 1981.
87. Tosato, G, et al: Abnormally elevated numbers of Epstein-Barr-virus-infected B cell precursors in patients with rheumatoid arthritis. J Clin Invest 73:1789, 1984.
88. Venables PJW, et al: Reaction to antibodies to rheumatoid arthritis nuclear antigen with a synthetic peptide corresponding to part of Epstein-Barr nuclear antigen-1. Ann Rheum Dis 47:270, 1988.
89. Roudier J, et al: The Epstein-Barr virus glycoprotein gp 110, a molecular link between HLA DR, HLA DR-1, and rheumatoid arthritis. Scand J Immunol 27:367, 1988.
88. Decker, JL, et al: Rheumatoid arthritis: Evolving concepts of pathogenesis and treatment. Ann Intern Med 101:810, 1984.
89. Venables PJW, et al: Reaction of antibodies to rheumatoid arthritis nuclear antigen with a synthetic peptide corresponding to partof Epstein-Barr nuclear antigen-1. Ann Rheum Dis 47:270, 1988.
90. Roudier, J, et al: The Epstein-Barr virus glycoprotein gp 100, a molecular link between HLA DR, HLA DR-1, and rheumatoid arthritis. Scand J Immunol 27:367, 1988.
91. Wilder, RL: Proinflammatory microbial products as etiologic agents of inflammatory arthritis. Rheum Dis Clin North Am 13:293, 1987.
92. Galelli, A, and Chedid, L: Induction of colony-stimulating activity (CSA) by a synthetic muramyl peptide (MDP): Synergism with LPS and activity in C3H/HeJ mice and in endotoxin-tolerized mice. J Immunol 137:3211, 1986.
93. Levy, RJ, et al: Bacterial peptidoglycan induces in vitro rheumatoid factor production by lymphocytes of healthy subjects. Clin Exp Immunol 64:311, 1986.
94. Koga, T, et al: Muramyl dipeptide induces acute joint inflammation in the mouse. Microbiol Immunol 30:717, 1986.
95. Heymer, B, et al: Detection of antibodies to bacterial cell wall peptidoglycan in human sera. J Immunol 117:23, 1976.
96. Lehman, THA, et al: Bacterial cell wall composition, lysozyme resistance, and the induction of chronic arthritis in rats. Rheumatol Int 5:163, 1985.
97. van Eden W, et al: Cloning of the mycobacterial epitope recognized by T lymphocytes in adjuvant arthritis. Nature 331:171, 1988.
98. Neame, TJ, Chrestner, JE, and Baker, JR: The primary structure of link protein from rat chondrosarcoma proteoglycan aggregate. J Biol Chem 261:3519, 1986.
99. Chirico, WJ, Waters, MG, and Blobel, G: 70 K heat shock related proteins stimulate protein translocation into microsomes. Nature 332:805, 1988.
100. Ananthan, J, Goldberg, AL, and Voellmy, R: Abnormal proteins serve as eukaryotic stress signals and trigger the activation of heat shock genes. Science 232:522, 1986.
101. Sargent, CA, et al: Human major histocompatibility complex contains genes for the major heat shock protein HSP70. Proc Natl Acad Sci USA 86:1968, 1989.
102. Minota, S, et al: Autoantibodies to the constitutive 73-kD member of the hsp70 family of heat shock proteins in systemic lupus erythematosus. J Exp Med 168:1475, 1988.
103. Holoshitz, J, et al: T lymphocytes of rheumatoid arthritis patients show augmented reactivity to a fraction of mycobacteria cross-reactive with cartilage. Lancet ii:305, 1986.
104. Res, PCM, et al: Synovial fluid T cell reactivity against 65 kD heat shock protein of mycobacteria in early chronic arthritis. Lancet ii:478, 1988.
105. Holoshitz, J, et al: Isolation of CD4- CD8- mycobacteria-reactive T lymphocyte clones from rheumatoid arthritis synovial fluid. Nature 339:226, 1989.
106. Young, D, et al: Stress proteins are immune targets in leprosy and tuberculosis. Proc Natl Acad Sci USA 85:4267, 1988.
107. Trentham, DE: Collagen arthritis as a relevant model for rheumatoid arthritis. Arthritis Rheum 25:911, 1982.
108. Stuart, JM, et al: Specificity of antibodies to types I, II, III, IV, and V collagen in rheumatoid arthritis and other rheumatic diseases as measured by radioimmunoassay. Arthritis Rheum 26:832, 1983.
109. Luthra, HS, et al: Immunogenetics of collagen-induced arthritis (CIA) in mice: A model of autoimmune disease. Ann NY Acad Sci 475:361, 1986.
110. Banerjee, S, et al: Possible role of V beta T cell receptor genes in susceptibility to collagen-induced arthritis in mice. J Exp Med 167:832, 1988.
111. David, CS, et al: Genes for MHC, TCR and Mls determine susceptibility to collagen induced arthritis. Acta Pathol Microbiol Immunol Scand 98:575, 1990.
111. Healey, LA, and Sheets PK: The relation of polymyalgia rheumatica to rheumatoid arthritis. J Rheumatol 15:750, 1988.
112. Larsen, EB: Adult Still's disease: Evolution of a clinical syndrome and diagnosis, treatment and follow-up of 17 patients. Medicine (Baltimore) 63:82, 1984.
113. Paget, SA: Joints, musculoskeletal and connective tissue problems. In: Samiy, AH (Ed): Textbook of Diagnostic Medicine. Philadelphia, Lea & Febiger, 1987, p 582.
114. Hurd, ER: Extraarticular manifestations of rheumatoid arthritis. Semin Arthritis Rheum 8:151, 1979.
115. Hollingsworth, JW, and Saykaly, RJ: Systemic complications of rheumatoid arthritis. Med Clin North Am 61:217, 1977.

116. Bacon, PA: Extraarticular rheumatoid arthritis. In: McCarty, DJ (Ed): Arthritis and Allied Conditions: A Textbook of Rheumatology. Philadelphia, Lea & Febiger, 1989, p 1967
117. Crowley, JP: Felty's syndrome. In: Utsinger, PD, Zvaifler, NJ, and Ehrlich, GE (Eds): Rheumatoid Arthritis. Philadelphia, JB Lippincott, 1985, p 393.
118. Geirsson, AJ, Sturfelt, G, and Truedsson, L: Clinical and serological features of severe vasculitis in rheumatoid arthritis: Prognostic implications. Ann Rheum Dis 46:727, 1987.
119. Hess, EV: Rheumatoid arthritis complicated by vasculitis. Hosp Pract 50, 1988.
120. Cathcart, ES, and Wohlgethan, JR: Amyloidosis. In: Utsinger, PD, Zvaifler, NJ, and Ehrlich, GE (Eds): Rheumatoid Arthritis. Philadelphia, JB Lippincott, 1985, p 495.
121. Baum, J, and Ziff, M: Laboratory abnormalities in rheumatoid arthritis. In: McCarty, DJ (Ed): Arthritis and Allied Conditions. Philadelphia, Lea & Febiger, 1989, p 744.
122. Youinou, P, et al: Relationship between rheumatoid arthritis and monoclonal gammopathy. J Rheumatol 10:210, 1983.
123. Thompson, PW, Kirwin, JR, and Moss, DW: Evidence supporting alkaline phosphatase as an acute phase protein in rheumatoid arthritis. Arthritis Rheum 325:16, 1989.
124. Linn, JE, Hardin, JG, and Halla, JT: A controlled study of ANA$^+$ RF$^-$ arthritis. Arthritis Rheum 21:645, 1978.
125. Lightfoot, RW: Treatment of rheumatoid arthritis. In: McCarthy, DJ (Ed) Arthritis and Allied Conditions. Philadelphia, Lea & Febiger, 1989, p 772.
126. Fries, J, et al: Discontinuation of treatment with nonsteroidal anti-inflammatory medications: Associated factors. Arthritis Rheum 325:66, 1989.
127. Fries, J: Arthritis: A Comprehensive Guide to Understanding Your Arthritis. Reading, Mass, Addison Wesley, 1988.
128. Rogers, MD, Liang, RH, and Partridge, AJ: Psychological care of adults with rheumatoid arthritis. Ann Intern Med 96:344, 1982.
129. Smith, RD, and Polley, HF: Rest therapy for rheumatoid arthritis. Mayo Clin Proc 53:141, 1978.
130. Spiegel, JS, et al: Rehabilitation for rheumatoid arthritis patients: A controlled trial. Arthritis Rheum 29:628, 1986.
131. Gerber, LH: Rehabilitation of patients with rheumatic diseases. In: Kelley, WN, et al (Eds): Textbook of Rheumatology. Philadelphia, WB Saunders, 1989, p 1904.
132. Harris, ED: Management of rheumatoid arthritis. In: Kelley, WN, et al (Eds): Textbook of Rheumatology. Philadelphia, WB Saunders, 1989, p 982.
133. Schlegal, SI, and Paulus, HE: Update on NSAID use in rheumatic disease. Bull Rheum Dis 36:1, 1986.
134. Paulus, HE: Non-steroidal anti-inflammatory drugs. In: Kelley, WN, et al (Eds): Textbook of Rheumatology. Philadelphia, WB Saunders, 1989, p 765.

135. Hardin, JG: Rheumatoid arthritis therapy: The slow-acting agents. Hosp Pract 24:163, 1989.
136. Kaplan, H, Weinblatt, ME, and Wilder, RL: Advances in arthritis drug therapy. Patient Care 23:31, 1989.
137. Ward, JR: The role of disease-modifying antirheumatic drugs versus cytotoxic agents in the therapy of rheumatoid arthritis. Am J Med 85 (suppl 4A):39, 1988.
138. Lipsky, P: Disease-modifying drugs. In: Utsinger, PD, Zvaifler, NJ, and Ehrlich, GE (Eds): Rheumatoid Arthritis. Philadelphia, JB Lippincott, 1985, p 601.
139. Alarcon, GS, et al: Methotrexate in rheumatoid arthritis: Toxic effects as the major factor in limiting long-term treatment. Arthritis Rheum 32:671, 1989.
140. Gottlieb, NL: Gold compounds. In: Kelley, WN, et al (Eds): Textbook of Rheumatology. Philadelphia, WB Saunders, 1985, p 789.
141. Blodgett, RC, Heuer, MA, and Pietrusko, RG: Auranofin: A unique oral chrysotherapeutic agent. Semin Arthritis Rheum 13:355, 1984.
142. Zvaifler, NJ: Update in rheumatology-focus on hydroxychloroquine. Am J Med 85(4A):68, 1988.
143. Easterbrook, M: Ocular effects and safety of antimalarial agents. Am J Med 85(4A):23, 1988.
144. Pinals, RS, et al: Sulfasalazine in rheumatoid arthritis: A double-blind placebo-controlled trial. Arthritis Rheum 29:1427, 1986.
145. Bax, DE, and Amos, RS: Suphasalazine: A safe, effective agent for prolonged control of rheumatoid arthritis. A comparison with sodium aurothiomalate. Ann Rheum Dis 44:94, 1985.
146. Jaffe, IA: Penicillamine. In: McCarty, DJ (Ed): Arthritis and Allied Conditions. Philadelphia, Lea & Febiger, 1989, p 593.
147. Kean, WF, et al: The toxicity pattern of D-penicillamine therapy: A guide to its use in RA. Arthritis Rheum 23:158, 1980.
148. De Silva, M, and Hazelman, BL: Long-term azathioprine in rheumatoid arthritis: A double-blind study. Ann Rheum Dis 40:560, 1981.
149. Anderson, PA, et al: Weekly pulse methotrexate in rheumatoid arthritis: Clinical and immunologic effects in a randomized double-blind study. Ann Intern Med 103:489, 1985.
150. Kremer, JM, Lee, RG, and Tolman, KG: Liver histology in rheumatoid arthritis patients receiving long-term methotrexate therapy. Arthritis Rheum 32:121, 1989.
151. Tugwell, P, Bennett, K, and Gent, M: Methotrexate in rheumatoid arthritis: Indications, contraindications, efficacy and safety. Ann Intern Med 107:358, 1987.
152. Klippel, JH, Strober, S, and Wofsy D: New therapies for the rheumatic diseases. Bull Rheum Dis 38:1, 1989.
153. Kinlin, LJ: Incidence of cancer in rheumatoid arthritis and other disorders after immunosuppressive treatment. Am J Med 78(1A):44, 1985.
154. Csuka, ME, Carrera, GF, and McCarty, DJ: Treatment of intractable rheumatoid arthritis with combined cyclophosphamide, azathioprine and hydroxychloroquine. JAMA 255:2315.

155. Lockshin, MD: Corticosteroids. In: Utsinger, PD, Zvaifler, NJ, and Ehrlich, GE (Eds): Rheumatoid Arthritis. Philadelphia, JB Lippincott, 1985, p 581.
156. Harris, ED, et al: Low-dose prednisone therapy in rheumatoid arthritis: A double-blind study. J Rheumatol 10:713, 1983.
157. Hess, EV, and Kammen, PL: Pulse therapy in rheumatoid arthritis. (Editorial) Ann Intern Med 94:128, 1981.
158. Pinals, RS: Felty's syndrome. In: Kelley, WN, et al (Eds): Textbook of Rheumatology. Philadelphia, WB Saunders, 1989, p 993.
159. Panush, R: Nutritional therapy for rheumatic diseases. Ann Intern Med 106:619, 1987.
160. Kremer, J: Fish-oil fatty acid supplementation in active rheumatoid arthritis: A double-blind, controlled, cross-over study. Ann Intern Med 106:497, 1987.
161. Cannon GW, Emkey RD, Denes A et al.: Prospective two year follow up of recombinant interferon-gamma in rheumatoid arthritis. J Rheumatol 17:304, 1990.
162. Lebsack, ME, Paul CC, Bloedow DC et al.: Subcutaneous IL-1 R antagonist in patients with rheumatoid arthritis. ACR annual meetings, Abstract 73, 1991.
163. Suzuki, H, Kamimura, J, Ayabe T et al: Demonstration of neutralizing antibodies against IL-1 in sera from patients with rheumatoid arthritis. J Immunol 145:2140–2146, 1990.
164. Seckinger P, Vey, E, Turcatti G, et al: Tumor necrosis factor inhibitor: Purification, NH_2-terminal amino acid sequence and evidence for anti-inflammatory and immunomodulatory activities. Eur J Immunol 20:1167–1174, 1990.
165. Sewell, KL, and Trentham, DE: Improvement in refractory rheumatoid arthritis by interleukin-2 receptor targeted therapy. ACR annual meetings, Abstract A141, 1991.
166. van der Lubbe, PA, Reiter, C, Reithmuller, G, et al: Treatment of RA with chimeric CD4 monoclonal antibody. ACR annual meetings, Abstract A143, 1991.
167. Strand, V, Lipsky PE, Cannon G, et al: Treatment of rheumatoid arthritis with an anti-CD5 immunoconjugate: Final results of phase II studies. ACR annual meetings, Abstract A155, 1991.
168. Paget, SA: Rheumatoid arthritis. In: Samiy, AH (Ed): Textbook of Therapeutic Medicine for Practicing Physicians. Philadelphia, Lea & Febiger (in press).

Appendix 3-1
Salicylates in the Treatment of Rheumatoid Arthritis

Type	Preparation	Clinically Important Characteristics
Acetylated Salicylates		
Plain aspirin	Tablets: 325 mgm Dosage: 600–1200 mg q.i.d. Maximum: 5–6 g/day Cost: $7.70/month	Inexpensive but dose schedule decreases compliance; can cause serious GI toxicity including gastritis, gastric ulcers, GI bleeding, and perforation; inhibit platelet function for 7–10 days.
Enteric coated aspirin (e.g., Ecotrin)	Tablets: 325–650 mg Dosage: 600–1200 mg q.i.d. Maximum: 5–6 g/day Cost: $9.15/month	Absorption in the small intestine decreases gastric toxicity; otherwise as above with aspirin.
Buffered aspirin (e.g., Bufferin, Ascripton)	Tablets: 300 mg Dosage: 600–1200 mg q.i.d. Maximum: 5–6 g/day Cost: $10.00/month	Inexpensive; formulated with insoluble calcium and magnesium antacids; no firm evidence of decreased gastric toxicity.
Time-release, enteric-coated, salicylates (e.g., Easprin)	Tablets: 900 mg Dosage: 900 mg q.i.d. Maximum: 3–4 g/day Cost: $26.95	Improved compliance with dosing schedule; decreased gastric toxicity with enteric coating; otherwise as above with aspirin.
Time-release, zero-order, aspirin (e.g., Zorprin)	Tablets: 800 mg Dosage: 2 tabs b.i.d. Maximum: 3.2 g/day Cost: $25.90/month	Improved compliance with b.i.d. dosing schedule; otherwise as above with aspirin.
Nonacetylated Salicylates		
Sodium salicylate[*†]	Tablets: 325 mg Dosage: 1 tab t.i.d. Maximum: 3 g/day Cost: $10.75/month	Less potent analgesic than aspirin; less gastric toxicity than aspirin; does not inhibit platelet function; watch sodium intake in heart failure or hypertension.
Choline salicylate[*†] (e.g., Arthropan)	Liquid formulation Dosage: 1 tsp q.i.d. Maximum: q.i.d. dosage Cost: $42.85/month	Very soluble; negligible gastric toxicity; probably less effective than aspirin and does not inhibit platelet function.

Type	Preparation	Clinically Important Characteristics
Choline magnesium salicylate*† (e.g., Trilisate)	Tablets: 500 mg Dosage: 2–3 tab b.i.d. Cost: $40.45	Convenient, well-accepted b.i.d. dosing schedule; long (9–17 hr) half-life; less gastric toxicity than aspirin; does not inhibit platelet function.
Salasate*† (e.g., Disalcid)	Tablets: 500 mg Dosage: 1000–1500 mg in a b.i.d. or t.i.d. dosing Maximum: 3 g/day Cost: $45.95/month	Convenient, well-accepted dose schedule; less gastric toxicity than aspirin; does not inhibit platelet function.
Diflunisal (e.g., Dolobid)	Tablets: 500 mg Dosage: 2 tabs initially, then 1 tab b.i.d. Maximum: 1–1.5 g/day Cost: $56.15/month	Well accepted b.i.d. dose schedule; employed both as an analgesic and anti-inflammatory agent; shares side effects with nonsalicylate NSAIDs and aspirin; more toxic and expensive than nonacetylated salicylates.

*Serum salicylate levels can and should be used to guide dosing (therapeutic salicylate level 15–25 mg%) and compliance.
†This drug can be considered in patients with a past history of NSAID-related gastrointestinal toxicity. The concomitant use of misoprostol should be considered in this group of patients.
NOTE: All of these drugs share the side effects profile of NSAIDS (see Appendix 3-2).[161]

Appendix 3-2
Profile of Nonsteroidal Anti-inflammatory Drugs (NSAIDs)

Indications

Salicylates are the first-line drugs for the treatment of rheumatoid arthritis because of their low cost and anti-inflammatory effects. Nonacetylated salicylates are a safe and convenient first choice, especially in patients with a history of NSAID-related gastrointestinal problems. Other NSAIDs can either be used as initial therapy or in patients who have been found to be unresponsive or intolerant to salicylates.

Pharmacokinetics

Currently available NSAIDs are rapidly and completely absorbed after oral administration, unless enteric coatings have been used to decrease gastric irritation. Essentially all available NSAIDs are converted by the liver to inactive metabolites that are excreted predominantly in the urine. Dosage reduction and extra care are advisable if NSAIDs are used in patients with impaired renal function, as well as the elderly. Indomethacin, meclofenamate, piroxicam, and sulindac are excreted in the bile and appear in the feces. Indomethacin, sulindac, and meclofenamate sodium display enterohepatic recirculation which enhances their gastrointestinal toxicity in the lower GI tract. **Physical and pharmacologic changes associated with aging may increase older patients' sensitivity to both the therapeutic and toxic effects of NSAIDs.**

Actions

All NSAIDs act by interrupting the arachidonic acid metabolism cascade, but therapeutic effects may involve actions other than, or in addition to, the inhibition of prostaglandin synthesis. There are significant but subtle differences in mechanisms of action, effectiveness in different diseases, and other properties of the NSAIDs. The unpredictable differences in effectiveness in different patients make it worthwhile to try a series of agents if the first drug does not work satisfactorily in a given patient. Nonacetylated salicylates do not appear to have significant anticyclooxygenase effect and yet are anti-inflammatory.

Dosage Regimen

Appendices 3-1 and 3-3 list the appropriate dosing for all of the NSAIDs. Salicylates are administered at dosages of 600–1200 mg q4–6h, usually with meals or with antacid to minimize gastric irritation. A salicylate blood level between 15–25 mg/ml is optimal and requires dosages between 3–5 g daily. Hepatic metabolic pathways may become saturated at higher salicylate levels. Therefore, a small dosage increase can result in a very large elevation of the serum salicylate level. Because of the marked individual variability in the dosage of salicylate needed to achieve therapeutic levels, serum concentrations must be monitored closely while initiating intensive salicylate therapy. Maximal dosages should be approached gradually over two to four weeks to allow time for self-induction of salicylate metabolism. Nonacetylated salicylates can be given in a b.i.d. dosing. The twice daily dosage regimens of these drugs improve patient compliance and these nonacetylated drugs have a lower potential for toxicity.

Adverse Effects of NSAIDs

Gastric Effects

All NSAIDs can cause gastric mucosal damage related to inhibition of prostaglandin synthesis and impairment of normal gastrointestinal protective mechanisms. The most common GI side effects include dyspepsia, nausea or vomiting, and GI bleeding due to gastritis and/or ulceration (gastric ulcers much more common than duodenal). Gastrointestinal upset is the most common adverse effect of both salicylate and nonsalicylate NSAIDs, and requires drug withdrawal in 5–20 percent of patients. Mucosal damage is more severe with aspirin, higher doses of NSAIDs, and combinations of NSAIDs. There is *no* persuasive evidence that there is less major gastrointestinal blood loss with nonsalicylate anti-inflammatory drugs than with aspirin. Nonacetylated salicylates are, however, associated with a significantly lower incidence of GI blood loss. In patients with a clear history of peptic ulcer disease or NSAID-related upper GI problems, the concomitant use of misoprostol (Cytotec) is indicated. Patients with active ulcer disease should avoid NSAIDs of all kinds.

Hematologic and Anticoagulant Effects

The NSAIDs decrease platelet adhesiveness and prolong the bleeding time by inhibiting a prostaglandin-initiated sequence that is necessary for platelet activation, thus interfering with coagulation. Their use in anticoagulated patients may increase the risk or severity of bleeding complications. With acetylated salicylates, an irreversible inhibition of platelet prostaglandin synthesis is produced that persists after drug withdrawal and body clearance. This effect lasts for as long as 10–12 days, while with other NSAIDs, in which the inhibition is reversible, the platelet effect persists only for as long as the drug is present (e.g., tolmetin and ibuprofen should be stopped at least 24 hours preoperatively, aspirin two weeks preoperatively, and other drugs at times relative to their half-lives). Nonacetylated salicylates have little or no effect upon platelets and sometimes may be used when other NSAIDs are contraindicated by an excessive risk of bleeding. NSAIDs may also displace warfarin from plasma protein binding sites and thus increase the anticoagulant effect (e.g., aspirin, phenylbutazone, meclofenamate, and sulindac can cause excessive prolongation of the prothrombin time while indomethacin, tolmetin and ibuprofen do not exert this effect). In general, all NSAIDs should be avoided while using Coumadin. However, when necessitated by the clinical situation, nonacetylated salicylates may be considered, with caution, in patients on oral anticoagulants. These agents can, like aspirin, displace Coumadin from binding sites, so that prothrombin time needs to be carefully monitored. An acute, reversible thrombocytopenia associated with the use of sulindac, ibuprofen, and other NSAIDs is probably due to peripheral, immune-mediated platelet destruction. All NSAIDs can lead to leukopenia although this is not common. The fact that phenylbutazone and oxyphenbutazone can lead to bone marrow aplasia or agranulocytosis in an unacceptably high incidence has led to strong FDA restrictions on the use of these drugs. These drugs should not be used in the treatment of rheumatoid arthritis, and should be used in spondyloarthropathies only in rare cases and after consultation with a rheumatologist who is well versed in the disease entity, other therapeutic options, and potential adverse effects of these two drugs. Aspirin and other NSAIDs all can induce acute hemolytic reactions in patients with glucose 6-phosphate dehydrogenase (G6PD) deficiency.

Hepatic Effects

All NSAIDs can lead to elevation in serum transminases. With aspirin, patients with JRA and SLE are particularly susceptible to developing this complication. In most patients, the abnormal liver function tests are asymptomatic and do not reflect significant liver damage. Liver function test abnormalities may revert to normal despite continuing the drug. If, on repeat testing, a patient is found to have SGOT or SGPT equal to or greater than three times the upper limit of normal, the NSAID should be stopped. When the tests return to normal, an alternative class of NSAID may be used, but with increased surveillance. A toxic hepatitis is a rare disorder. NSAIDs should generally not be used in patients with known hepatic disease.

Renal Reactions

Because prostaglandins exert a protective compensatory role in maintaining renal function in patients with renal failure, hepatic cirrhosis, cardiac ventricular failure, or volume depletion (e.g., patients on diuretics), NSAIDs should be avoided or used with caution in patients with these disorders. All NSAIDs have the potential to mediate drug-induced nephrotoxicity via their inhibition of prostaglandin synthesis. In patients with underlying renal dysfunction, NSAIDs sometimes produce a mild to moderate increase in serum creatinine. Acute renal failure may present as prerenal azotemia, acute tubular insufficiency, or acute allergic interstitial nephritis with nephrotic syndrome (most common with fenoprofen). Although renal insufficiency is usually reversible upon discontinuation of the offending NSAID, at times short-term dialysis may be needed. While drugs containing phenacetin have been implicated in the development of chronic interstitial nephritis and papillary necrosis, the risk of clinically significant renal damage with salicylates seems small. Nonacetylated salicylates do not appear to suppress renal prostaglandin synthesis and thus may be the preferred analgesic, anti-inflammatory drugs for patients with rheumatoid arthritis and underlying renal disease or poorly controlled hypertension. Prostaglandin inhibition from NSAIDs also can cause fluid retention with resistance to diuretics, aggravation of preexisting hypertension and hyporeninemic hypoaldosteronism with hyperkalemia.

Mucocutaneous Reactions

Urticaria and other allergic skin reactions can occur with all NSAIDs. Fortunately, ereythema multiforme, Stevens-Johnson syndrome and exfoliative dermatitis are rarely encountered.

Allergic Reactions and Asthma

Salicylates and the newer NSAIDs inhibit the biosynthesis of bronchodilating prostaglandins and may therefore exacerbate asthma. Such acute bonchospastic reactions are more common in patients with a history of nasal polyps and asthma. Cross-hypersensitivity may exist among all of the NSAIDs and extreme caution must be used when introducing a new NSAID to a patient with a past history of a significant reaction to a previous one. Once a patient with asthma is on a NSAID, he can be switched to another without problem (presumably desensitized). While anaphylactoid reactions have been reported with various NSAIDs. Tolmetin has accounted for a large proportion of such cases.

Cardiovascular Reactions

NSAIDs should be used with caution in patients with significant coronary artery disease or impaired ventricular function. NSAIDs may cause coronary vasoconstriction in some patients. NSAIDs may aggrevate congestive heart failure and hypertension. Patients on diuretics (especially aldactone) for congestive heart failure are at increased risk for NSAID-induced renal dysfunction.

Neuropsychiatric Reactions

Headaches, dizziness and psychic disturbances can occur with all NSAIDs but are more frequently seen with indomethacin, less so with tolmetin and meclofenamate. Cognitive dysfunction may be subtle, especially in the elderly. In the elderly, Indocin may lead to psychosis and may aggrevate underlying seizure disorder and parkinsonism. Indocin should, thus, be used with caution in the elderly.

Ocular Reactions

Rarely, NSAIDs can cause blurred vision, amblyopia, maculopathy, retinal edema, corneal deposits, and optic neuritis. For this reason, ophthalmologic examinations should be performed yearly and whenever patients complain of ocular symptoms.

Auditory Reactions

Reversible sensorineural hearing loss and tinnitus can develop in patients treated with salicylates and all other NSAIDs. This is particularly important in the elderly because tinnitus is not a reliable signal of salicylism because of their already impaired hearing.

Pregnancy and Teratogenic Reactions

All NSAIDs should be considered potentially teratogenic and should be discontinued when patients are trying to conceive and during pregnancy. If severe polyarthritis is present during pregnancy and a NSAID is needed (as opposed to a short course of steroids), aspirin is preferred to the newer NSAIDs. Salicylates should be stopped in the final month of pregnancy because of potential postpartum maternal hemorrhage. If the patient is breast feeding, an avoidance of all NSAIDs is appropriate.[161]

Appendix 3-3
Nonsalicylate Nonsteroidal Anti-inflammatory Drugs (NSAIDs) in the Treatment of Rheumatoid Arthritis

Type	Preparation	Clinically Important Characteristics
Indoleacetic Acid Series		
Indomethacin (Indocin)	Capsules: 25 mg, 50 mg, 75 mg (slow release [SR]) Dosage: Acute: 25–50 mg t.i.d.–q.i.d. Chronic: 75–100 mg per day in divided doses or 75 mg slow release formula once per day. Maximum: Acute: 200 mg/day Chronic: 75–100 mg per day in divided doses. Cost: Indocin 50 mg t.i.d.—$69.85/month brand, $18.55/month generic Indocin SR—$35.00/month brand; $20.75/month generic	GI and CNS side effects; single daily dose (SR) formula improves compliance; favored use in spondyloarthropathies, not RA; some use this as an h.s. dose along with other NSAIDs; helpful in crystal-induced disorders and in tendonitis and bursitis.

Type	Preparation	Clinically Important Characteristics
Sulindac (Clinoril)	Tablets: 150 mg, 200 mg Dosage: 400 mg/day Cost: $61.40/month	Convenient, well-accepted b.i.d. dose schedule; possibly less renal toxicity; enterohepatic circulation.
Tolmetin	Tablets: 200 mg Dosage: 1 tab t.i.d. Maximum: 1,200 mg/day Cost: $61.94/month	t.i.d. dose schedule less convenient; FDA approved for JRA.
Proprionic Acids		
Naprosyn (Naproxen)	Tablets: 250 mg, 375 mg, 500 mg Dosage: 1 tab b.i.d. Maximum: 1,000 mg/day Cost: $60.35/month.	Long half-life allowing for convenient b.i.d. dosing; FDA approved for JRA.
Ibuprofen (Motrin, Advil, Nuprin)	Tablets: 200 mg (OTC), 400 mg, 600 mg, 800 mg Dosage: t.i.d.–q.i.d. schedule Maximum: 2,400 mg/day Cost: $36.05/month	t.i.d.–q.i.d. dosing less convenient; available in over-the-counter 200 mg. analgesic dose; long-term safety established.
Fenoprofen (Nalfon)	Tablets: 300 mg, 600 mg Dosage: t.i.d.–q.i.d. schedule Maximum: 2,400 mg/day Cost: $72.60/month	t.i.d.–q.i.d. dosing less convenient
Ketoprofen (Orudis)	Capsules: 50 mg, 75 mg Dosage: t.i.d.–q.i.d. schedule Maximum: 300 mg/day Cost: $58.00/month	t.i.d.–q.i.d. dosing less convenient; lower dose used for pain control.
Anthranilic Acids		
Meclofenamate sodium (Meclomen)	Tablets: 50 mg, 100 mg Dosage: t.i.d. Maximum: 300 mg/day Cost: $65.35/month	t.i.d. dosing less convenient; second line drug for RA due to occasional colitis and diarrhea in 20% of patients.
Benzothiazine Series		
Piroxicam (Feldene)	Capsules: 10 mg, 20 mg Dosage: 1 cap/day Maximum: 20 mg/day Cost: $55.45/month	Convenient and well accepted single daily dosing; long half-life (30 hr) lends it to tissue accumulation in patients with compromised renal function; close monitoring in the elderly, cardiovascular/renal compromised population. Might be avoided in the elderly where a shorter half-life drug is available.
Pyrazoles		
Phenylbutazone (Butazolidin)	Tablets: 100 mg Dosage: t.i.d.–q.i.d. Maximum: 400 mg/day for chronic therapy Cost: $17.00	FDA requires listing as a second line RA drug to be used after other NSAIDs have failed; potential hematologic suppression limits the use to 2 weeks in spondyloarthropathies and RA only after all else has failed; potentiates warfarin, tolbutamide, and sulfonamides; not recommended for RA.[161]

Appendix 3-4
Gold Salt Therapy in the Treatment of Rheumatoid Arthritis

Name

Parenteral Gold Preparations

Aurothioglucose (Solganal) and gold sodium thiomalate (myochrysine)

Oral Gold Preparation

Auranofin (Ridaura)

Chemistry

Parenteral Gold Preparations

The two parenteral gold preparations are aurous salts, contain 50% gold by weight, and are attached to a sulfur moiety.

Oral Gold Preparation

Auranofin, a conjugated gold compound with two ligands, contains sulfur, is 29% gold by weight, and is distinctly different physicochemically from the parenteral compounds.

Distribution

Parenteral Gold Preparations

With parenteral gold, the kidneys, adrenals and reticuloendothelial system organs achieve the highest gold concentrations. Gold concentrations in body fluids are much lower than most tissues. Synovial fluid levels of gold generally are about 50% of serum concentrations. Gold preferentially localizes in the synovial membrane during gold therapy.

Oral Gold Preparation

With oral gold, tissue levels appear to be much lower than is found with parenteral gold preparations.

Pharmacokinetics

Parenteral Gold Preparations

With parenteral preparations, gold levels rise gradually and plateau after 6-8 weeks. Serum gold concentrations correlate directly with the administered gold dose. Upon termination of treatment, low levels exist for many months, and gold is detectable as long as one year later. Gold diffuses from serum to synovial fluid rapidly. With IM therapy, after 20 weekly injections of 50 mg, approximately 300 mg of elemental gold is retained.

Oral Gold Preparation

With oral gold, levels plateau after three months of therapy. Approximately 40% of the administered dose of gold is eliminated, 70% in the urine and 30% in the feces. Forty percent of the excreted gold derives from the current dose and 60% from previous doses. After 20 weeks of therapy with oral gold, 73 mg of elemental gold is retained.

Clinical-Pharmacologic Correlates

No relationship has been defined between serum gold levels and clinical efficacy. Further, serum gold levels are not helpful in monitoring adverse reactions.

Mechanism of Action

Parenteral Gold Preparations

The mechanism responsible for the favorable action of parenteral gold in rheumatoid arthritis is unknown. Possible mechanisms of action include alteration of macrophage function and complement function.

Oral Gold Preparation

Oral gold exhibits anti-inflammatory action, suppresses humoral immune mechanisms, alters cell-mediated immunity, and alters polymorphonuclear leukocyte and mononuclear leukocyte activity. One or more of these functions may explain the efficacy of Auranofin in RA despite the low blood and tissue levels.

Clinical Efficacy

Parenteral Gold Preparations

Many clinical trials have demonstrated the efficacy of gold salt therapy in the treatment of rheumatoid arthritis. Not only do patients benefit clinically, but laboratory manifestations of disease activity (sedimentation rate, hemoglobin) improve and some studies show that gold results in a significantly beneficial effect upon radiographic progression of bone defects. At least two thirds of patients with RA who receive therapeutic amounts of gold show significant improvement of synovitis. Because of its toxicity, gold is not the initial therapy for RA. It is reserved for patients who have active synovitis and constitutional symptoms or who develop erosions on a conservative regimen of NSAIDs, rest, and physical therapy. In general, gold is not indicated for mild disease, pauciarticular (2 or 3 joints involved) disease or end-stage noninflammatory disease.

Oral Gold Preparation

This agent has been shown to be more effective than placebo in two double-blind, 6-month multicenter trials, and similar in efficacy to gold sodium thiomalate in both double-blinded and unblinded controlled multicenter trials. However, while oral gold is considered to be less toxic than parenteral gold, it is also felt to be somewhat less effective in disease control.

Selection of Gold Compound

In view of the 55 years of experience of rheumatologists with parenteral gold and its positive and negative effects, IM gold remains the agent of choice for active, erosive, systemic disease. However, because of the advantageous safety profile of oral gold and ease of administration, both patients and physicians may choose this drug for the treatment of active disease with the understanding that if the drug fails to improve the patient's status, parenteral gold can then be instituted. Rheumatologists are also using IM and oral gold as separate remittive drugs to be employed either before or after the other. The long-term "track record" for oral gold remains to be defined.

Note

The release of restraints implicit with many years of parenteral use should in no way result in broadening the indications of gold usage in RA patients over those mentioned previously. Similarly, despite the more rapid excretion of oral gold, there must be no decrease in vigilance with which patients are followed regarding potential toxicity. Patients must also be aware that no self-determined increase in dosage should be carried out to bring about a more rapid clinical response!

Supply

Parenteral Gold Preparations

Gold thioglucose, 50 mg/ml in 10-ml vials. Gold sodium thiomalate, 10, 25, 50, 100 mg/ml in 1-ml ampoules; 50 mg/ml in 10-ml ampoules.

Oral Gold Preparation

Auranofin, 3-mg capsules.

Cost of Medication

Parenteral Gold Preparations

The cost of administering and monitoring the initial phase (20 weeks) of parenteral gold is considerable. A survey conducted in 1976 indicated that the expense varies from $300–800, depending on the frequency and number of laboratory tests and physician visits. This cost does not even consider the expense of travel and lost time at work. The price of the injectable gold is approximately $50.00 for a 10-ml vial of aurothioglucose or gold sodium thiomalate.

Oral Gold Preparation

Two 3-mg tablets per day for one month—$54.55.

Dosage

Parenteral Gold Preparation

These preparations are given by deep IM injection. The initial dose should be small (10 mg) to test for drug idiosyncracy (e.g., rash, thrombocytopenia). If this dose is tolerated, 25 mg should be given 1 week later, and then 50 mg weekly if tolerated. The therapeutic response begins in most (80%) patients when the cumulative dose is 300–700 mg. Improvement is gradual but appears to increase with time. When improvement plateaus, usually at doses ranging from 500–1000 mg, the dosage frequency of gold can be decreased to 50 mg once every two weeks for 1–2 months, then gradually to 50 mg once a month. If gold is discontinued, the condition flares in some patients within several months. Therefore, if tolerated, it is recommended to continue gold injections indefinitely (some physicians reassess gold therapy at the 5-year point). The degree of improvement is proportional to the duration of treatment. However, if improvement does not occur after 1,000 mg, the drug should be discontinued. Future courses of parenteral gold in such patients are unlikely to be effective.

Oral Gold Preparation

The initial dose is one 3-mg capsule twice a day. If, after 9 months of therapy, there is no clinical response, a final dosage increase to one capsule three times a day is recommended.

Note

Gold-induced thrombocytopenia and proteinuria occurs many times more frequently than anticipated in RA patients possessing HLA-DR3 and DRW3. Although HLA typing is not recommended prior to the institution of gold, a strong family history of such gold reaction should direct the physician to HLA type or be very cautious in the administration of gold.

Adverse Reactions

Parenteral Gold Preparations

Adverse reactions develop in approximately one third of patients receiving parenteral gold salts. Toxicity usually appears after 300–500 mg of gold has been administered. However, undesirable reactions may occur at any time during the course of therapy. Approximately four times as many patients were withdrawn from intramuscular gold treatment (20%) because of drug intolerance as from oral gold (5%) in most studies comparing the two drugs in RA patients.

Oral Gold Preparation

With oral gold, the type and severity of complications differ greatly from injectable gold and most are mild, transient, affect the lower GI tract, and are dose-related. It must be mentioned that patients receiving oral gold have developed serious mucocutaneous, hematopoietic system and kidney complications but their incidence appears to be less than that found with parenteral gold.

Mucocutaneous Reactions (10–15% of patients or 60–80% of all adverse gold reactions with injectable gold)

The most common manifestations of gold toxicity is dermatitis, which may be heralded by pruritis (in

85%) or eosinophilia, and is almost always reversible. Stomatitis is another side effect and can be painful or painless. The development of these side effects is an indication to withhold gold until at least 3-4 weeks after the lesions clear. (Topical steroids can be used along with antihistamines, e.g., hydroxyzine 25 mg t.i.d. for the treatment of skin rash). Then, beginning at very low doses (5 mg), a slow and gradual increase in dosage is indicated with close observation for reoccurrence of rash, stomatitis, or other side effect. Exfoliative dermatitis is an uncommon but serious potential reaction. Corticosteroids (40-60 mg/day) are beneficial for instances of exfoliation. Isolated eosinophilia is also noted frequently and should merely alert the physician to watch more carefully for side effects. Chrysiasis of the skin and nails has been reported rarely in patients on long-term gold therapy and presents as an asymptomatic gray or blue skin discoloration.

Renal (4-10%)

Proteinura is detectable at some time in at least 10% of patients receiving gold injections. Urinalysis should be performed before each gold injection. Nephritis and nephrotic syndrome (0.2-2.6% of patients) are much less common. The most common histologic lesion is a membranous glomerulonephritis with deposits of immunoglobulin and complement in the glomerulus. Renal failure is very rare. If minor urinary abnormalities occur (proteinuria less than 500 mg/day), therapy should be interrupted until the urine is normal, then reinstituted at lower doses. If the abnormalities recur, gold must be stopped. At times, nephrotic syndrome demands treatment with 40-60 mg/day of prednisone. Treatment with heavy-metal chelators such as dimercaprol or penicillamine is usually unnecessary. The prognosis of gold-induced nephrotic syndrome is favorable, 70% of patients recovering fully within months to years.

Hematologic Reactions (2-3%)

The most serious side effects of gold therapy are hematologic disorders, including thrombocytopenia, agranulocytosis, and aplastic anemia. These complications are rare. Granulocytopenia may be noted incidentally on routine blood tests or may present with fever and pharyngitis. Thrombocytopenia is not dose-related and may occur after very low cumulative doses of gold compounds. Aplastic anemia is a rare complication and has been reported even after the cessation of gold therapy. Management of severe hematologic gold toxicity includes the administration of prednisone, 60 mg/day in three divided doses; anabolic steroids, such as testosterone proprionate, 200 mg IM, three times weekly; and chelating agents, such as dimercaprol (BAL), penicillamine, and ethylenediaminetetraacetic acid (EDTA) (these drugs are used either in patients unresponsive to steroids or in combination with them). The recent demonstration of the usefulness of *N*-acetylcysteine for leukopenia and/or thrombocytopenia due to gold is an important advance. GSCF has been effective in the setting of leukopenia. *Note:* If any of these severe, life-threatening side effects occur, it is best to consult with the drug manufacturer in order to report the adverse reaction and to discuss the most recent therapeutic approaches.

Gastrointestinal Reactions (2% with parenteral gold, 40% with oral gold with 6% discontinuing therapy because of these side effects).

Parenteral gold—Cholestatic jaundice may occur early in the course of therapy, is often associated with eosinophilia, and resolves with drug discontinuation. Enterocolitis, an uncommon complication, may occur in middle-aged females after small doses of gold. The presentation is abdominal pain, severe diarrhea (with or without blood), and fever. The mortality remains 50% despite corticosteroids and other therapeutic measures. *Oral gold*—In a recent study, 30% of patients developed diarrhea or loose stools and 4% had to be withdrawn from the study due to this side effect. If diarrhea is mild, dosage decrease to 3 mg/day may improve the GI complaint; if severe, discontinuation is indicated. Severe enterocolitis is rare. Extensive GI studies in most patients with oral gold-related GI irritation have not demonstrated significant pathologic change.

Cardiopulmonary Reactions

Vasomotor (nitritoid) reactions due to peripheral vasodilatation occur predominantly with gold sodium thiomalate, and are characterized by weakness, dizziness, vomiting and nausea, tongue swelling, sweating, and facial flushing. It may occur in as many as 34% of patients, and, rarely, can result in myocardial infarction or CNS injury (especially in the elderly). Management includes switching to another gold compound or decreasing the dosage and administering the drug with the patient supine. Rarely, parenteral gold has been associated with the development of pulmonary infiltrates with associated dyspnea and restrictive lung disease. This problem usually responds to drug discontinuation and the institution of corticosteroids.

Ophthalmic Reactions

Corneal chrysiasis occurs in 75% of patients receiving more than 1,500 mg of parenteral gold but does not lead to ocular disease. Rarely, conjunctivitis, iritis, and corneal ulcers have been attributed to gold.

Musculoskeletal Reactions

Myalgias, joint pains, and inflammation are relatively common and may occur just after each injection. These may be severe enough that cessation of therapy may be necessary. A change to aurothioglucose may be associated with a decreased incidence of this problem.

Miscellaneous Reactions

Metallic taste is common, while peripheral neuropathy and headaches are rare.

Retreatment

Patients with severe toxicity such as thrombocytopenia, asplastic anemia, exfoliative dermatitis, or nephropathy should *not* be retreated with gold. With milder side effects, especially mucocutaneous reactions, it may be possible to restart gold, beginning with low doses (e.g., 5 mg for 3–4 weeks then slowly increasing by 5–10 mg increments over the next months) 4 weeks after total resolution of the skin reaction.

Remember

Some studies claim that patients who have had specific side effect with gold have an increased propensity for the same side effect with penicillamine.

Appropriate Surveillance for Side Effects

Parenteral Gold Preparations

For the first few months of therapy, complete blood and platelet counts should be done before each gold injection is given. If no changes have occurred after 3–4 months, the tests can be done at 2-week intervals and, ultimately, at monthly intervals or (when on monthly maintenance therapy) before every fourth injection. A trend toward progressive cytopenia may be observed by making a flow sheet of the patient's laboratory data. A urinalysis should precede each gold injection.

Oral Gold Preparation

For the first three months, complete blood and platelet count and urinalysis every two weeks, then monthly.[161]

Cautions and Contraindications

Gold is contraindicated in patients with a history of a previous severe skin, bone marrow, or renal reaction to gold. Significant functional impairment of the kidneys or liver is a relative contraindication to gold therapy, but toxicity to these organs is rare, and with careful clinical and laboratory monitoring, serious problems can be avoided. Leukopenia was previously considered a relative contraindication, but gold-induced improvement of leukopenia has been demonstrated in patients with Felty's syndrome. As a rule, phenylbutazone, oxyphenylbutazone, or immunosuppressive drugs, such as azathioprine and cyclophosphamide, are not given concomitantly with gold because, like gold, they may suppress the bone marrow. The concomitant administration of warfarin anticoagulants and parenteral gold salts is problematic because of potential local bleeding with the IM injection and also the potential thrombocytopenia. Patients who have proteinuria due to other diseases (such as diabetes) should generally not be given gold because of the difficulty in surveillance and the potential for membranous nephropathy.

Appendix 3-5
Sulfasalazine Therapy in the Treatment of Rheumatoid Arthritis

Name

Sulfasalazine (Azulfidine, Azulfidine EN-tabs)

Chemistry

Sulfasalazine (SSZ) is synthesized through the linkage of 5-amino salicylic acid (5-ASA) and sulfapyridine (SP) via an azo bond.

Absorption, Metabolism and Distribution

Thirty percent is absorbed in the upper intestinal tract; 70% is subjected to azo-reduction cleavage in the colon by intestinal flora. Up to 80% of intact sulfasalazine is recovered in the bile. Colon reduction yields 5-ASA and SP, both of which are metabolized. The rate at which SP is acetylated is genetically determined. Most of 5-ASA is excreted unchanged in the stool. Serum levels of salicylates are negligible. SSZ and 5-ASA concentrate in the intestinal wall as well as peritoneal, pleural and synovial fluids. SP is distributed in body tissues and fluids.

Mechanism of Action

While in ulcerative colitis, the likely mechanism of action is local colonic anti-inflammatory effect by 5-ASA via prostaglandin inhibition, the action in rheumatoid arthritis is probably different, but undefined. In colitis, 5-ASA given alone has the same effect as SSZ. In RA, the "antirheumatic" effect may be due to either SSZ, SP, or both; 5-ASA alone is clinically ineffective. While the exact mechanism of action in RA is unknown, there is evidence for anti-inflammatory, immunomodulatory, antibacterial (in the colon), and folate metabolism actions.

Clinical Efficacy

In open and double-blind, placebo-controlled trials, suppression of rheumatoid synovitis may be induced by SSZ within two months after full maintenance doses are reached. Because of its convenience, relative safety, and fairly rapid onset of action, SSZ may be an appropriate choice for early and mild cases of RA, prior to the use of gold salts and penicillamine, and with the same clinical indications as antimalarial drugs. Further experience with this drug in RA is needed to define its place in the armamentarium for RA and also to define its long-term side effect profile in this group of patients. Avoidance of SSZ in patients with ANA+, latex− rheumatoid-like polyarthritis is appropriate because such patients could have systemic lupus erythematosus.

Supply

500 mg EN-tabs.

Cost of Medication

Four 500-mg tablets per day for one month—$28.90.

Dosage

One 500-mg tablet is started with breakfast for the first week, then one 500-mg tablet is added weekly with each meal, then with meals and before bed to attain, after four weeks, a dose of one tab with meals and h.s. Dosing with meals decreases gastrointestinal side effects. Some studies reach a maximum of 3 g/day in divided doses in both RA and seronegative spondyloarthropathies (Reiter's syndrome, reactive arthritis, ankylosing spondylitis, psoriatic arthritis, and colitic arthropathies). While most studies recommend doses of 2 g/day or more, some have demonstrated efficacy at 1 g/day in divided doses.

Adverse Reactions

Two major categories are noted: (1) dose-related and related to acetylator phenotype—Nausea, vomiting, headache, malaise, hemolytic anemia, and (2) idiosyncratic—Rash, toxic, hepatitis, pneumonitis, aplastic anemia.

Gastrointestinal and Hepatic Reactions

Nausea, vomiting, anorexia, and abdominal pain account for two thirds of treatment discontinuation. Transient elevation of liver function tests are noted in 2%; rarely a toxic hepatitis with fever, rash, eosinophils, and marked liver function test abnormalities can occur. Liver changes occur in initial weeks of therapy. Upper GI symptoms are managed empirically with dose reduction or discontinuation according to the severity.

Mucocutaneous Reactions

These account for 15% of withdrawals. Most are nonspecific maculopapular rashes which clear with drug discontinuation. Rarely, toxic epidermal necrolysis and Stevens-Johnson syndrome occurs. Buccal ulcerations are rare.

Hematologic Reactions (0.3%)

Agranulocytosis, leukopenia, aplastic anemia, megaloblastic anemia, methemoglobinemia, sulfhemoglobinemia.

Pulmonary Reactions

Allergic interstitial pneumonitis reported, but not in RA.

Central Nervous System Reactions

Depression, irritability, headache, and/or dizziness in < 5%.

Autoimmune Reactions

Systemic lupus-like disorders reported, but not in RA.

Male Infertility and Teratogenicity

Reversible. Possible association with teratogenicity.

Appropriate Surveillance for Side Effects

Complete blood count, chemistry profile and urinalysis prior to therapy. CBC every week for the first month of therapy, then every 4 weeks thereafter. Chemical profile with half the frequency of the CBC, unless there is a clinical indicator of abnormality. Urinalysis every 4–6 months. Fever and rash should stimulate immediate testing in view of their association with hepatic and blood disorders.

Cautions and Contraindications

This drug should be avoided in patients with a history of sulfa or sulfasalazine allergy, and in patients with a possible diagnosis of SLE (there is an increased potential for severe drug reactions to sulfa in patients with SLE).[161]

Appendix 3-6
D-Penicillamine Therapy in the Treatment of Rheumatoid Arthritis

Name

D-Penicillamine (Cuprimine, De-Pen)

Chemistry and Biochemical Properties

D-Penicillamine is a trifunctional amino acid with a sulfhydryl group attached to one carbon atom. The D-isomer has less toxicity than the L-isomer. Biochemical properties include:

1. Capacity to form stable chelates with various metals and thus promote their excretion. This is the basis for its use in Wilson's disease and heavy metal poisoning.
2. Ability to participate in thiol-disulfide interchange reactions. This is the basis for use in cystinuria and D-penicillamine's ability to dissociate pentameric IgM into monomeric units. This action and D-penicillamine's ability to decrease circulating immune complexes and rheumatoid factor was the initial rationale for use in rheumatoid arthritis.
3. Capacity to react with aldehyde-containing compounds. D-Penicillamine inhibits cross-linking of collagen. In animals this leads to change seen in lathyrism. This is the rationale for its use in scleroderma.

Mechanism of Action

The exact mechanism is unknown but probably involves immunosuppressive actions working at the level of T lymphocyte function.

Clinical Efficacy

Controlled, double-blind clinical trials have demonstrated statistically significant clinical improvement with this drug. Low dose (<375 mg per day) therapy may be associated with fewer side effects but it also has less therapeutic efficacy. There is no strong evidence that D-penicillamine can prevent the development of bone erosions or facilitate their healing once present. Because of its profile of side effects, this drug is less commonly employed as a remittive agent in rheumatoid patients.

Supply

Capsules, 125 mg, 250 mg.

Cost of Medication

Three 250-mg tablets per day for one month—$62.50.

Dosage

The drug is given orally by Jaffe's rule: "Go low, go slow." Start at 125–250 mg/day, and advance in 125-mg increments at 8–12 week intervals. Doses less than 375 mg are associated with only minimal benefits. Maximum dosage is 1,000 mg/24 hours. Absorption is affected by food and drugs and thus it is given as a single dose 1½ hr before meals and 1 hr after administration of other medications, including vitamins and iron. Doses above 500 mg are given in a b.i.d. dosage.

Adverse Reactions

The side-effects rate is 30–65% with 25–40% of treated patients stopping therapy because of the severity of the side effects. Some studies note an increased propensity for a recurrence of the same side effects seen with prior parenteral gold salt therapy.

Mucocutaneous Reactions (10–40%)

Rashes usually occur early in the course and are morbilliform, maculopapular, and pruritic. These often respond to topical steroids and antihistamines but do not necessitate discontinuation. Stomatitis can be a persistent problem. Late lesions, such as pemphigus vulgaris, necessitate drug discontinuation. There is no clinically significant increase in wound healing time.

Gastrointestinal Reactions (5–20%)

Taste abnormalities occur in 12%, usually early in the course, and clear despite continued drug use. Anorexia, nausea, vomiting, dyspepsia, early satiety, diarrhea, abdominal cramps, flatus, and transaminitis are reported.

Renal Reactions (6–9%)

Proteinuria may occur in 6–9%, usually late in the course (>7–12 months), and can lead to nephrotic syndrome due to membraneous nephritis. This renal lesion is almost always reversible, but proteinuria may last for months or years. If proteinuria of 2+ or more has persisted for 30 days and other causes of renal disease or infection have been ruled out, a 24-hour urine protein determination should be done and repeated at monthly intervals. As long as the protein excretion does not exceed 1g/24 hr and the creatinine clearance is stable, the drug may be continued. Proteinuria may clear completely with only a 125-mg reduction in the daily dose. Development of hypoalbuminemia, nephrotic syndrome, or significant hematuria requires discontinuation of the drug. Rechallenge will usually lead to recurrence of proteinuria.

Hematologic Reactions (9%)

Thrombocytopenia occurs in 4–7% of patients, usually between the 10th and 20th weeks of therapy. Hematologic toxicity is potentially dangerous and dictates the need for close followup: complete blood counts, including platelet count, at 2-week intervals for the first six months of therapy and then at least monthly thereafter. Recording laboratory data on flow sheets permits early detection of downward trends in white blood cell counts and platelet count. Onset of hematologic toxicity may be sudden and may occur in the interval between scheduled laboratory studies; thus patients must be alerted to report skin or mucous membrane bleeding, infection or fever. Leukopenia of ≤3000 cells/mm^3, platelet count <100,000, or a rapidly falling platelet count require immediate and permanent discontinuation of D-penicillamine therapy. Leukopenia associated with thrombocytopenia, or thrombocytopenia alone may indicate impending aplastic anemia. There is no good therapy for aplastic anemia other than discontinuation of the medication. Increased doses of steroids only increase the risk of infection.

Pulmonary Reactions (rare)

Obliterative bronchiolitis may be progressive and lead to pulmonary insufficiency. Close observation for dyspnea, cough, or bonchospasm symptoms is important.

Autoimmune Reactions (rare)

Myasthenia gravis, pemphigus vulgaris, Goodpasture's syndrome, drug-induced lupus syndrome, hemolytic anemia, polymyositis, and thrombotic thrombocytopenic purpura are uncommon but potentially dangerous problems associated with this drug. Discontinuation of the drug usually leads to disappearance of the autoimmune syndromes.

Appropriate Surveillance for Side Effects

Complete blood count, with differential counts and platelet counts, and urinalysis are mandated every two weeks for the first six months of therapy and then on a monthly basis. Recording laboratory data on flow sheets allows for early recognition of downward or abnormal trends in test results. Questioning the patient about rash, itching, mouth ulcers, GI upsets, fever, easy bruising, and so forth is important during each visit. Patients should receive prescriptions for only the amount of medication needed until the next visit; this will prevent self-treatment without appropriate medical followup.

Cautions and Contraindications

A history of allergy to penicillin is not a contraindication to penicillamine, but institution of therapy in such patients should be carried out under close observation and using low doses. Contraindications include pregnancy, renal failure, patients who are unreliable, and patients who have poor ability to communicate their symptoms. Women of childbearing age should be told to use contraception and be warned of the small but indeterminate risk of adverse effects from this drug. They should notify the physician if pregnancy is suspected and the drug should be stopped immediately.[161]

Appendix 3-7
Azathioprine Therapy in the Treatment of Rheumatoid Arthritis

Name

Azathioprine (Imuran).

Chemistry

Azathioprine is a nitroimidazole derivative of 6-mercaptopurine.

Drug Action

This is a cycle-specific antimetaboite that suppresses synthesis of adenine and guanine. Azathioprine and its metabolites modify mainly T cell function and inhibit DNA synthesis. It is also anti-inflammatory.

Metabolism

Azathioprine is metabolized by the liver by several enzymes, including xanthine oxidase. 6-Mercaptopurine, the most active metabolite of azathioprine, is oxidized by this enzyme to 6-thiouric acid, which is excreted in the urine. Plasma half-life is 90 minutes.

Mechanism of Action

The drug probably functions both as an immunosuppressive and anti-inflammatory drug.

Clinical Efficacy

Several well-performed studies demonstrate efficacy and low toxicity at doses of 50–200 mg/day with steroid-sparing effect. This drug may retard the progression of bone erosions. This immunoregulatory drug is approved by the FDA for the treatment of RA refractory to other DMARDs, such as antimalarials, gold salts, and D-penicillamine.

Supply

50-mg tablets.

Cost of Medication

Two 50-mg tablets per day for one month—$47.40.

Dosage

Oral dose of 1–2.5 mg/kg/day. The initial dose is 50 mg. If there is no response or toxicity after six weeks, the dose is increased by 0.5 mg/kg/day every four weeks up to a maximum of 2.5 mg/kg/day. If azathioprine is used with allopurinol (this combination should be avoided), the dose of azathioprine should be reduced by 75%. If the creatinine clearance is less than 15 ml/min, a 50% reduction in dosage is indicated. This is a slow-acting, remittive agent and thus treatment should not be abandoned as ineffective before three or four months of treatment.

Adverse Reactions

1. Hematologic Reactions (25%). Leukopenia, neutropenia, thrombocytopenia, and macrocytic anemia are all seen and are dose-related, and usually clear with discontinuation or a change in dosage. Idiosyncratic acute agranulocytosis may occur.
2. Gastrointestinal Reactions (12–20%). Nausea, vomiting, hepatotoxicity, hepatic fribrosis, and pancreatis.
3. Dermatologic Reactions (1–2%). Dermatitis, hair thinning, stomatitis.
4. Central Nervous System Reactions (rare). Aseptic meningitis.
5. Lung Reactions (rare). Restrictive lung disease, cough.
6. General Reactions (rare). Fever.
7. Infections. There is a general increase in the propensity for infection.
8. Oncogenesis. Although an increased incidence of lymphoma and leukemia have not been demonstrated in RA patients taking azathioprine, such an increased risk of tumor development must be considered to exist in RA in view of the 30× increased risk in azathioprine-treated renal transplant patients who were concurrently treated with other immunosuppressive agents.
9. Hypersensitivity Reactions. Two types exist: (a) acute allergic hepatitis and (b) systemic illness manifested by fever, rash, polyarthralgia, and meningismus.
10. Teratogenicity. Not thought to exist with this drug.

Appropriate Surveillance for Side Effects

Initially, weekly complete blood counts and platelet counts are indicated. If hematologic status is stable for 1–2 months, then biweekly counts are appropriate. Counts should never be performed less than monthly. Liver function tests should be done monthly. General screening for infection and tumor is indicated.

Cautions and Contraindications

1. Dosage reductions must be made when azathioprine is used concomitantly with allopurinol to avoid prior severe side effects (see Dosage).
2. Avoid rechallenge in patients with prior severe side effects to this drug.
3. Cautious use in patients with history of infection or joint prosthesis.
4. These drugs should be used with great caution in patients with hepatic or renal impairment, and should not be used in patients with a history of malignant tumors.

Appendix 3-8
Methotrexate Therapy in the Treatment of Rheumatoid Arthritis

Name

Methotrexate (Rheumatrex)

Metabolism, Absorption, Interactions

Methotrexate can be give orally, intramuscularly or intravenously. It is well absorbed after oral administration and peak levels are reached within 2 hr. The major portion of the dose is excreted, unchanged, in the urine by 8 hr, and by 24 hr, more than 80% of the dose has been excreted. Approximately 50% of circulating methotrexate is protein-bound and thus displaceable by other drugs that have affinity for serum proteins, such as salicylates and other NSAIDs. NSAIDs and other weak acids diminish renal tubular transport. Of the total administered dose, 80-90% reappears in the urine. Thus, adjustments in dose must be made in patients with impaired renal function. Drugs that increase toxicity include salicylates, oral contraceptives, barbiturates, diphenylhydantoin, phenylbutazone, probenecid, and colchicine.

Drug Reactions

Methotrexate binds to the enzyme dihydrofolate reductase, blocking the conversion of dihydrofolic acid to tetrahydrofolic acid. This prevents the one-carbon transfer necessary in important cellular synthetic reactions, including amino acid and DNA synthesis. Methotrexate is phase specific, with effects on proliferating cells in the S phase of the cell cycle. Folinic acid (leucovorin calcium) overcomes the metabolic block induced by methotrexte and is used to counteract some of its toxic effects in the setting of high-dose therapy in malignancies. In animals, it suppresses both humoral and cell mediated responses.

Mechanism of Action

It is unclear as to whether methotrexate acts as an anti-inflammatory drug, an immunosuppressive (anti-metabolite), or both. There is some evidence that the drug alters the natural history of rheumatoid arthritis or decreases the rate of new erosions.

Clinical Efficacy

Clinical studies have defined methotrexate as an effective drug in the treatment of rheumatoid arthritis. The initial stimulus for use in RA was the drug's efficacy in psoriatic arthritis and psoriasis. Clinical improvement begins within 4-6 weeks after institution of therapy, plateaus at 6 months but remains effective (with continued use) for 2-4 years or more. It is important to remember that clinical flares occur within 4 weeks of stopping Methotrexate, even after 40 weeks of therapy. These flares can be quite severe and the potential for them should be understood by the physician and the patient prior to the drug's institution. One study demonstrated that the probability of continuing therapy for up to 6 years is nearly 50%, which is better than other DMARDs including gold salts, D-penicillamine, and sulfasalazine. This drug is approved by the FDA for the treatment of rheumatoid arthritis. However, it should be used only *after* the patient has failed or had unacceptable side effects from other DMARDs, including antimalarial drugs, gold salts, and D-penicillamine.

Supply

Tablets, 2.5 mg, or liquid for parenteral use.

Cost of Medication

Three 2.5-mg tablets per week for 1 month—$33.85.

Dosage

Oral therapy: 0.1–0.2 mg/kg once a week. Starting dose: 7.5 mg given as three 2.5-mg tablets together once a week (preferred) or 2.5 mg every 12 hours for three doses. (The rationale for the q12 hour dosing was "borrowed" from the treatment of psoriasis and based upon the of psoriatic cell division of once every 37.5 hours.) Doses can be increased by 2.5 mg every 4–6 weeks to a high of 15 mg depending on clinical response. Staring dose in the elderly: 5 mg. Parenteral therapy: The same dose can be given either IV or IM once a week to attempt to avoid unacceptable GI side effects from the medication. We recommend beginning with oral therapy.

Adverse Reactions

The probability of developing a major or minor toxic event is significant, especially during the first year of administration. The toxic effect, rather than lack of response, is the main limiting factor in maintaining a patient on therapy. In one study, the overall probability of continuing to take methotrexate was 71% at 1 year, 55.5% at 3 years, 50% at 5 years, and 49% at 6 years. In six of the patients in whom it was permanently stopped (7.7%), withdrawal was due to lack of efficacy, whereas in 47 (60.3%), the reason for discontinuation was the occurrence of toxic events.

1. Gastrointestinal Reactions (50%). Nausea, vomiting (these can be so severe that the drug may have to be discontinued; alternatives include decreasing the dose or considering parenteral route), dyspepsia, diarrhea, may exacerbate a prior ulcer, and may cause gastric ulcerations and stomatitis (30%).
2. Alopecia. Occurs in up to 5%.
3. Pulmonary Reactions. Acute hypersensitivity pneumonitis occurs but is uncommon; more likely if doses are greater than 15 mg/week.
4. Blood and Bone Marrow Reactions. Leukopenia occurs in 4%, thrombocytopenia in 3%. Anemia is rare.
5. Teratogenicity and Carcinogenicity. The drug is teratogenic and its use should be restricted to sterile women, postmenopausal females, or reliable patients practicing birth control. If fertile, counsel on birth control. This drug may cause oligospermia but permanent sterility is not linked to it. There is no evidence that this drug causes cancer, whether low or high doses are used.
6. Liver. Up to 60% of patients develop elevated transaminases but this does not correlate with liver biopsy-demonstrated fibrosis or cirrhosis. Minor fibrosis occurs in 40% of RA patients with cumulative doses of >2 g. In psoriasis, there is a correlation between duration of therapy, age of patient and cirrhosis. In general, histologic changes are low grade, but long-term biopsy information is not available and surveillance is mandatory. There are two types of liver changes: (a) Acute elevation of SGOT and SGPT due to inflammation—This hypersensitivity hepatitis is acute and reversible and occurs in high-dose therapy. Some acute changes in liver enzymes can occur due to the concomitant use of NSAIDs. (b) Fibrosis and cirrhosis–not reflected by liver function tests or liver scans.

Therapy for Toxicity

For life-threatening toxicity (e.g., pancytopenia or exfoliative mucositis) use leucovorin rescue with folinic acid, as is used in cancer chemotherapy. No routine folic acid is recommended.

Appropriate Surveillance for Side Effects

Blood and Bone Marrow. Complete blood count and platelet count every 2 weeks for the first 6 months, every 2–4 weeks for the next 6 months, and then monthly thereafter. Decrease in white blood cell count to $<3,500/mm^3$ or a decrease in the platelet count to $<150,000/mm^3$ is cause to discontinue methotrexate until values return to normal.

Liver Function Tests

Monthly liver function tests including SGOT, SGPT, GGTP, alkaline phosphatase, bilirubin, and albumin. If enzymes continue to rise (especially to greater than 3 times the upper limits of normal) or albumin falls despite control of RA, discontinue methotrexate until levels normalize and then restart at half dosage.

Liver Biopsy

After a cumulative dose of 1.5 g (approximately 3 years) and then after each additional 1–1.5 g or for patients with persistently elevated liver function tests, hepatomegaly, or persistent, unexplained gastrointestinal symptoms.

Chest x-Ray

Pre-methotrexate and yearly while on the drug. Any pulmonary symptoms should stimulate a repeat chest x-ray.

Cautions and Contraindications

1. Use with caution in obese and elderly patients and patients with diabetes. While not all studies have demonstrated it, these patients may have an increased incidence of liver toxicity.
2. In patients with renal compromise, use with great caution in reduced dosage, if at all.
3. Trimethoprim/sulfamethoxazole is relatively contraindicated.
4. Increased toxicity (e.g., bone marrow suppression) can occur with methotrexate if combined with NSAIDs and aspirin. Thus, increased caution is needed with these drugs.
5. Active alcoholism is an absolute contraindication to methotrexate therapy. With a history of alcohol abuse, a pre-methotrexate liver biopsy is recommended. If fibrosis or cirrhosis is found, no drug should be given.
6. Vigilance is needed in RA patients with pre-existing pulmonary disease because of an increased propensity to lung toxicity due to methotrexate in this group. Low PO_2 or significant x-ray or pulmonary function test abnormalities may contraindicate this drug.
7. Teratogenicity—See adverse effects.[161]

Chapter 4
Septic Arthritis, Lyme Disease, and Prosthetic Joint Infection

BARRY D. BRAUSE, M.D.

Septic Arthritis

The interaction of microorganism and host inflammatory response with underlying synovial tissue, cartilage, and bone determines the clinical presentation, course, and prognosis in patients with septic arthritis. Prompt recognition of the pathologic process as well as timely, appropriate medical and surgical intervention can neutralize the destruction and provide a favorable functional outcome. This chapter outlines the pathogenesis, microbiology, and therapy of infected native joint spaces to assist clinical decision making in their management.

Pathogenesis

The initial event in all pyogenic arthritides involving native (nonprosthetic) joints is invasion of the synovial membrane by microorganisms. Infection subsequently extends into the joint space where a paucity of phagocytes, antibodies, and complement permits a closed space infection to be established. When the pathologic process continues, the avascular cartilage is degraded by the combined action of bacterial and leukocytic enzymes. The progression of these events is determined by the virulence of the pathogen, the nature and extent of the inflammatory reaction, as well as the vulnerability of the underlying host tissue. Recruitment of polymorphonuclear leukocytes by microbial chemotactic factors appears to be essential for the evolution of the tissue destructive component in septic arthritis. This component is most fulminant when the involved articular tissue has been damaged by prior injury. The inflamed hypertrophic synovium evolves into an aggressive form of granulation tissue (pannus), which spreads to involve the entire articulation. Irreversible loss of joint function is related to the extent of cartilaginous dissolution and the subsequent overgrowth of adjacent osseous tissue.

Routes of Infection

Etiologic organisms can invade intra-articular tissue by hematogenous seeding, by extension from infection in adjacent tissue, and by implantation. Infection of the skin and soft tissues, the genitourinary tract, the respiratory tract, and the gastrointestinal tract can spread to the synovial membrane through the bloodstream. Local septic processes in tissue contiguous to the joint such as cellulitis, infected skin ulcerations, paronychia, infected synovial cysts, and osteomyelitis can involve synovial tissue by direct extension. Contamination associated with traumatic injury, arthrocentesis, intra-articular injections, and orthopedic surgery can introduce bacteria into articular tissue.

Predisposing Factors

Most patients who develop septic arthritis have associated conditions that predispose them to joint infection.[1] Discovery of these pathogenetic potentials by history and physical examination offers great assistance in diagnosing the nature of the articular disease and in predicting the causative pathogen. Twenty-five to 50 percent of patients have extra-articular infection of the skin, respiratory, or genitourinary tracts. Microorganisms from these remote sites reach the synovium by way of the bloodstream. Chronic diseases associated with impaired immunologic defenses, such as malignancies, diabetes mellitus, and hepatic cirrhosis, predispose patients to frequent, severe bacterial infections including pyarthrosis. Patients receiving immunosuppressive therapy (systemic or intra-articular corticosteroids and cytotoxic chemotherapy) have an enhanced risk for these septic processes. Parenteral drug abuse often is accompanied by bacteremic synovial seeding.

Chronic arthritic conditions predispose affected joints to infection.[2] Patients with rheumatoid arthritis have an increased frequency of pyarthrosis compared with control populations. This clinical observation may be caused by preexistent articular damage, immunologic impairment mediated by rheumatoid factor and corticosteroid therapy, or the increased incidence of bacterial infection seen with rheumatoid arthritis. Other types of articular disease, such as systemic lupus erythematosus, gout, pseudogout, degenerative joint disease and neuropathic arthropathy, have been reported to be complicated by joint sepsis. Approximately 30 percent of patients with septic arthritis have previous joint disease.

Clinical Manifestations and Diagnosis

Bacterial arthritis presents with the cardinal signs of inflammation. The acute onset of joint pain is most characteristic with increasing severity upon flexion, extension, or weight bearing. Articular pain is induced by even minimal degrees of joint motion. Arthralgia produced only by extreme flexion or extreme extension is suggestive of periarticular inflammation, as seen in septic bursitis. Local soft tissue swelling, tenderness, erythema, and warmth accompany a restricted range of motion in the involved articulation. Fever is an almost constant feature of pyarthrosis, and systemic sepsis can occur with particularly virulent pathogens in vulnerable patients. Synovial effusions are present in 90 percent of cases. Bacterial arthritis usually affects only one joint; however, polyarticular infection is seen in 10 percent of patients and frequently reflects concomitant bacteremia. The knees and hips are the most commonly infected joints, although septic arthritis in parenteral drug abusers often affects the sternoclavicular, sacroiliac, or shoulder articulations.[3] Hip joint sepsis can be very difficult to diagnose since symptoms may be minimal and effusions may be undemonstrable.[2] In viral arthritis, multiple joint involvement is common especially in the hands and wrists. More subacute and chronic presentations occur with mycobacterial and fungal arthritis.[4-6]

Certain pyarthroses are accompanied by dermatologic manifestations as well as articular involvement (dermatitis-arthritis syndromes). This presentation is most commonly recognized with septic arthritis caused by Neisseria gonorrhoeae and Hemophilus influenzae. Gonococcal arthritis often is associated with prodromal or concomitant tenosynovitis, erythematous papules, and vesiculopustular or petechial skin rashes characteristic of the disseminated stage of gonococcemia.[7] Frequently the pathogen can be demonstrated in these lesions by Gram stain or culture. Hemophilus influenzae pyarthrosis also can be associated with tenosynovitis and erysipeloid, pustular, or petechial rashes.[8] Dermatitis-arthritis syndromes have been described due to other bacteria such as Neisseria meningitidis and Streptobacillus moniliformis (rat-bite fever). The characteristic appearance of the erythema chronicum migrans rash can be essential to the diagnosis of early Borrelia burgdorferi arthritis (Lyme disease), which is discussed in the next section of the chapter. Viral arthritides due to rubella and hepatitis B infections also are associated with exanthems as important features in their presentation.

Although blood cultures are positive in approximately 50 percent of patients, synovial fluid analysis is the basis for initiation of therapy and confirmation of the specific microbiologic diagnosis (Table 4-1). Normal joint fluid contains a paucity of leukocytes (mainly lymphocytes and monocytes) with a glucose level at least 80 percent that of serum. Inflamed (but nonseptic) joints have turbid effusions with a moderate number of polymorphonuclear leukocytes and

Table 4-1. Synovial Fluid Analysis

	Normal	Inflammation	Bacterial Infection
Color	Colorless, pale yellow	Yellow	Yellow
Turbidity	Slight	Turbid	Turbid, purulent
Leukocyte count	200–1000	1000–10,000	10,000–over 100,000
Cell type	Mononuclear	Neutrophils	Neutrophils
Synovial fluid/blood glucose	0.8–1.0	0.5–0.8	Less than 0.5
Gram stain	Negative	Negative	Positive (65%)
Culture	Negative	Negative	Positive

a slight reduction in glucose concentration. Infected synovial fluid usually contains high polymorphonuclear counts and a substantially decreased glucose level. However, these features are not sufficiently distinctive to permit an absolute diagnosis since they can be indistinguishable from uninfected, inflammatory effusions. For example, the synovial fluid glucose level is reduced in only 50 percent of infected patients. Gram stains of joint fluid can be diagnostic when positive (65 percent of cases) and can provide adequate data to institute appropriate antibiotic therapy promptly. Counterimmunoelectrophoretic techniques can rapidly detect antigens from pneumococci, meningococci, and H. influenzae in joint fluid and urine, but these pathogens are seen mainly in the pediatric population. Cultures of synovial fluid confirm the specific causative microorganism in all bacterial arthritides except in gonococcal infection, in which only 50 percent positivity is found and the diagnosis is then made on the basis of urethral, cervical, pharyngeal, and rectal cultures, the presence of tenosynovitis, or the characteristic skin lesions of disseminated gonococcemia.

Radiologic evaluation of the infected joint is helpful but is not diagnostic since the anatomic changes seen are not specific for septic processes. The earliest radiographic sign of joint infection is periarticular soft tissue swelling with displacement of the adjacent fat pads by synovial edema or an articular effusion during the first week of pyarthrosis. After this period, periarticular osteopenia (subchondral bone rarefaction) develops from local hyperemia, as well as bone atrophy secondary to relative immobility. With more fulminant infection, uniform joint space narrowing becomes visible by x-ray study as a consequence of articular cartilage dissolution. Subsequently osseous erosions, induced by the pannus formation, can be seen subchondrally or in peripheral areas between the joint capsule insertion and the joint cartilage where the synovium is in direct contact with bone. Eventually, fibrous or bony ankylosis may develop in chronic infections.[9]

Bacteriology

Since Staphylococcus aureus is a frequent cause of septic arthritis in all age groups, it should be considered a potential pathogen in clinical decision making for all patients. The incidence of other bacterial causative agents is age related (Table 4-2).[10-13] Infants under 1 month old develop group B streptococcal and gram-negative bacillary joint sepsis as a result of the frequent bacteremias with these organisms experienced by neonates. Young children are prone to H.

Table 4-2. Age-Related Bacteriologic Causes of Septic Arthritis

Microorganism	Under 2 Yr	2-15 Yr	16-50 Yr	over 50 Yr
Staphylococcus aureus	40%	50%	15%	70%
Streptococci	25	30	5	15
Hemophilus	30	9	—	—
Neisseria gonorrhoeae	—	5	75	—
Gram-negative bacilli	3	5	5	8

influenzae respiratory tract infections until they develop sufficient specific antibody activity against this pathogen (usually by age 8). As a result, hematogenous Hemophilus arthritis is prominent in the youngest age group. Streptococci are important pathogens in children under age 15 on the basis of upper respiratory tract infections with Pneumococcus pneumoniae and Streptococcus pyogenes. The gonococcus is the most common cause of septic arthritis in the United States and is the causative agent in 75 percent of these infections during the most sexually active years. The population at risk for gram-negative bacillary pyarthroses reflects those predisposed to gram-negative bacteremia. Two thirds of these patients have debilitating chronic diseases and most of their joint infections are caused by hematogenous spread from pathologic processes in the urinary tract.[14] Parenteral drug abuse is also strongly associated with gram-negative bacillary infections including septic arthritis due to Pseudomonas aeruginosa.

Treatment

Treatment of bacterial arthritis requires antimicrobial therapy, adequate drainage, and avoidance of weight bearing on the involved articulation. After obtaining necessary cultures, appropriate (usually parenteral) antibiotics should be instituted promptly. The antimicrobial regimen is designed on the basis of synovial fluid Gram stain observations and the clinical setting in which the infection developed (patient's age, preceding septic processes, associated conditions, and physical examination findings). After culture results identify the causative pathogen, the antimicrobial regimen is modified when necessary to include only the most appropriate agent(s). Most antibiotics achieve effective synovial fluid levels with parenteral administration; therefore, intra-articular instillation or irrigation is not indicated and may be hazardous.[15-17] Injection of antibiotics directly into the joint space can cause chemical synovitis and can be absorbed systemically resulting in potentially toxic serum levels.[13]

The duration of antimicrobial therapy varies with different types of bacterial arthritis. Gonococcal arthritis can be treated with parenteral ceftriaxone, ceftizoxime, or cefotaxime for 7 days. Other bacterial pathogens require 2 to 4 weeks of antibiotic therapy depending on the pathogen, the response to therapy, and the health of the underlying articular tissues. Treatment of infections in prosthetic total joint arthroplasties is discussed in the last section of the chapter.

Initially, the involved joint should be immobilized (usually in extension) until symptoms begin resolving. Weight bearing should be avoided to reduce the risk of damage to the involved articular cartilage. Subsequently, range of motion exercises should be employed (without weight bearing) since this technique may enhance nutritional diffusion to cartilage and assist in restoring natural cartilage repair mechanisms inhibited by immobilization.[18]

Since septic arthritis is a closed space infection, drainage procedures are essential to decrease intraarticular pressure and to reduce leukocyte enzyme activity. Simple arthrocentesis is commonly adequate to accomplish this aspect of therapy, and serial aspirations are necessary as prompted by reaccumulations of inflammatory effusions. Surgical drainage, often with synovectomy, is indicated in the treatment of hip infections (particularly with Staphylococcus aureus or gram-negative bacilli) because of the mechanical difficulty encountered in percutaneous needle aspiration of this deep articulation. Operative débridement is essential when pyarthrosis is inadequately responsive to less invasive drainage procedures due to loculation of infection by intraarticular adhesions or underlying joint disease. The response to therapy can be monitored by serial synovial fluid leukocyte counts. After 5 to 7 days of effective treatment, the joint fluid white blood cell count should decline by 50 to 75 percent.[1] Failure to achieve such a reduction should be viewed as an indication of inadequate therapy, and surgical drainage should be considered. Recently arthroscopic techniques have been employed, instead of open arthrotomy, for débridement in these situations, especially when the knee is involved.[19] Arthroscopy provides for more complete visualization of the tissue (by magnification and access to posterior compartments), decreases morbidity (lower complication rate), increases joint mobility (earlier postoperative motion because there is decreased incision size and its associated pain), and is more economical (allows a shorter hospitalization period).

Prognosis

A successful outcome in treatment of an infected joint is measured by the restoration of full articular function. Incomplete recovery indicates irreversible articular damage to some degree and is related to (1) the duration of symptoms prior to institution of therapy; (2) the specific causative microorganism in the infection; (3) serial decreases in synovial leukocyte counts during therapy; and (4) the rapidity in achieving synovial fluid sterility. Complete functional recovery is observed in two thirds (67 percent) of patients treated within 7 days of initial symptoms but in less than one third (27 percent) receiving therapy after more than 7 days' delay.[20] Different pathogens are associated with varying therapeutic success rates.[1] Whereas treatment of pyarthrosis caused by N. gonorrhoeae is over 95 percent successful and Pneumococcus pneumoniae infection is associated with full recovery in 94 percent, Streptococcus pyogenes infection (group A streptococcus) has an 85 percent success rate, Staphylococcus aureus has a 73 percent success rate, and in infection with gram-negative bacilli, only 21 percent completely recover joint function. A decline in the synovial fluid leukocyte count by 50 to 75 percent within 5 to 7 days of initiating therapy is usually associated with complete recovery of articular function.[1] A good therapeutic outcome is also related to timely elimination of the pathogen, with the best results obtained when synovial fluid cultures are sterilized within 5 days of treatment.[21]

Lyme Disease

Lyme disease (Lyme borreliosis) is a worldwide multisystem disorder about which our knowledge is rapidly expanding. It is an emerging disease in that our presently limited understanding of its pathogenesis, spectrum of manifestations, diagnostic criteria, and therapeutic adequacy is growing significantly each year.

Although elements of Lyme disease were described as discrete entities during the first half of this century, a geographic clustering of acute pediatric arthritis in Lyme, Connecticut, during 1977 triggered the present surge of investigations that has led to our present incomplete comprehension of this infection. Lyme borreliosis is the most common vector-borne infection in the United States. Its geographic incidence corresponds to the distribution of the vector, the Ixodes tick. Ninety percent of the cases in this country have been seen in Massachusetts, Rhode Island, Connecticut, New York, New Jersey, Wisconsin and Minnesota, but the disease is also prominent in the western states (California and Oregon).

Pathogenesis

The infection is caused by the spirochete, Borrelia burgdorferi, a fastidious microaerophilic organism found in ticks of the Ixodes ricinus complex. These vectors are represented by Ixodes dammini in the northeast and midwest United States, Ixodes pacificus in the western states, I. ricinus in Europe, and Ixodes persulcatus in Asia. Borrelia burgdorferi has been demonstrated in other tick species, mosquitoes and deer flies, but only ticks of the I. ricinus group appear to be important in transmission of the spirochete to humans. Ixodes dammini ticks are dependent on rodent hosts (white-footed mice) to complete their life cycle during their larval and nymphal stages, but the white-tailed deer is the preferred host for the adult stage. The deer is not involved in the life cycle of the tick and if deer are removed from the environment, the tick may be able to survive on other animal hosts.

Transmission of Borrelia to humans is usually by the aggressive nymphal forms that feed between May and July. Adult ticks, which feed in the autumn, also transmit the spirochete. The nymphal forms are so small that only a minority of patients with Lyme disease recall the bite. It appears that tick attachment for 24 hours may be necessary for transfer of the pathogen to humans.[22] Development of Lyme disease after spirochetal transfer seems to be a complex host-parasite interaction with tropism for the skin, joints, nervous system, and heart. In addition to direct borrelial tissue invasion, immune mechanisms involving the host inflammatory response may be important in disease pathogenesis.

Clinical Manifestations

With clear similarities to another spirochetal infection, syphilis, Lyme borreliosis evolves through sequential phases of disease with different symptomatic presentations. Stage 1 is the localized form of "early" infection, stage 2 is the disseminated form of "early" infection and stage 3 represents the "late" or persistent infection.[23]

Early, Localized Disease (Stage 1)

The principal manifestation of early local infection (stage 1) is the appearance of the skin lesion, erythema chronicum migrans (Fig. 4-1). This rash is a red macule or papule that expands to form a large annular zone of erythema, occasionally 60 cm in area, at the presumed tick-bite site.[24] The border is often a bright red with partial clearing of erythema in the central, occasionally indurated portion. Erythema chronicum migrans is reported in 60 to 80 percent of patients and appears 3 to 30 days after tick exposure. Spirochetes have been seen in tissue sections and cultured from these lesions. The rash usually fades within 3 to 4 weeks but may persist for as long as 14 months and can recur. Other dermatologic manifestations include malar rashes, diffuse erythema, urticaria, and rarely panniculitis with tender subcutaneous nodules. Patients may experience fever, regional lymphadenopathy, arthralgias, and minor constitutional symptoms during this phase of illness. Often the differential diagnosis includes mononucleosis and other viral infections, secondary syphilis, and connective tissue diseases in the clinical evaluation at this stage.

Early, Disseminated Disease (Stage 2)

Borrelia organisms appear to spread by way of the bloodstream or lymphatics to many sites over several days or weeks following inoculation. In stage 2 Lyme disease patients develop severe malaise and fatigue with episodic headaches and migratory pains in joints, bursae, tendons, muscles, and bones. Single or multiple annular skin rashes of erythema chronicum migrans may appear but are usually much smaller than the primary lesion.

An episodic, asymmetric, oligoarticular arthritis (Lyme arthritis) is seen in 60 percent of patients 2 weeks to 2 years (average of 6 months) after disease onset. The large joints are primarily involved with the knee being most common, then the shoulder, elbow, temporomandibular joint, ankle, wrist, and hip. Each attack usually resolves after about 1 week with a symptom-free period of approximately 4 weeks between migratory recurrences. Synovial fluid analysis during these episodes reveals leukocyte counts in the thousands (range 500 to 110,000) with predominantly polymorphonuclear cells.[23] The differential diagnoses entertained in this stage of Lyme borreliosis include juvenile rheumatoid arthritis, crystal-induced arthritis (gout, pseudogout), and Reiter's syndrome.

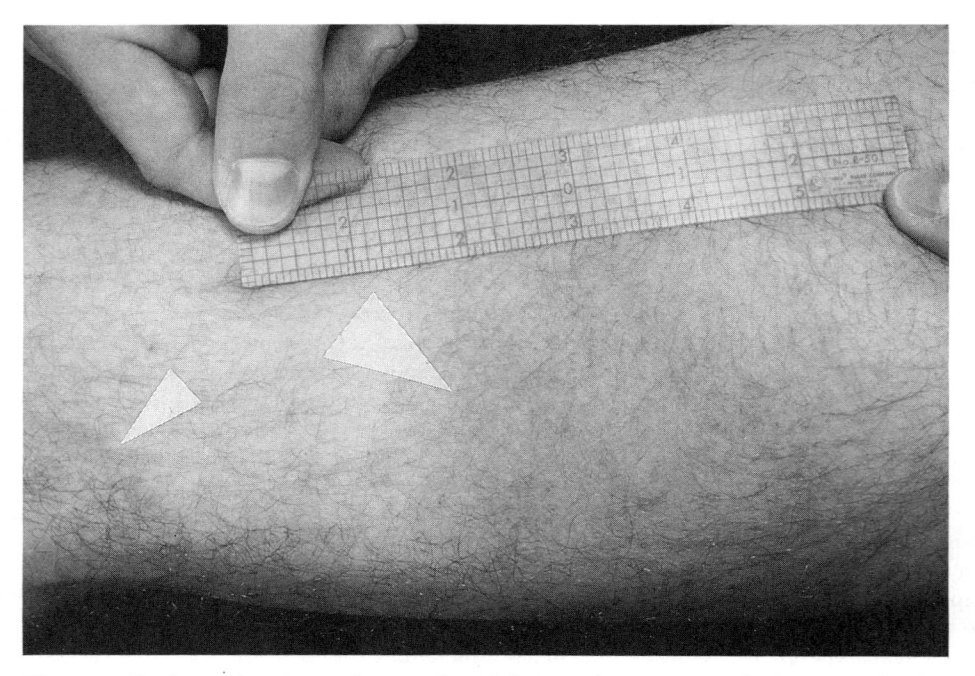

Figure 4-1. Erythema chronicum migrans rash with large erythematous macule (*large arrowhead*) and bright red margin at a separate lesion (*small arrowhead*)

Neurologic symptoms develop in 15 to 20 percent of patients several weeks or months after inoculation (usually 2 to 10 weeks after erythema chronicum migrans). Frequently a subacute meningitis with cranial or peripheral neuropathy is observed.[25,26] Unilateral or bilateral facial nerve palsy is the most common cranial neuropathy. Peripheral neuropathies are usually asymmetric involving the limbs or trunk. Occasionally patients manifest subtle encephalitic signs with confusion, decreased memory, and emotional lability. Cerebrospinal fluid appears similar to aseptic meningitis, revealing a lymphocytic pleocytosis and elevated protein (oligoclonal banding may be present) with normal glucose levels. Borrelia organisms have been cultured from the cerebrospinal fluid during this phase of illness. Symptoms frequently last for several weeks; or months and they may recur or become chronic.

Cardiac involvement is seen in 4 to 8 percent of cases, occurring within 3 to 21 weeks after erythema chronicum migrans. Fluctuating degrees of atrioventricular conduction blockage are the most common abnormalities including first-degree heart block, Wenckebach phenomena, and complete heart block.[27] Patients may complain of palpitations or syncope requiring temporary cardiac pacemaker insertion but since the defect resolves within 3 days to 6 weeks, permanent pacemaker implantation is not necessary. Occasionally an acute myopericarditis is seen. The differential diagnosis often includes acute rheumatic fever, viral myopericarditis, and connective tissue diseases.

Late, Persistent Lyme Disease (Stage 3)

If Lyme borreliosis becomes a persistent infection (stage 3), the recurrent arthritis progresses. Episodes become longer, lasting months rather than weeks, and symptoms can be continual.[28] Generally only one or a few joints are affected, with the knee remaining the most commonly involved. Whereas polymorphonuclear cells were most prominent in synovial fluid during stage 2 of Lyme arthritis, mononuclear cells predominate in this later phase. There appears to be an increased incidence of late Lyme arthritis in patients carrying the HLA-DR4 histocompatibility complex. In severe cases, erosion of cartilage and bone can be observed but permanent joint disability is only rarely seen. Symptoms resolve in 10 to 20 percent of patients in each year of illness.

Persistent Lyme disease can also be associated with chronic neurologic dysfunction. In Europe a progressive encephalomyelitis has been described with spastic paraparesis, bladder dysfunction, ataxia, cognitive impairment (including dementia), and seventh and eighth cranial neuropathies.[29] Of the small number of patients extensively evaluated in the United States to date, 89 percent have had mild encephalopathy characterized by memory loss, mood changes and sleep disturbance, and 70 percent have had polyneuropathy with radicular pain or distal paresthesias.[30] Associated complaints in these persons include fatigue, headache, and hearing loss. The symptoms appear to be nonprogressive but responsive to anti-Borrelia antibiotic therapy in a majority of cases. Cerebrospinal fluid examination reveals elevated protein levels, evidence of antibody production to B. burgdorferi, or both in 67 percent of patients.

A chronic dermatologic manifestation of Lyme disease, acrodermatitis chronica atrophicans, has been observed primarily in Europe.[31] Developing an average of 3 years after erythema chronicum migrans, this lesion is a bluish red swelling (plaque or nodule) usually on an extremity (most often the dorsal surface of the hand or foot). The abnormality lasts for many years with gradual skin atrophy occurring. The site of this pathologic process may be the same as the original erythema chronicum migrans years earlier. Occasionally joint and bone involvement emerges beneath the skin lesions including periostitis and small joint subluxation. Spirochetes have been recovered from acrodermatitis chronica atrophicans tissue.

Diagnosis

Establishing the presence or absence of Lyme disease in an individual patient can be problematic. Culture of B. burgdorferi from human tissues and fluids is very difficult because of the paucity of spirochetes present and the specialized techniques required to cultivate this fastidious pathogen. Visualization of Borrelia in pathologic tissue is also too difficult to be used for routine diagnosis. Therefore serologic testing has been employed with the enzyme-linked immunosorbent assay (ELISA) generally available. With this method anti-Borrelia IgM is detectable only after 3 to 4 weeks of infection and IgG is often demonstrable only after 2 to 3 months of infection.[32] Unlike the Venereal Disease Research Laboratory (VDRL) serologic test for syphilis which is standardized and reproducible, the ELISA test for Lyme disease provides results that vary significantly among different laboratories due to lack of reagent standardization and quality control.[33] The present ELISA test also has inadequate sensitivity and to a lesser extent, specificity. False-negative results occur during the initial weeks of infection, as noted above; therefore the diagnosis of early Lyme disease is based mainly on clinical findings (appropriate signs or symptoms in a patient with potential tick exposure). Early administration of anti-Borrelia antibiotics is likely to abort the antibody response (as detected by current methods), thereby interfering with post-treatment confirmation of the diagnosis. Untreated patients who develop arthritic, neurologic, or cardiac involvement uniformly test positive serologically.[34] Some patients with treated Lyme disease have continued chronic symptoms including fatigue, paresthesias, memory loss, and arthralgias. Whether these symptoms are actually related to persistent infection in the absence of a demonstrable antibody response is unknown. False positivity is also seen with the ELISA assay in patients with other spirochetal infections (syphilis, relapsing fever, yaws, and pinta), Rocky Mountain spotted fever, and autoimmune disorders. Immunoblotting serologic methods are advocated to delineate these falsely positive results but are not generally available because they are labor-intensive and costly. Present efforts are directed at applying the polymerase chain reaction technique to the diagnosis of Lyme disease by detecting B. burgdorferi antigen (DNA sequence). Hopefully this novel technology will provide a method to follow the disease course and quantitate the effect of therapy serologically, which has not been possible before.

Treatment

Borrelia burgdorferi is very sensitive to tetracycline, ampicillin, ceftriaxone, and imipenem and moderately sensitive to penicillin, oxacillin, chloramphenicol, and erythromycin. The duration of treatment and the route of administration have not been delineated due to the lack of controlled efficacy trials and the absence of serologic markers for adequacy of therapy. *The Medical Letter* has published a consensus view of recommended schedules for treating the various presentations of Lyme disease.[35] Their recommendations are based on limited data and should be considered tentative. In adults, early Lyme borreliosis is treated with doxycycline or amoxicillin, orally for 10 to 21 days. Erythromycin has been used as an alternative in patients who cannot take doxycycline or amoxicillin. Mild neurologic involvement (Bell's palsy) is treated with oral doxycycline or amoxicillin for 1 month, and more serious central nervous system disease is treated with ceftriaxone for 14 days or penicillin G for 10 to 14 days intravenously. Mild cardiac involvement is treated with oral doxycycline or amoxicillin for 21 days, and more serious cardiac disease with ceftriaxone or penicillin G intravenously for 10 to 21 days. Lyme arthritis is treated orally with doxycycline or amoxicillin for 1 month or intravenously with ceftriaxone or penicillin G for 14 to 21 days. Obviously more data is needed on the therapeutic modalities for these infections to provide confidence in the adequacy of these regimens. Ten percent of patients with Lyme borreliosis experience worsening of their symptoms within 24 to 72 hours of initiating antibiotic therapy. This phenomenon has been attributed to the Jarisch-Herxheimer reaction seen with syphilis treatment and appears to respond to salicylates and acetaminophen.

Prevention

Prevention of Lyme borreliosis is of paramount importance in view of the difficulties present in establishing timely diagnoses and in delineating adequacy of treatment in this serious, prevalent disease. Attempts at eliminating Ixodes ticks have met with only small success using aerial spraying and acaricide (permethrin)-impregnated cotton batting. Substantial reductions in the deer population have not markedly decreased tick densities and total removal of deer is impractical at this time. Moreover, eliminating the deer may not affect the Ixodes tick since the deer is not essential to the tick life cycle. Therefore, present efforts to prevent Lyme disease are limited to the use of tick-repellent sprays such as DEET (*N,N*-diethyl-3-methyl-toluamide) applications to skin and permethrin applications to clothing. Public education regarding the dangers of Lyme borreliosis will need to continue with additional emphasis on protective clothing to cover exposed skin when in Ixodes territory and on early recognition of disease. It appears that early Lyme infection is far more predictably responsive to antibiotic therapy than late Lyme disease. This clinical observation is similar to that found with another spirochetal infection, syphilis. The similarities between these two diseases are probably not coincidental.

Prosthetic Joint Infection

Due to the magnificent success of prosthetic total joint replacement in restoring function to those disabled with arthritis, virtually millions of people worldwide now have these devices implanted. One to 5 percent of these arthroplasties become infected, representing a calamity for the patient and associated with significant morbidity and occasionally death. This section traces the pathogenesis of these infections, their diagnosis, and approaches to their treatment and prevention.

Pathogenesis

Patients with a predisposition toward prosthetic joint infection include those with prior surgery at the site of implantation, rheumatoid arthritis patients, those on corticosteroid therapy, persons with diabetes mellitus, poor nutritional status and obesity, and those of extremely advanced age.[36,37] These conditions all share a potential for slow or poor wound healing. Prosthetic joint sepsis is actually a special form of osteomyelitis, usually occurring in osseous tissue adjacent to the foreign body. Because most prostheses are cemented in place with polymethylmethacrylate, infection develops at the bone-cement interface. Sepsis involving cementless implants develops in the bone contiguous with the metallic alloy.

These prostheses become infected by the introduced route or the hematogenous route of infection. The introduced form is the result of wound sepsis overlying the implant or operative contamination. Any factor or event that delays wound healing increases the risk of infection. During the early post-implantation period, the fascial layers have not yet healed and the deep, periprosthetic tissue is not protected by the usual anatomic barriers. Any superficial soft-tissue infection occurring at or near the surgical wound can spread rapidly to involve the underlying bone. Infections by this route are generally caused by a single pathogen, but polymicrobial sepsis with as many as five different microorganisms is also seen. Staphylococcus epidermidis is the most common causative agent in this setting. Occasionally latent foci of quiescent chronic osteomyelitis are reactivated by the tissue disruption inherent in this type of surgery. Although bone cultures are sterile at the time of implantation, old staphylococcal or tuberculous infection can recrudesce postoperatively.

Any bacteremia can produce infection in a joint prosthesis.[38] Dentogingival infections and manipulations are known causes of streptococcal and anaerobic infections in total joint replacements. Pyogenic skin processes can cause staphylococcal and streptococcal infections of prosthetic arthroplasties. Genitourinary and gastrointestinal tract procedures or infections are associated with gram-negative bacillary, enterococcal, and anaerobic infections of prostheses. Twenty to 40 percent of prosthetic joint infections arise by the hematogenous route, the remainder being of the introduced type.

The bacteriology of prosthetic joint sepsis varies among the published studies but a representative view of the spectrum of these organisms and the prominence of certain microbial groups is seen in Table 4-3. Staphylococci are the principal causative agents, but the spectrum of organisms capable of causing prosthetic joint infection is unlimited and includes organisms ordinarily considered "contaminants" of cultures, such as corynebacteria (aerobic diphtheroids), propionibacteria (anaerobic diphtheroids), and members of the Bacillus genus. Rarely, infections with fungi and mycobacteria have been reported.

Polymethylmethacrylate cement, which binds the metal alloy to adjacent bone, appears to predispose toward infection to an extent beyond that of other foreign bodies. The cement in unpolymerized form has been shown to inhibit phagocytic, lymphocytic, and complement function in vitro.[39] In an effort to provide total joint arthroplasty without polymethylmethacrylate, cementless prostheses have been designed but the performance and durability of these arthroplasties is uncertain.

Microbial products may assist the development and persistence of infection in association with prosthetic materials. In the presence of artificial substrates, many bacteria elaborate a material called glycocalyx ("slime"). Organisms grow within this exopolysaccharide matrix forming thick biofilms. The glycocalyx modifies the local tissue environment in favor of the pathogen by protecting the organism from surfactants, opsonic antibodies, phagocytes, and antimicrobial agents. These conditions enhance the density of colonization on the surface of metallic prostheses in vivo and may play a role in predisposing toward tissue invasion.[36,40] The presence of these protective biofilms also may result in persistence of infection despite treatment with systemic antibiotic therapy (especially in the absence of meticulous débridement of material at the bone-cement interface).

Clinical Manifestations

Most patients present with a long indolent course characterized by progressively increasing joint pain and occasionally the formation of cutaneous draining sinuses but no fever, soft tissue swelling, or systemic toxicity. Others develop an acute, fulminant illness with high fever, intolerable joint pain, local swelling, and erythema. The frequencies of these presenting symptoms are listed in Table 4-4.[41] Staphylococcus aureus, beta-hemolytic streptococci, and aerobic gram-negative bacilli are capable of producing the acute, fulminant clinical picture, occasionally with septic shock. Staphylococcus epidermidis is consistently associated with the indolent form of infection. Wound hematomas, and ischemic wounds and tissues in diabetic and steroid-treated patients all enhance the ability of bacteria to multiply and promote an acute, fulminant process. Joint pain is the principal symptom of prosthetic joint infection irrespective of the mode of presentation and suggests either inflammation of periarticular tissue or loosening of the prosthesis due to slow erosion of bone at the bone-cement interface.

Diagnosis

The clinical manifestations of prosthetic joint infection reflect an underlying inflammatory process in the surrounding tissues but are not specific for infection. Painful prostheses accompanied by fever or purulent drainage from an overlying cutaneous sinus may be presumed to be infected, but in the vast majority of cases infection must be differentiated

Table 4-3. Bacteriology of Prosthetic Joint Infection

Pathogens	Frequency (%)
Staphylococci	53
Staphylococcus epidermidis	28
Staphylococcus aureus	25
Streptococci	20
Beta-hemolytic streptococci	12
viridans streptococci	8
Gram-negative aerobic bacilli	20
Anaerobes	7

Table 4-4. Presenting Symptoms of Prosthetic Joint Infection

Symptom	Frequency (%)
Joint pain	95
Fever	43
Periarticular swelling	38
Wound or cutaneous sinus drainage	32

from aseptic, mechanical problems (e.g., bland loosening, hemarthrosis, gout) which are more common causes of pain and inflammatory symptoms in these patients.

Radiographic evaluation can reveal wide or long lucencies at the bone-cement interface (Fig. 4-2).

X-ray abnormalities are found in 50 percent of septic prostheses and are generally related to the duration of infection, since it may require 3 to 6 months to manifest such changes. However, these radiologic findings are not specific for infection since they can be observed frequently with aseptic processes.

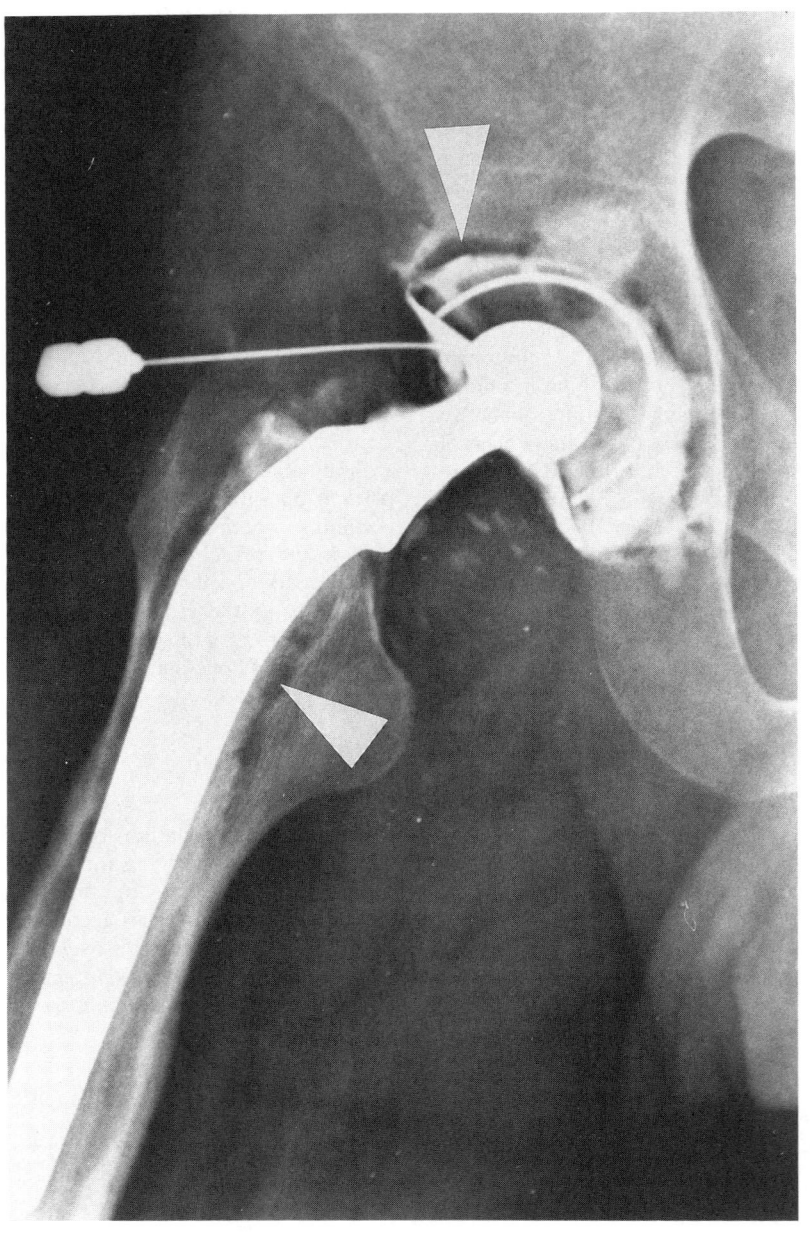

Figure 4-2. Infected total hip replacement prosthesis. Arrowheads indicate lucencies at the bone-cement interfaces of both the acetabular and femoral components. A needle has been inserted in the joint space using fluoroscopy in preparation for an aspiration.

Radioisotopic scans with technetium diphosphonate demonstrate increased uptake in areas of bone with enhanced blood supply or heightened metabolic activity. Increased technetium uptake is seen routinely around normal prostheses for 6 months after implantation. A positive scan after this interval is abnormal but is not specific for infection. Sequential technetium-gallium scanning and indium-labeled leukocyte scans are also nonspecific.[42,43] Therefore, a negative technetium or indium leukocyte scan can be considered strong evidence against the presence of infection, but they are not definitive in making the diagnosis.

To establish the diagnosis of joint replacement infection, the pathogen must be isolated by aspiration of joint fluid or by culture of tissue obtained at arthrotomy.[44] Analysis of joint fluid frequently reveals large numbers of neutrophils, high protein levels and low glucose concentrations, but these findings are neither prerequisites for making the diagnosis of sepsis nor specific for the entity in this setting. Histopathologic examination of periprosthetic tissue often reveals infiltration of neutrophils indicative of an acute inflammatory reaction, but this parameter is positive in only 55 percent of infected patients and also may not be sufficiently specific. Therefore, the sole observation that defines the presence of implant infection is isolation of the pathogen by arthrocentesis or surgical débridement (Table 4-5).

Arthrocentesis demonstrates the pathogen in 85 to 98 percent of cases.[44,45] Fluoroscopic guidance and arthrography are useful in documenting accurate needle insertion. When difficulty is encountered in obtaining intra-articular fluid, irrigation with normal saline (without antiseptic additives) can be employed to provide the necessary material for culture. If initial cultures reveal a relatively avirulent organism (Staphylococcus epidermidis, diphtheroids, Bacillus sp.), a second aspirate should be considered to reconfirm the bacteriologic diagnosis and to eliminate the possibility that the isolate is a "contaminant." Operative cultures are definitely diagnostic, therefore, the patient should not receive antimicrobial therapy for several weeks prior to the procedure. Multiple specimens of tissue and fluid should be retrieved for culture. In the uncommon situation when the clinical suggestion of sepsis is strong but the cultures are sterile, fastidious organisms (particularly anaerobes) should be suspected. In order to design effective and the least toxic antimicrobial therapy, the patient's infecting strain of bacteria must be available for in vitro evaluation, which is described later in the chapter.

Treatment

Meticulously complete surgical débridement and efficacious antimicrobial therapy are essential for successful treatment of a total joint arthroplasty infection. Surgical drainage alone (with retention of the prosthesis) followed by nonstandardized antibiotic therapy has been unsuccessful.[46] Two different approaches to more effective treatment have evolved, both of which require total removal of all foreign materials (metallic prosthesis and cement).

The most successful protocol incorporates standardized antimicrobial therapy with a two-stage surgical procedure. Removal of the prosthesis and cement is followed by a 6-week course of intravenous, bactericidal antibiotics designed on the basis of quantitative in vitro sensitivity studies (minimum bactericidal concentrations) performed with the particular pathogen isolated from the patient. Adequate antimicrobial therapy is defined as a serum bactericidal titer of at least 1:8 in postpeak blood samples (drawn 1, 1.5, 2, or 3 hours after infusion of antibiotics given every 4, 6, 8, or 12 hours, respectively). A new prosthesis is implanted at the conclusion of the 6-week antibiotic regimen. With this protocol a 90 percent success rate has been achieved for hip prostheses and a 97 percent success rate for knee prostheses.[47-49] Employing a similar two-stage, removal-reimplantation approach with a 4-week (average, unstandardized) antibiotic course, a 93 percent success rate has been obtained for total hip arthroplasties, if reimplantation is delayed for 1 year.[50]

An alternative method of treating total joint sepsis involves complete prosthesis and cement extraction with immediate reimplantation of a new prosthesis

Table 4-5. Examinations to Establish the Diagnosis of Prosthetic Joint Infection

Examination	Sensitivity(%)*
Arthrocentesis fluid Gram stain	32
Frozen section histopathology (leukocytic infiltrate in nonosseous periprosthetic tissue)	55
Arthrocentesis fluid culture	85-98
Operative culture (osseous and nonosseous periprosthetic tissue)	100

*Frequency of positivity in subsequently proven infection.

in a one-stage procedure (exchange operation). Systemic antibiotic therapy is not used in this approach; instead methylmethacrylate cement impregnated with an antibiotic (usually gentamicin or tobramycin) is employed during reimplantation. The antimicrobial agent diffuses from the hardened cement producing variable but high initial release and protracted low levels of antibiotic into surrounding tissues at the bone-cement interface.[51] This technique is effective in 70 to 80 percent of cases.[52,53] It has been suggested that this mode of therapy should be used only for infections with relatively avirulent organisms (e.g., Staphylococcus epidermidis), since high failure rates are experienced when Staphylococcus aureus or gram-negative bacilli are the pathogens.[54] Future therapeutic protocols will likely include the specific, standardized, 6-week antibiotic regimen and two-stage prosthesis removal-reimplantation surgery with the incorporation of antibiotic-loaded cement during arthroplasty reinsertion. In those clinical situations in which adequate antimicrobial potency cannot be achieved, arthrodesis or resection arthroplasty is recommended rather than attempting prosthesis reimplantation. However, with the further development of antibiotic-impregnated cements, even these difficult patients may be candidates for another total joint arthroplasty.

Suppressive Antibiotic Therapy

Occasionally, surgical extraction of an infected joint prosthesis is contraindicated due to medical conditions, surgical problems, or patient refusal. Since it is likely that the pathogen will persist at the undébrided bone-cement interface despite a high-dose, finite course of systemic antimicrobial therapy, lifelong oral antibiotic treatment can be considered to suppress the infection and retain the usefulness of the total joint replacement. Suppressive therapy is an option for selected cases when all of the following criteria are met: (1) prosthesis removal is not possible, (2) the pathogen is relatively avirulent, (3) the pathogen is exquisitely sensitive to an orally absorbed antibiotic, (4) the patient can tolerate an appropriate oral antibiotic, and (5) the prosthesis is not loose. Successful retention of the functioning joint replacement has been seen in 63 percent of patients in this unusual setting.[55] This suppressive approach is not without risk. Serial x-ray films are needed over the course of therapy to monitor for progressive bone resorption at the bone-cement interface, which could reduce the success of any future revision surgery. Despite continual antibiotic treatment, the localized septic process could spread into adjacent tissue compartments or become a systemic infection. Moreover, the patient would be exposed to the potential side effects of chronic antibiotic administration.

Prevention of Joint Prosthesis Infection

In view of the catastrophic effects of prosthetic arthroplasty infection, prevention of these septic processes is of prime importance. In anticipation of elective total joint implantation, the patient should be evaluated for the presence of pyogenic dentogingival pathology, obstructive uropathy, and dermatologic conditions that might predispose to infection and bacteremia. Consideration should be given to reducing the risks represented by these factors before insertion of the prosthesis. Perioperative antibiotic prophylaxis has been shown to effectively decrease wound infection rates in total joint replacement.[56] Cefazolin, oxacillin, or vancomycin are commonly administered as antistaphylococcal agents immediately preoperatively and for 1 to 2 days thereafter. Filtered laminar air flow systems in the operating room further reduce infection rates, especially when whole-body, exhaust-ventilated suits are worn by all members of the surgical team.[57,58]

Early recognition and prompt treatment of infection in any location is critical to decrease the risk of seeding the joint implant hematogenously. Circumstances likely to cause bacteremia should be avoided. The use of prophylactic antibiotics in anticipation of bacteremic events (e.g., dental surgery, cystoscopy, colonoscopic biopsy, and surgical procedures on infected or contaminated tissues) has been suggested on the same empiric basis as endocarditis prophylaxis is recommended.[37,59-61] This approach to prevention is controversial at the present time and no data are available to determine the adequacy or cost-effectiveness of such measures. Clinical decisions regarding prophylactic antibiotics for expectant bacteremias in patients with indwelling prosthetic joints should be made on an individual basis.

References

1. Goldenberg, DL, and Cohen, AS: Acute infectious arthritis. Am J Med 60:369, 1976.
2. Ward, JR, and Atcheson, SG: Infectious arthritis. Med Clin North Am 61:313, 1977.
3. Gifford, DB et al: Septic arthritis due to Pseudomonas in heroin addicts. J Bone Joint Surg (Am) 57:631, 1975.

4. Hyer, FH, and Gottlieb, NL: Rheumatic disorders associated with viral infection. Semin Arthritis Rheum 8:17, 1979.
5. Wallace, R, and Cohen, AS: Tuberculous arthritis. Am J Med 61:277, 1976.
6. Goldenberg, DL, and Cohen, AS: Arthritis due to tuberculous and fungal microorganisms. Clin Rheum Dis 4:211, 1978.
7. Holmes, KK, Counts, GW, and Beaty, HN: Disseminated gonococcal infection. Ann Intern Med 74:979, 1971.
8. Krauss, DS et al: Hemophilus influenzae septic arthritis. Arthritis Rheum 17:267, 1974.
9. Bjorkengren, A, Resnick, D, and Sartoris, DJ: Radiographic changes in pyogenic arthritis. IM 7:119, 1986.
10. Cooper, C, and Cawley, MID: Bacterial arthritis in an English health district: A 10 year review. Ann Rheum Dis 45:458, 1986.
11. Fink, CW, and Nelson, JD. Septic arthritis and osteomyelitis in children. Clin Rheum Dis 12:423, 1986.
12. Kelly, PJ, Martin, WJ, and Coventry, MB: Bacterial arthritis in the adult. J Bone Joint Surg (Am) 52:1595, 1970.
13. Argen, RJ, Wilson, CH Jr, and Wood, P: Suppurative arthritis. Arch Intern Med 117:661, 1966.
14. Goldenberg, DL et al: Acute arthritis caused by gram-negative bacilli: A clinical characterization. Medicine (Baltimore) 53:197, 1974.
15. Nelson, JD: Antibiotic concentrations in septic joint effusions. N Engl J Med 284:349, 1971.
16. Parker, RH, and Schmid, R: Antibacterial activity of synovial fluid during therapy of septic arthritis. Arthritis Rheum 14:96, 1971.
17. Chow, A, Hecht, R, and Winters, R: Gentamicin and carbenicillin penetration into the septic joint. N Engl J Med 285:178, 1971.
18. Mahowald, ML: Animal models of infectious arthritis. Clin Rheum Dis 12:403, 1986.
19. Broy, SB, Stulberg, SD, and Schmid, FR: The role of arthroscopy in the diagnosis and management of the septic joint. Clin Rheum Dis 12:489, 1986.
20. Goldenberg, DL, Reed, JI: Bacterial arthritis. N Engl J Med 312:764, 1985.
21. Ho, G Jr, and Su, EY: Therapy of septic arthritis. JAMA 247:797, 1982.
22. Piesman, J et al: Duration of tick attachment and Borrelia burgdorferi transmission. J Clin Microbiol 25:557, 1987.
23. Steere, AC: Lyme disease. N Engl J Med 321:586, 1989.
24. Berger, BW: Dermatologic manifestations of Lyme disease. Rev Infect Dis 11 (Suppl 6):S1475, 1989.
25. Reik, L et al: Neurologic abnormalities of Lyme disease. Medicine (Baltimore) 58:281, 1979.
26. Pachner, AR, and Steere, AC: The triad of neurologic manifestations of Lyme disease: Meningitis, cranial neuritis and radiculoneuritis. Neurology 35:47, 1985.
27. Steere, AC et al: Lyme carditis: Cardiac abnormalities of Lyme disease. Ann Intern Med 93:8, 1980.
28. Steere, AC, Schoen, RT, and Taylor, E: The clinical evolution of Lyme arthritis. Ann Intern Med 107:725, 1987.
29. Ackerman, R et al: Chronic neurologic manifestations of erythema migrans borreliosis. Ann NY Acad Sci 539:16, 1988.
30. Logigian, EL, Kaplan, RF, and Steere, AC: Chronic neurologic manifestations of Lyme disease. N Engl J Med 323:1438, 1990.
31. Asbrink, E, and Hovmark, A: Early and late cutaneous manifestations of Ixodes-borne borreliosis. Ann NY Acad Sci 539:4, 1988.
32. Berardi, VP, Weeks, KE, and Steere, AC: Serodiagnosis of early Lyme disease: Analysis of IgM and IgG antibody responses by using an antibody-capture enzyme immunoassay. J Infect Dis 158:754, 1988.
33. Schwartz, BS et al: Antibody testing in Lyme disease. JAMA 262:3431, 1989.
34. Duffy, J et al: Diagnosing Lyme disease: The contribution of serologic testing. Mayo Clin Proc 63:1116, 1988.
35. Treatment of Lyme disease. Med Lett 31:57, 1989.
36. Gristina, AG, and Kolkin, J: Total joint replacement and sepsis. J Bone Joint Surg (Am) 65:128, 1983.
37. Brause, BD: Infections associated with prosthetic joints. Clin Rheum Dis 12:523, 1986.
38. Brause, BD: Infected orthopedic prostheses. In: Bisno, AL, and Waldvogel, FA (eds): Infections Associated with Indwelling Medical Devices. Washington, DC, American Society for Microbiology, 1989, p 111.
39. Petty, W: The effect of methylmethacrylate on bacterial phagocytosis and killing by human polymorphonuclear leukocytes. J Bone Joint Surg (Am) 60:752, 1978.
40. Costerton, JW, Irvin, RT, and Cheng, K-J: The bacterial glycocalyx in nature and disease. Ann Rev Microbiol 35:299, 1981.
41. Inman, JN et al: Clinical and microbial features of prosthetic joint infection. Am J Med 77:47, 1984.
42. Merkel, KD, Brown, MK, and Fitzgerald, RH: Sequential technetium-99m HMDP-gallium-67 citrate imaging for the evaluation of infection in the painful prosthesis. J Nucl Med 27:1413, 1986.
43. Pring, DJ et al: Autologous granulocyte scanning of painful prosthetic joints. J Bone Joint Surg (Br) 68:647, 1986.
44. O'Neill, DA, and Harris, WH: Failed total hip replacement: Assessment by plain radiographs, arthrograms and aspiration of the hip joint. J Bone Joint Surg (Am) 66:540, 1984.
45. Eftehar, NS: Wound infection complicating total hip joint arthroplasty. Orthop Rev 8:49, 1979.
46. Fitzgerald, RH et al: Deep wound sepsis following total hip arthroplasty. J Bone Joint Surg (Am) 59:847, 1977.
47. Callaghan, JJ et al: Reimplantation for salvage of the infected hip. In: Fitzgerald, RH (ed): The Hip, Proceedings of the 14th Open Scientific Meeting of the Hip Society. St. Louis, CV Mosby, 1986, p 65.

48. Windsor, RE et al: Two-stage reimplantation for the salvage of total knee arthroplasty complicated by infection. J Bone Joint Surg (Am) 72:272, 1990.
49. Salvati, EA et al: Reimplantation in infection. Clin Orthop 170:62, 1982.
50. McDonald, DJ, Fitzgerald, RH, and Ilstrup, DM: Two-stage reconstruction of a total hip arthroplasty because of infection. J Bone Joint Surg (Am) 71:828, 1989.
51. Trippel, SB: Antibiotic-impregnated cement in total joint arthroplasty. J Bone Joint Surg (Am) 68:1297, 1986.
52. Buchholz, HW et al: Management of deep infection of total hip replacement. J Bone Joint Surg (Br) 63:342, 1981.
53. Carlsson, AS, Josefsson, G, and Lindberg, L: Revision with gentamicin-impregnated cement for deep infection in total hip arthroplasties. J Bone Joint Surg (Am) 60:1059, 1978.
54. Fitzgerald, RH, and Jones, DR: Hip implant infection. Am J Med 78 (Suppl 6B):225, 1986.
55. Goulet, JA et al: Prolonged suppression of infection in total hip arthroplasty. J Arthroplasty 3:109, 1988.
56. Norden, C: A critical review of antibiotic proplylaxis in orthopedic surgery. Rev Infect Dis 5:928, 1983.
57. Lidwell, O, Lowbury, E, and Whyte, E: Effect of ultraclean air in operating rooms on deep sepsis in the joint after total hip or total knee replacement. Br Med J 285:10, 1982.
58. Salvati, EA et al: Infection rates after 3175 total hip and total knee replacements performed with and without a horizontal unidirectional filtered air-flow system. J Bone Joint Surg (Am) 64:525, 1982.
59. Cioffi, GA, Terezhalmy, GT, and Taybos, GM: Total joint replacement: A consideration for antimicrobial prophylaxis. Oral Surg Oral Med Oral Pathol 66:124, 1988.
60. Maderazo, EG, Judson, S, and Pasternak, H: Late infections of total joint prostheses: A review and recommendations for prevention. Clin Orthop 229:131, 1988.
61. Nelson, JP et al: Prophylactic antimicrobial coverage in arthroplasty patients. J Bone Joint Surg (Am) 72:1, 1990.

Chapter 5
Osteoarthritis

LEE D. KAUFMAN, M.D., F.A.C.P.
LEON SOKOLOFF, M.D.

Introduction

Osteoarthritis (OA) is not a single disease but a heterogeneous group of mechanically determined disorders of joints that have in common remodeling of articular cartilage, subchondral bone, and capsular structures. The underlying pathologic events are both productive and degenerative. Secondary inflammatory processes contribute to disease progression both by their destructive mechanisms and also by creating new intra-articular forces.[1] Osteoarthritis is generally progressive, although its clinical course is variable and unpredictable. The appendicular as well as the axial skeleton is involved.

A clear distinction must be made between radiographic and clinical findings because they often are discordant. Clinically the disease is characterized by pain, deformity, and limitation of motion[2]; radiographically, by joint space narrowing, subchondral sclerosis, and osteophyte formation. By both measures OA occurs with great frequency throughout the world. Radiographic surveys have demonstrated a prevalence of between 40 and 60 percent for the population over age 35.[3,4] In peripheral joints the figures range from 4 percent in those below age 24 to as high as 85 percent in persons more than age 75. Women predominate over men.[4-6] Ninety percent of persons by age 50 manifest lumbosacral spinal changes by autopsy or radiographic criteria, but only 20 percent have clinical complaints.[7] The large disparity between the radiographic findings and clinical manifestations of lumbar disease applies to the apophyseal as well as the intervertebral disk lesions.[4]

Current Concepts of Pathogenesis

Multiple biochemical and biomechanical factors act in concert to effect the tissue changes seen in OA. Degradation of cartilage and hypertrophic remodeling represent the characteristic lesion. Although the precise mechanism by which these alterations develop is uncertain, there are three principal theories[1,8,9]: (1) abnormal mechanical forces induce failure and loss of cartilage; (2) increased bone stiffness precedes and causes the cartilage damage; and (3) chondrocyte dysfunction represents the primary process. These mechanisms may be modulated by age, sex hormones, diet, obesity, physical activity, heredity, and metabolic aberrations to produce a variety of clinical subsets (Table 5-1). These interrelationships and the inflammatory mediators of cartilage degradation are shown schematically in Figure 5-1.

Local Metabolic and Environmental Factors

Mechanical Force

In 1892 Wolff postulated that the form of the skeleton is influenced by functional stresses in bone.[10] These physical stimuli lead to adaptive bone formation and resorption that minimizes the strain (remodeling). Changes in the alignment, stability, or neural control of a given articulation can induce remodeling. Hence, preexisting acetabular dysplasia or internal derangement, for example, severing a cruciate ligament or medial meniscectomy, lead to premature OA of the hip or knee, respectively.[9]

Table 5-1. Classification of Osteoarthritis (OA)

I. Primary (Idiopathic) OA
   1. Localized OA
   2. Generalized OA
   3. Diffuse Idiopathic Skeletal Hyperostosis
   4. Erosive Inflammatory OA

II. Secondary OA
   1. Mechanical aberrations
      a. Meniscectomy
      b. Anterior cruciate ligament transection
      c. Previous fracture
      d. Hip dysplasia
      e. Slipped femoral epiphysis
      f. Following avascular necrosis

   2. Pre-existing inflammatory arthritis
      a. Crystal-induced arthritis
      b. Septic arthritis
      c. Rheumatoid Arthritis

   3. Occupation-related

   4. Metabolic Disease
      a. Hemochromatosis
      b. Acromegaly
      c. Ochronosis
      d. Wilson's Disease
      e. Hemophilia
      f. Tophaceous gout

   5. Neuropathic arthropathy

III. Endemic OA
   1. Kashin-Beck Disease
   2. Mseleni Disease

Similarly, peripheral neuropathies of several types predispose to the articular disruption seen in a Charcot joint.[9]

Mechanical stress has often been invoked to explain occupation-related OA. Osteoarthritis of the hip, knee, and shoulder has been found to be more prevalent in miners than porters.[2] In foundry workers using long tongs to lift hot metal, increased leverage produced severe OA of the elbow.[11] Analogous mechanisms of overuse are associated with OA in the fingers, elbows and knees of dock workers,[12] the distal interphalangeal joints of cotton workers,[13] and the hands of women weavers after many years of repetitive motion.[14] Data on this theme have not been concordant. Although heavier hand use is associated with greater radiographically documented OA, a recent study found no increase in the prevalence of OA in dominant hand use among persons in occupations involving light labor.[15] Pneumatic drill operators were reported to have excessive OA of the elbow in some studies[16] but not in others.[17] Enthesopathic lesions have also been described in excessively used joints,[18] and increased numbers of osteophytes and bony sclerosis have been noted in radiographs in the absence of significant functional impairment.[19] The knee bending demanded by certain occupations (carpentry, farming, etc.) has been implicated in OA of this joint.[20]

Views about prolonged or vigorous sport and exercise causing OA have also been controversial. Difficulties in clarifying this point arise from selection bias. Several retrospective investigations have demonstrated no increase in OA among long distance runners.[19,21] By contrast, another study revealed radiographically more advanced hip OA among elite long distance runners compared with bobsled riders or healthy, untrained men.[22] In fulfillment of Wolff's law, bone density was greater in marathon runners.[19] Although it has been accepted for many years that OA and osteoporosis do not coexist, one recent study challenges this view.[23]

Age, Sex, Race, and Heredity

Radiographic and clinical evidence of OA increases after age 45 in many populations.[3,4,24] By the ages of 55 to 64, 85 percent of patients have radiographic changes in one or more joints.[25] It is seen in the first metatarsophalangeal joint after age 25; between ages 35 and 45 in the first carpometacarpal joint and spine; after age 45, distal interphalangeal joint disease appears. Osteoarthritis of the knee and hip follow, generally after age 50.[3] The radiographic findings are in apparent contrast to those of the autopsy. Autopsy findings indicate that degenerative changes in the knee and hip antedate those in the first metatarsophalangeal joint.[26]

Several age-related changes in articular cartilage have been reported, including decreased water content, decreased chondroitin sulfate chain length, fragmentation of link protein, and normal protease activity.[27] These changes differ from those of OA. In practice it is difficult to separate the two phenomena sharply. Whether the development of OA with advancing years is related to the aging of cartilage or to age-related changes in biomechanics, or both, is not clear at this time.

Racial and ethnic differences in OA have also been noted. Racial differences may be attributed to occupation, lifestyle, or genetic factors.[25] Southern Chinese, South African blacks, and East Indians have a lower frequency of hip OA than white Americans or Europeans. Histocompatibility antigen predilections have been described for nodal OA:

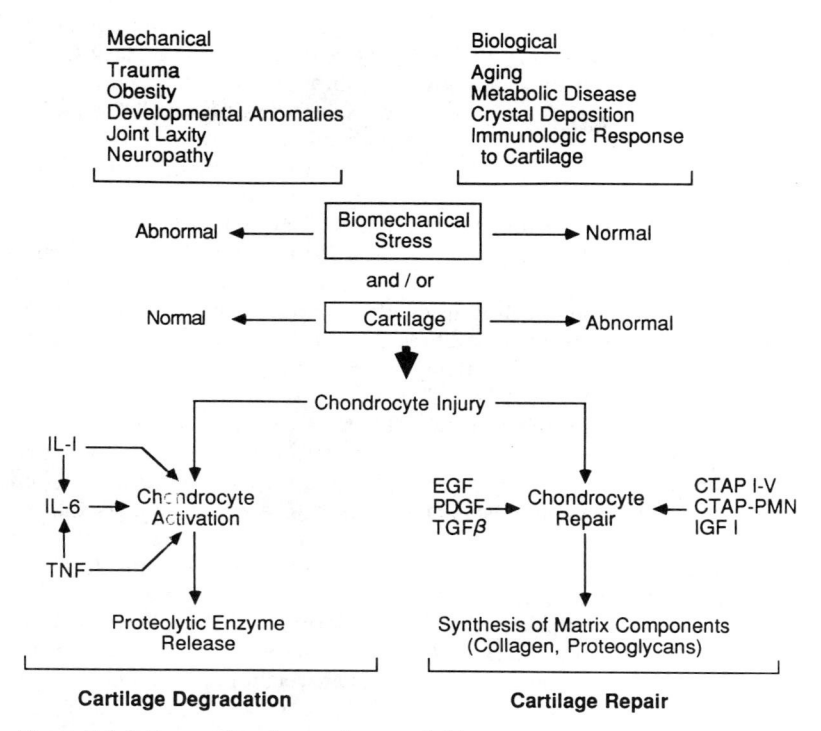

Figure 5-1. Pathogenetic schema of osteoarthritis.

HLA-DR2 with Heberden's nodes[28]; and HLA-AIB8 and the MZ alpha$_1$-antitrypsin phenotype for generalized nodal OA.[29] Recent studies have identified a single base mutation in the type II procollagen gene in a family of patients with primary OA.[30]

After age 55, OA is more common in women than in men.[25] Polyarticular involvement (four or more joints) was seen in 47 percent of women ages 55 to 64 and in 29 percent of men in this age range.[4,25] The distribution of joint involvement also differs with sex. Interphalangeal, first carpometacarpal, and knee joints are affected more often in women, whereas hip and axial involvement predominate in men.[3,24]

The influence of sex hormones is controversial. The therapeutic efficacy of hormonal manipulation has not been demonstrated in humans, although there is some experimental support for the idea. In one strain of mouse that spontaneously develops OA, orchiectomy or administration of estrogen lessens the severity of lesions[31]; this did not hold true in another strain.[32] Estrogens increased OA severity in an experimental model of OA in rabbits, whereas the estrogen antagonist tamoxifen lessened it.[33]

Obesity

The intuition that obesity is a factor in the development of OA is supported primarily by epidemiologic evidence. The link between the two phenomena in population studies is based only on radiographic examination.[4,20,34–38] The relationship to symptoms is less clear. The information is most extensive in knee OA. Obesity and knee OA coexist in 10 to 20 percent of persons ages 65 to 80, and produce significant disability.[38] Current data favor obesity as the factor causing the OA rather than being the consequence of inactivity.[37] Knee pain is associated with advanced OA seen radiographically.[35,36]

There is evidence for obesity increasing OA of non-weight-bearing joints too, for example, the distal interphalangeal joints.[39] Obesity as an individual variable was associated with hand pain in one study.[36] Interpretation of these data is made more difficult because socioeconomic factors (specifically lower education and income levels) were significant covariables related to hand pain. These observations point out the difficulty of ascribing the effect of obesity simply to mechanical overloading. Associated metabolic derangements might theoretically be at fault. In humans, OA has not been associated with such metabolic aberration as hyperuricemia,[34] diabetes,[20] hyperlipidemia,[40] or with hypertension.[35]

Role of the Chondrocyte, Inflammation, and Immunologic and Biochemical Factors

Multiple factors play a role in the chondrocyte injury seen in OA (Figure 5-1). Matrix breakdown results from release of chondrocytic enzymes. Proliferation of chondrocytes follows along with remodeling of bone. In certain forms of secondary OA the degradative events are initiated by products of metabolism, for example, homogentisic acid in ochronosis, monosodium urate in gout, and possibly degraded hemoglobin in hemophilia.

Cartilage consists of water (approximately 70 percent), chondrocytes (5 percent), and matrix molecules (25 percent). The dry substance, in turn, is made up of proteoglycan (35 percent), collagen (60 percent), and noncollagenous-nonproteoglycan proteins (5 percent). Proteoglycans are enormous, complex molecules composed of proteoglycan subunits, hyaluronic acid, and link proteins. The subunits (Figure 5-2) are arrayed noncovalently along a hyaluronic acid backbone. The attachment is stabilized by link glycoproteins. Linear chains of glycosaminoglycans (predominantly chondroitin-6-sulfate and keratan sulfate and, to a lesser extent, chondroitin-4-sulfate[27] are bound covalently to a core protein to comprise the subunits. The entire aggregate with its water content are constrained by the collagen framework. This composite nature confers viscoelasticity and compressive strength on the cartilage. The collagen is the source of the tensile strength. It is primarily (90 percent) of type II species. There also is some type IX collagen, a variety that also contains a glycosaminoglycan domain. Type IX collagen may stabilize the type II meshwork.[27,41] A chondrocyte membrane receptor for type II collagen, anchorin C-II, and another glycoprotein, chondronectin, also contribute to the cellular-matrix interactions of articular cartilage.[41] The type II collagen has a nearly unmeasurably long half-life.[27] Proteoglycans, however, have a turnover time of 200 to 800 days in human articular cartilage.[42] The tissue can, therefore, reconstitute proteoglycan more readily than it can collagen destroyed in an inflammatory process. Splitting of proteoglycans by chondrocytic enzymes (metalloproteases and cathepsins) occurs predominantly at the hyaluronic acid-binding region of core protein. The matrix also contains tissue inhibitors of metalloproteases and serine proteases that participate in regulating the degradation and replenishment of its components.

Biochemical changes in articular cartilage vary with the duration and degree of pathologic alteration in OA. They include (1) an increase in water content; (2) a reduction in the width of the collagen fibrils; and (3) a decrease in the total proteoglycan content. Proteoglycan aggregates are smaller, glycosaminoglycan chain lengths shorter, and the ratio of keratan sulfate and chondroitin-6-sulfate to chondroitin-4-sulfate reduced.[9,35] These changes are in contrast to those of aging (Table 5-2). The early morphologic lesion is metabolically active. Thus proteoglycan and DNA synthesis by chondrocytes is increased in affected foci. As the process advances chondrocyte failure ensues and metabolic activity decreases.[2,27] The end result is an overall decrease in proteoglycan content.

Matrix metabolism is affected by various growth factors and cytokines. These are generally low molecular weight proteins produced by other cell populations. Table 5-3 lists the presently recognized molecules of this kind, as well as hormones and vitamins that also influence connective tissue metabolism.[43]

The connective tissue-activating peptides (CTAP) I, III, IV, and V augment proteoglycan and glycosaminoglycan synthesis by synovial fibroblasts in culture. Prostaglandin E_2 (PGE_2) and collagenase, produced by interleukin-1 (IL-1)-stimulated chondrocytes in vitro, promote bone resorption. Prostaglandin E_2 also potentiates CTAP I and III. It thus has the potential to mediate both degradation and production of matrix. Interleukin-1 also increases types I and III collagen synthesis by cultured chondrocytes, at the expense

Table 5-2. Contrasting Features of Cartilage in Osteoarthritis and Aging*

	OA	Aging
Water content	Increased	Decreased
Proteoglycan aggregates	Decreased	Normal
Chondroitin sulfate	Increased C4S:C6S	Normal
Link protein	Normal	Fragmented
Protease activity	Increased	Normal

C6S = Chondroitin-6-sulfate.
C4S = Chondroitin-4-sulfate.
*Data compiled from references 9 and 27.

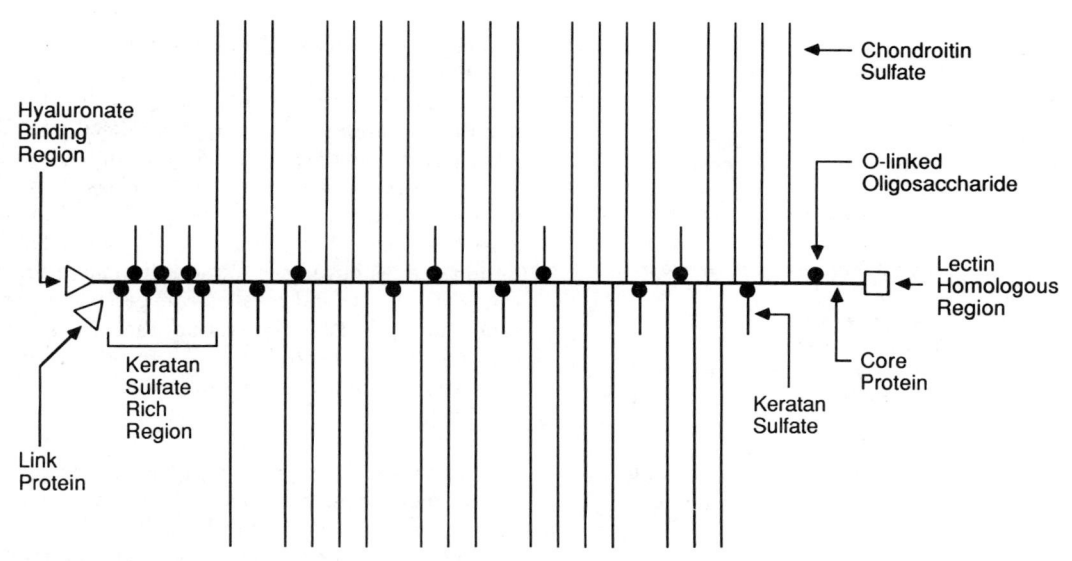

Figure 5-2. Structure of a proteoglycan monomer.

of type II collagen.[44] Osteoarthritic synovial fluid contains levels of neutral-active and lysosomal enzymes[2,9] that may effect tissue breakdown during inflammatory episodes (Figure 5-1).

Physical factors also are important. Temperature elevation augments collagenase activity.[45] It also increases synovial cell responsiveness to CTAP I.[43] Chondrocytes modulate proteoglycan synthesis in response to compressive loading.[27] These effects of heat and pressure may have implications for the modalities of physical therapy.

There is some interest in a possible role for a crystal-associated inflammatory component in OA. From 40 to 60 percent of knee synovial fluids in OA contain calcium pyrophosphate dihydrate (CPPD) or basic calcium phosphate (apatite) crystals.[46] Deposition of CPPD is found six times as often in knees subjected to total arthroplasty as in age- and sex-matched controls.[47] At times these crystals clearly cause acute inflammatory episodes and a case can be made for their potentiating the development of OA. They stimulate IL-1 production in vitro, and this cytokine is present in OA synovial fluid.[48] Levels of collagenase, IL-1 driven, correlate with the severity of the inflammatory reaction.[49] Bone resorption is also modulated in a differential manner by inflammatory mediators. Hydroxyapatite crystal effects are mediated by PGE_2, while those of monosodium urate are mediated by PGE_2 and IL-1.[50] Against the hypothesis that crystals are the important factor in the synovitis of OA is the empirical observation that CPPD deposition occurs only infrequently in OA of the hip joint.

Immunoreactants have been identified in the cartilage of some OA subsets.[51] IgG, IgM, and C3 deposits were present on the surface of cartilage in 40 percent of inflammatory OA patients and 16 percent of patients whose OA is caused by structural joint abnormalities. Immune events associated with this deposition may augment the inflammatory changes.

Clinical Manifestations

Osteoarthritis is classified clinically into primary and secondary forms. These refer respectively to idiopathic disease and disease that occurs in the setting of structural, inflammatory, or metabolic abnormalities (see Table 5-1).[52] Radiographic changes and clinical manifestations generally parallel each other in primary OA of the knee,[36] but the two are often discordant in the spine, hands, and feet.[7]

The principal clinical complaint is pain. It usually follows activity and is relieved by rest. Sometimes, however, it leads to an abnormal sleep pattern as well.[53] Morning stiffness occurs frequently but is usually of short duration (less than 30 minutes), unlike that seen in rheumatoid arthritis. Cartilage is devoid of a nerve supply and the sources of pain are in periarticular and capsular tissues and subchondral bone.[54] Multiple mechanisms are involved.

Pain Mechanisms. The joint capsule contains stretch and pain receptors. Pain increases linearly with intra-articular[55] and intraosseous[56] pressure.

Table 5-3. Factors Influencing Cartilage Matrix Formation and Breakdown in Vitro

Factors Upregulating Proteoglycan and Glycosaminoglycan Synthesis
1. Epidermal growth factor—platelet derived*
2. Platelet-derived growth factor—platelet derived*
3. Connective tissue activating peptides (CTAP)
    CTAP I—Lymphocyte derived
    CTAP II—Derived from laryngeal carcinoma cell line
    CTAP III—Platelet derived
    CTAP IV—Platelet derived
    CTAP V—Isolated from urine of normal persons
    CTAP-PMN—Derived from polymorphonuclear leukocytes (PMNs)
4. Insulin-like growth factor-1 (IGF-1) or somatomedin-C
5. Transforming growth factor-1 (TGF-beta-1)—derived from platelets, kidney, placenta, tumor cells
6. Insulin
7. Ascorbic acid

Factors Downregulating Proteoglycan and Glycosaminoglycan Synthesis
1. Interleukin-1 (IL-1)—produced by monocytes/macrophages and chondrocytes
2. Tumor necrosis factor-alpha (TNF-alpha)—derived from monocytes/macrophages and chondrocytes
3. PGE$_2$*
4. Glucocorticoids*
5. Thyroid hormone*
6. Retinoic acid—vitamin A metabolite

*The effects reported for these growth factors are not always concordant, may be dose-dependent, and may vary with experimental design. Their clinical relevance remains to be established.

Stretch receptors are the source of muscle spasm. Atrophy of adjacent muscle in advanced disease is a component of the stiffness observed.

Mild to moderate synovitis is found in more than half of hip specimens resected for OA.[57] The inflammatory infiltrate, predominantly mononuclear, resembles that of low-grade rheumatoid arthritis, but represents a secondary phenomenon. It, nevertheless, shares with other inflammatory arthropathies a variety of mediators of pain: neuropeptides, cytokines, prostaglandins, and vasoactive substances. The principal pain afferents are the thin myelinated (A delta) and nonmyelinated (C) fibers. These can be activated by prostaglandin E$_2$, bradykinin, histamine, and serotonin. Bradykinin also stimulates production of PGE$_2$ and potentiates the contribution to pain of PGE$_2$ and serotonin.[58]

Type C fibers also have a secretory function. These afferent neurons produce a peptide, substance P, which is transported antidromically to articular tissues, among others. When these sensory neurons are stimulated, substance P and other nerve products, such as vasoactive intestinal polypeptide, somatostatin, and the calcitonin gene-related peptide, are released from the peripheral nerve endings. Substance P degranulates mast cells, releasing histamine, and also stimulates synovial cells and monocytes to secrete other proinflammatory mediators.[59] Neuropeptides have been found in human arthritic synovial fluids[58] and localized in periosteum and synovium.[60,61] The observation that Heberden's nodes develop only on the unaffected side following a stroke may conceivably be related to an action of neuropeptides.

Joints Involved. Low-grade degenerative changes occur in many joints and increase linearly with age. They are more marked in the knee than in the hip joint. For the most part, the alterations are far milder than those seen in surgically removed, presumably more symptomatic, lesions. Furthermore, the brunt of the changes in the latter is borne by different parts of the joints, for example, the femorotibial rather than the patellofemoral compartments of the knee; and the superolateral rather than the perifoveal portions of the femoral head. These features underlie the concept of nonprogressive vs. progressive forms of degenerative joint disease, that is, asymptomatic aging changes vs. osteoarthritis.

Primary OA can be divided into different clinical subsets based on the distribution and extent of articular involvement: (1) localized OA; (2) generalized OA—that in which three or more regional areas as defined by Kellgren and Moore[63] are affected; (3) diffuse idiopathic skeletal hyperostosis (DISH); and (4) erosive, inflammatory OA. Endemic forms of OA and the metabolic secondary forms of OA are quite different from the preceding (see Table 5-1). They suggest clues to the pathogenesis of OA and its heterogeneity. Osteoarthritis secondary to metabolic derangement must be considered particularly in persons with premature OA, associated chondrocalcinosis, or atypical locations, for example, metacarpophalangeal, wrist, elbow, or shoulder joints.

Types of Osteoarthritis

Localized or Generalized Osteoarthritis

The joints most frequently involved in primary OA are the distal interphalangeal (DIP), proximal interphalangeal (PIP), first carpometacarpal (CMC), trapezioscaphoid, first metatarsophalangeal (MTP), knee, hip, and the spine. Heberden's and Bouchard's nodes represent the dorsal osteophytic components of DIP and PIP joint OA respectively.[25] Heberden's nodes are usually multiple, but they sometimes affect only a single joint. They are most prominent after age 45[3,24] and affect women more than men.[24,25] In women, there is a familial distribution. These nodes usually cause no pain. At times they become painful in association with the development of a gelatinous, subcutaneous cyst or an inflammatory process. The inflammation in some instances is a consequence of gouty or other crystal depositions.[46,64] Heberden's nodes may be part of generalized OA. In this setting, the pattern of hip involvement differs from that of secondary OA: it has a concentric migration pattern in x-ray films rather than the usual eccentric lateral or medial form.[65]

Wrist involvement is usually restricted to the first CMC joint. This former is characterized by a sudden dropoff or "shelf" at the base of the thumb.[25] It commonly is associated with OA of the DIP and PIP joints of other fingers. Typical radiographic features are shown in Figure 5-3. Isolated MCP or trapezioscaphoid joint disease should arouse suspicion of chondrocalcinosis, even in the absence of radiographic evidence of the latter.[66]

Osteoarthritis of the knee is the most common cause of disability in the elderly. Radiographic and clinical findings generally parallel each other[35,38]; both increase with age.[24,35,38] Obesity is a risk factor.[34,37,39] Women are more often affected than men.[24,38] Criteria for the diagnosis, recently established by the American College of Rheumatology (previously known as the American Rheumatism Association), include knee pain in a person over age 50; morning stiffness for less than 30 minutes; crepitus; and radiographic evidence of osteophytes.[52] The sensitivity of these criteria is 91 percent; the specificity, 86 percent. Serum rheumatoid factor levels are low (less than 1:40), erythrocyte sedimentation rate less than 40 mm per hour, and synovial fluid white blood cell count less than or equal to 2000 per mm^3.

The portion of the knee most affected is the medial femorotibial compartment (Figure 5-4); hence, the common finding of a varus deformity. The other compartments are involved less frequently. When

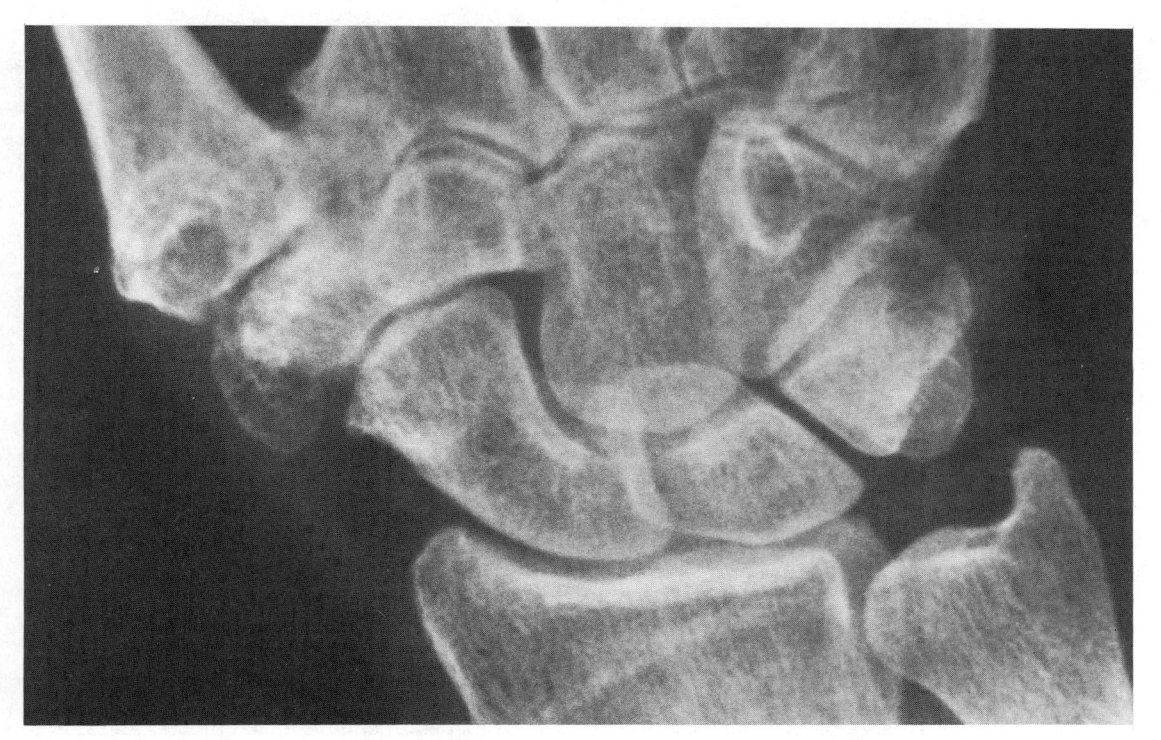

Figure 5-3. Radiographic abnormalities of the first carpometacarpal joint in osteoarthritis. Evident is joint space narrowing, subchondral sclerosis, and osteophyte formation.

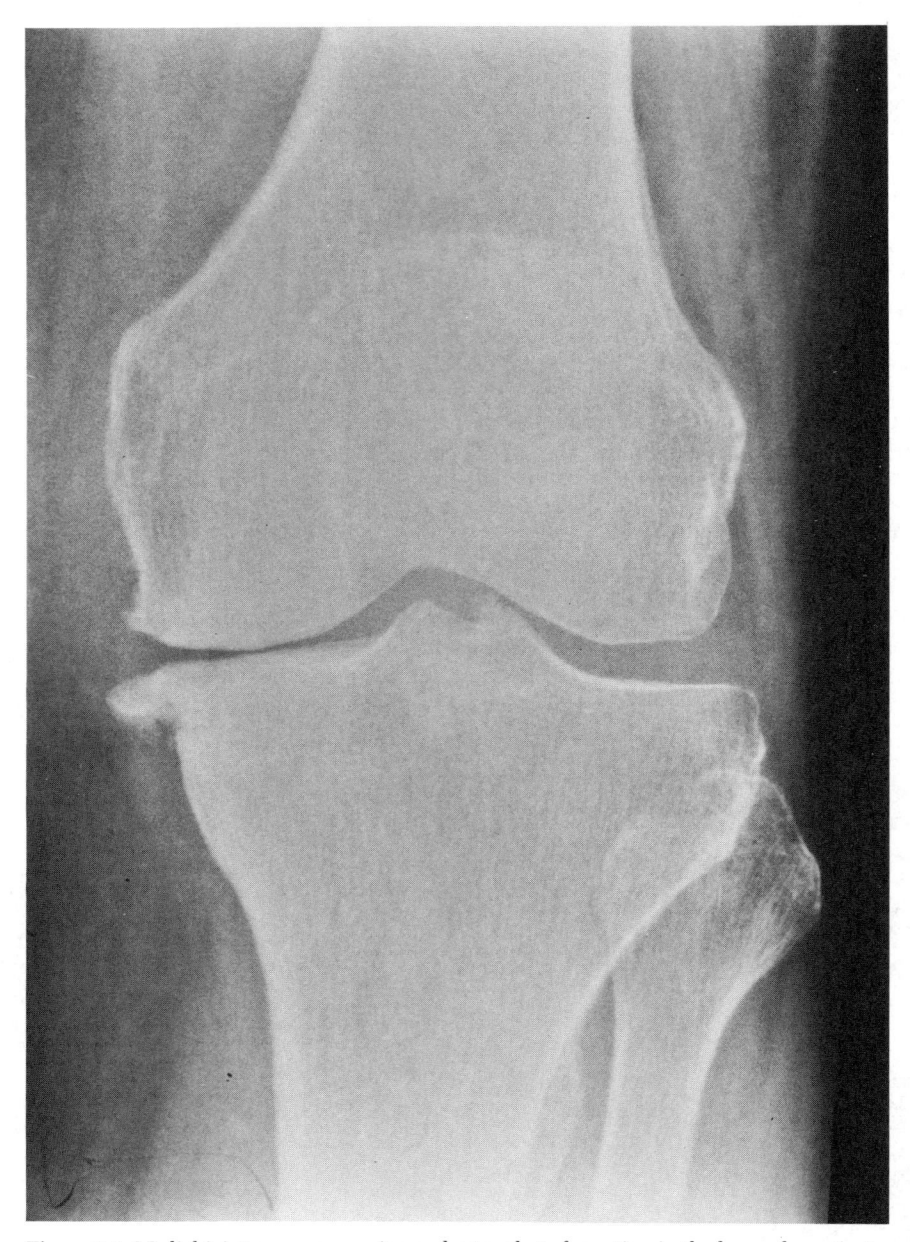

Figure 5-4. Medial joint space narrowing and osteophyte formation in the knee of a patient with osteoarthritis.

these other compartments predominate, the possibility of chondrocalcinosis should be considered.[66]

Coxarthrosis (hip OA), when unilateral is typically a secondary, localized form. Superolateral joint space narrowing suggests a predisposing acetabular dysplasia, slipped capital epiphysis, old fracture, or Legg-Calvé-Perthes disease.[25,52] Although avascular necrosis of bone is frequently listed among the factors predisposing to secondary OA, foci of ischemic necrosis commonly develop not as a cause, but as a consequence of the OA.[67] The basis for this contention is that eburnation is a vital process and cannot therefore arise in dead bone. This in no way argues against development of osteoarthritic remodeling of the acetabulum as a late sequela of osteonecrosis of the femoral head.

Pain in hip OA begins insidiously and leads to an antalgic gait. It is increased by weight bearing and is decreased by maneuvers that decrease intra-articular pressure: mild flexion, abduction, and external rotation. Extension and medial rotation increase the pressure and pain.[55] The pain often presents with inguinal or anterior thigh discomfort. It may be referred to the buttock or knee. Occasionally the complaint is in the low back when a flexion contracture of the hip accentuates lumbosacral lordosis. If pain is located laterally and hip motion is normal, some other source should be considered, for example, the trochanteric bursa or ipsilateral sacroiliac joint.

Degenerative disease of the axial skeleton occurs both at the level of the intervertebral disk (spondylosis) and the synovial joints. In spondylosis the x-ray changes are disk space narrowing, vacuum disk phenomenon, and anterolateral osteophytosis. Schmorl's nodes represent intrusions of disk substance through the vertebral end plate into the subjacent bone marrow. There is little correlation between these radiographic findings and clincal syndromes of back pain.[7]

Involvement of the movable joints, by contrast, does cause symptoms. The uncovertebral joints of Luschka are acquired rather than natural structures of the cervical spine. They arise in the intervertebral disks in front of the neural foramina and have a joint cavity. They are thus prone to result in syndromes of foraminal narrowing. Facet joint OA produces symptoms of spinal stenosis. The structures primarily responsible for low back pain include the facet joints, interspinous and longitudinal ligaments, and periosteum of the vertebral arch. These structures have different nerve supplies.[68]

Diffuse Idiopathic Skeletal Hyperostosis

In its classic form diffuse idiopathic skeletal hyperostosis (DISH) is an ankylosing hyperostosis of the vertebral bodies in which the disk space is preserved. Coexistent spondylosis, however, often blurs the distinction between the two spinal diseases. The classification of DISH as a primary entity rather than a subset of OA thus is uncertain at this time. Vertebral bodies T7-T11 are most often affected. DISH is recognized largely by radiographic means and the following criteria have been proposed for the differential diagnosis[69]: (1) flowing ossification along the anterolateral aspect of at least four contiguous vertebral bodies; (2) preservation of disk space height, along with absence of vertebral end plate sclerosis or vacuum disk phenomenon; and (3) absence of apophyseal or sacroiliac joint involvement. These criteria are meant to exclude typical spondylosis and ankylosing spondylitis. The classic bamboo-spine appearance of ankylosing spondylitis in anteroposterior films is not seen in DISH. Contrasting radiographic findings between the osteophytes of OA and syndesmophytes of ankylosing spondylitis are summarized in Table 5-4. The different radiographic appearances of DISH and spondylosis are illustrated in Figure 5-5A and B. Appendicular joint involvement occurs in 38 percent of cases. The usual manifestation is a symmetric enthesopathy of the posterior calcaneum, olecranon, or superior pole of the patella.[70]

DISH occurs twice as often in men as women. Stiffness, primarily in the thoracic region, is the most frequent clinical manifestation (over 80 percent). It is usually aggravated by rest and relieved by the activity of daily living. Different complaints, sometimes nonarticular, result from involvement of the cervical spine. Here posterior longitudinal ligament ossification or osteophytes may give rise to myelopathic complaints. Ventral osteophytes at times cause dysphagia.

Laboratory abnormalities are uncommon. The most consistent one is glucose intolerance. The prevalence of diabetes ranges from 9 to 40 percent in different series. Levels of growth hormone, somatomedins, and parathormone are normal. There is no relation to fluoride exposure. Obesity is common. Hypervitaminosis A has been suggested as a causative factor in some studies. Radiographic changes simulating DISH have been reported from the use of cis-retinoic acid.[71]

Table 5-4. Contrasting Features of Osteophytes and Syndesmophytes

	Osteophytes	Syndesmophytes
Origin	Several mm from the discovertebral margin	At the discovertebral margin
Mechanism	New bone originating in periosteum	Ossification of annulus fibrosus
Course	Initially horizontal then vertical	Vertical from origin
Associated Condition	Spondylosis	Ankylosing spondylitis and related spondyloarthropathies

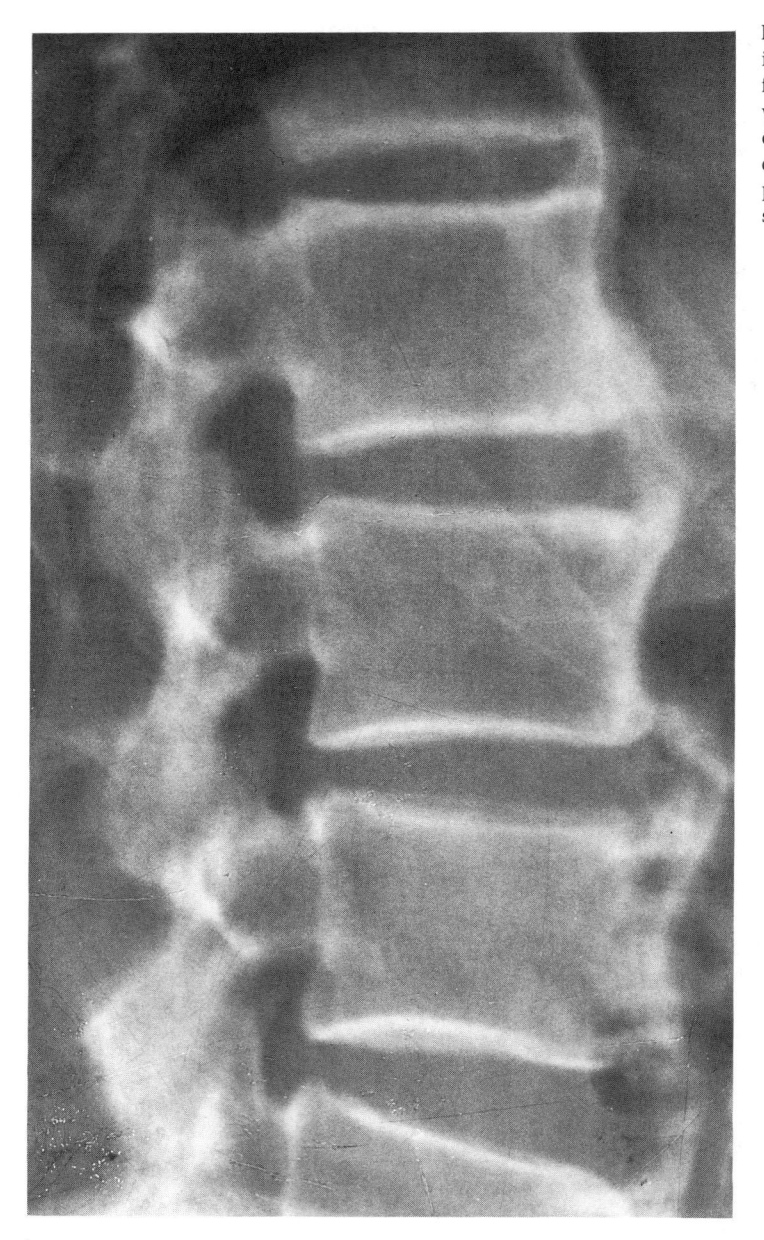

Figure 5-5. Preservation of the intervertebral disk space and anterior flowing ossification from a patient with DISH (A) are contrasted with the disk space narrowing, anterior osteophyte lipping, and vacuum disk phenomenon that characterize spondylosis (B).

A

Erosive Inflammatory Osteoarthritis

Inflammatory OA occurs predominantly in women. The mean age is 52.[72] The disease is symmetric and polyarticular. DIP, PIP, and MCP joints are affected in 75, 50, and 25 percent of cases respectively. Knees, hips, and spine are commonly affected concurrently. Periarticular warmth and erythema occur, unlike classic OA uncomplicated by crystal deposition. Many patients who present with inflammatory manifestations at the onset evolve an erosive variety of disease. The latter is characterized by central and peripheral erosions in the smaller joints. Deformity and instability are common accompaniments in the hands.[73] Ankylosis sometimes supervenes. The presence of the sicca syndrome in some patients further separates erosive from ordinary OA,[74] but this is unrelated to rheumatoid arthritis.

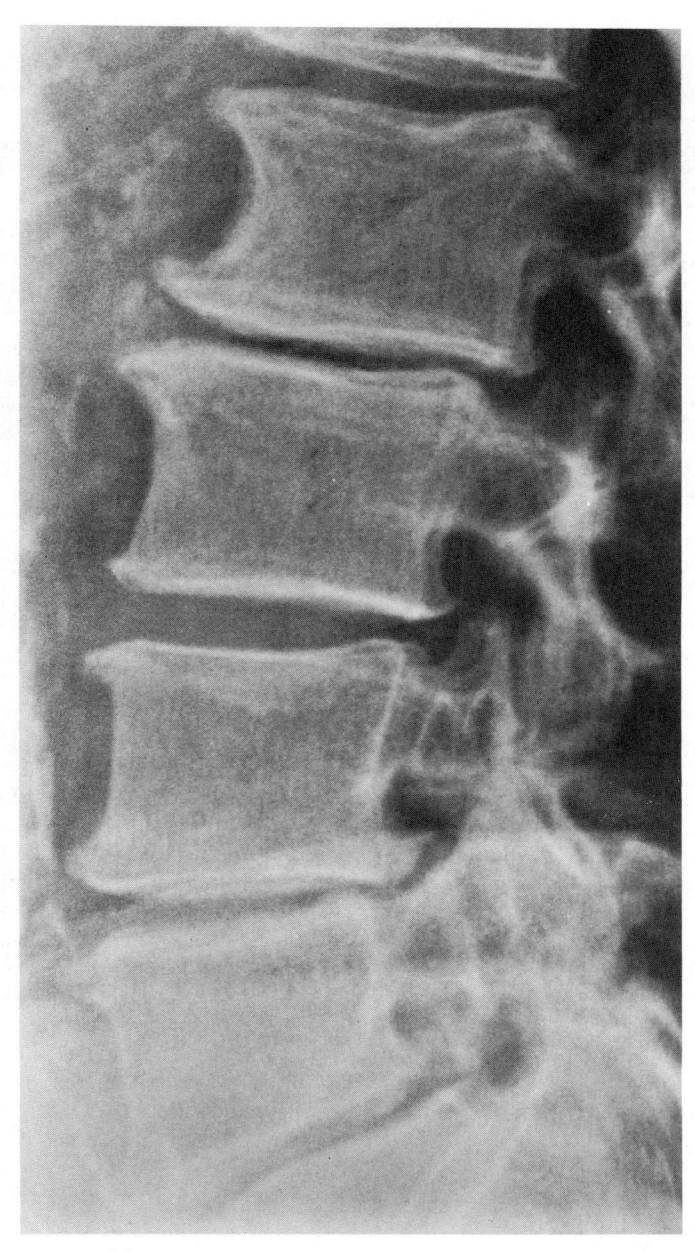

B

Endemic Forms of Osteoarthritis

In remote parts of the world two types of endemic polyarticular degenerative joint disease occur and share several features: (1) onset during the first 2 decades of life; (2) disease is acquired rather than inherited; (3) occurrence in impoverished rural communities; and (4) causes growth restriction.[75] The possible clinical significance for OA is the demonstration that articular cartilage is subject to selective environmental damages.

Kashin-Beck disease is the most extensively studied endemic form of OA. It is found mostly in northern China and adjacent portions of Siberia and North Korea.[75] Initially patients present with symmetric pain, stiffness, and enlargement of finger and wrist joints. More advanced instances involve elbows, knees, and ankles. The distinctive pathologic feature is zonal necrosis of chondrocytes in the articular and growth plate cartilages. In time, segments of damaged joint cartilage split off, form loose bodies, and lead to locking. Osteophytes are prominent, but unlike ordinary OA, eburnation is not characteristic. The cause is totally unknown. Evidence that selenium deficiency is the culprit is not persuasive, although this theory has been advanced. Chondrocytes in vitro do not have a selective requirement for selenium. Other theories include mycotoxicoses, trace element excesses, and abnormal organic components in water and soil.

In a small region of South Africa there is another osteoarthritic endemic disorder, Mseleni disease. It affects the hip primarily. Severe disability, resembling banal coxarthrosis, occurs by the fourth decade of life.[75] Again, there is no agreement on the cause of this endemic form of OA.

Metabolic Disorders Associated with Osteoarthritis

Hemochromatosis. Articular involvement occurs in approximately half of patients with hemochromatosis.[76] It is seen most often in the MCP and PIP joints, where the radiographic changes mimic OA. Knee involvement is also common followed by the hips, shoulders, and wrists. These patients are often misdiagnosed as having seronegative rheumatoid arthritis. Advanced degenerative changes occur in the cartilage and up to 60 percent of patients have chondrocalcinosis. Iron is found both in synoviocytes and chondrocytes. It is not related spatially to the CPPD crystals. The mechanism by which the iron damages the cartilage is not known. Ferric iron impairs the elasticity of cartilage.[77] Other possibilities include stimulation of collagenase production by synovial fibroblasts[78] and free radical formation.[79] Ferric ions also inhibit pyrophosphatase and may promote CPPD deposition.[80] The arthropathy usually peaks between ages 40 and 60. Phlebotomy is of little or no value for articular disease in the majority of patients.[76]

Acromegaly. Peripheral articular complaints are seen in approximately 60 percent of patients, principally in the knees, hips, shoulders, and elbows.[81] The severity varies from mild swelling to disablement. Acromegalic arthropathy is characterized by an early phase of hypermobility, joint effusions, and widening of the radiologic joint space. Bony hypertrophy and loss of motion follow.[81] Hip lesions resemble primary OA and at times require total joint replacement. In the hands, mild soft-tissue swelling and carpal tunnel syndrome are frequent. Although the widening of the distal phalangeal tuft is a characteristic feature, Heberden's and Bouchard's nodes are not seen. Back pain is common. It is usually associated with normal or increased mobility and may be related to ligamentous laxity. The increase in the apparent joint space and intervertebral disk height reflect hypertrophy of the respective cartilages produced by the excess of growth hormone-dependent somatomedin C (insulin-like growth factor-1, IGF-1).[82] Synovial effusions are noninflammatory. Chondrocalcinosis is an occasional feature.[81] Although soft tissue swelling and carpal tunnel syndrome often remit with therapy, the chronic articular changes do not.

Ochronosis. Ochronotic arthropathy results from deposition of polymerized homogentisic acid (HGA) in cartilage matrix. The pigment is also deposited in intervertebral disk and, to a lesser extent, sclera. Most often it results from hereditary deficiency of HGA oxidase. As a consequence, large concentrations of HGA accumulate in body fluids. When excreted in the urine, the HGA is converted under alkaline conditions to a black pigment and so gives rise to alkaptonuria. The axial skeleton is affected before the appendicular skeleton. Typically, spinal disease is manifested by back pain, spondylosis, and disk calcification.[83] In peripheral joints the pigmented cartilage becomes friable, and premature OA ensues. Chondrocalcinosis is sometimes found.[83] Synovial effusions occur in up to half of affected knees. Hips and shoulders are the other commonly involved joints.[83] Synovial fluids are noninflammatory and occasionally contain small fragments of pigmented cartilage ("ground pepper sign").[84]

The aortic and mitral valves are also sometimes pigmented and perhaps 20 percent of patients have heart murmurs. The affinity of HGA for chondroid tissues is unexplained. In a rat model, ascorbic acid inhibited binding of polymerized HGA to tendon and xiphoid cartilage,[85] but in humans high doses have not been helpful.

Wilson's Disease. In this condition, a deficiency of the serum copper-binding protein, ceruloplasmin, results in copper deposition in many tissues. It produces cirrhosis, basal ganglion degeneration, brown pigment at the corneal margin (Kayser-Fleischer ring), and joint disease. Articular manifestations include early-onset OA. Wrist joint involvement is prominent, followed by elbows, shoulders, hips, and knees. The synovial fluid has a noninflammatory character.[86] Hypermobility also has been reported. Radiographic changes include joint space narrowing, sclerosis, fragmentation of subchondral bone, and pseudocysts. The mechanism responsible for these changes is unknown. Pyrophosphatase activity is inhibited by Cu^{++} ions in vitro and this may be responsible for the chondrocalcinosis that has been reported at times.[80]

Hemophilia. Hemarthrosis occurs in 75 to 90 percent of patients with major hemophilias.[87] The bleeding may be acute or chronic and leads to progressive joint disease in approximately one third to one half of patients.[87] The precise mechanism of articular damage is uncertain. Cytokine release, lysosomal and other protease activities, toxicity from iron, and organic breakdown products of hemoglobin, have all been invoked without proof. Large amounts of hemosiderin accumulate in synovium as well as in chondrocytes. Inflammatory cells are few, and stains for immunoglobulin deposits are uniformly negative.

The joints most commonly affected are the knee, elbow and ankle, less often the hip and shoulder. It is unusual to see disease in the hands, feet, and spine.[87] Bleeding occurs in periarticular as well as articular tissues; it extends into muscle and fascial planes. In the forearm this produces Volkmann's contracture; in the iliopsoas, femoral entrapment neuropathy.[87] Large expansive lesions are referred to as hemophilic pseudotumors. Subperiosteal and intraosseous bleeding distort trabecular architecture.

Patients with factor VIII or factor IX levels of greater than 20 percent rarely develop major joint disease. As a consequence of early replacement therapy, younger hemophiliacs appear to have less severe disease.[87,88] The number of joints affected, radiographic changes, development of joint restriction, and contracture increase with age and the degree of factor VIII or IX deficiency. Chronic pain, however, is unrelated to the level of factor VIII or IX present.[82] Advancing x-ray changes in the knee parallel the loss of joint motion and decreased extensor muscle torque.[89] Involvement of the ankle and elbow, however, may be extensive but result in little functional disability.

Radiographic changes are distinctive. Early there may be only soft tissue swelling accompanied by synovial shadows of hemosiderin deposition. As the process progresses to involve the cartilage, joint space narrowing, erosion and subchondral cysts, reminiscent of OA, become prominent. In the knee, a characteristic widening of the intercondylar notch follows hemorrhage around the cruciate ligaments. Magnetic resonance imaging is effective in evaluating the synovial hypertrophy and cartilaginous changes.[90]

Therapy depends on the stage of the disease. For acute hemarthrosis, factor VIII or IX replacement and physical therapy are indicated.[91] At times, percutaneous evacuation of the joint space is required. For advanced disease with recurrent hemarthrosis in the face of adequate factor VIII or IX levels, synovectomy has been advocated to achieve pain relief and decrease the frequency of rebleeding.[92] Synovectomy does not, however, significantly alter radiographically evidenced progression of disease. It often leads to a decreased range of motion postoperatively. Arthroscopic synovectomy may offer the same benefit yet preserve the range of motion. Intra-articular steroids may be useful adjunctive therapy for ongoing synovitis. Total joint replacement may be required for disabling end-stage disease. Arthrodesis is preferred for the ankle.

Gout. In tophaceous gout monosodium urate crystals deposit in cartilage, subchondral bone, and periarticular tissue. Secondary osteoarthritis often supervenes.[8]

Neuropathic Joint Disease (Charcot's Joint)

In these disorders sensory defects allow excessive and repetitive mechanical insults to disintegrate the affected joints. Neuropathic arthropathy most commonly arises in the context of defective proprioception, but also at times from congenital or acquired absence of pain sensibility. In the former circumstance many patients complain of pain.[93] It is most often seen at the present time in patients with diabetic neuropathy. Here the tarsal and metatarsal regions are the sites of predilection. Unlike classic neuroarthropathy, in the diabetic foot the bony structures rather than the joint surfaces proper are affected. The Charcot joint of tertiary syphilis (tabes dorsalis) typically affects the knee. Upper extremity disease (shoulder, elbow, wrist) results from syringomyelia, and hand lesions from leprosy.[94] Forefoot lesions, resembling the diabetic type, occasionally follow alcoholic neuropathy. Rare cases have been reported with amyloidosis. A picture rather similar to neuropathic joint disease occurs at times after use of intra-articular steroids, but a neural mechanism is not apparent.

The patients present clinically with a wide spectrum of complaints. Swelling, deformity and instability are usual, but pain is also a common initial complaint. Ulcers of the skin are found in acral areas and the process is occasionally mistaken for septic arthritis or osteomyelitis. Radiographic examination discloses varying degrees of articular disorganization, bone resorption, and osteophytosis, changes that resemble exaggerated OA. Gallium (^{67}Ga) and technetium (^{99m}Tc-MDP [methylene diphosphonate]) scintigraphy may be positive but indium (^{111}In) labeled white blood cell imaging is negative.[95] Synovial fluid is usually noninflammatory but may be bloody or xanthochromic. CPPD deposition occurs at times in Charcot's joints, but chondrocalcinosis may itself produce a destructive pseudoneuroarthropathy.

Treatment is supportive and directed to the underlying disease. Orthotics are useful. Surgical management is difficult. Total joint replacement is occasionally successful, but generally is not recommended because of loosening and subluxation. Arthrodesis at times offers relief of pain.

Therapeutic Intervention: Evolving Concepts

General Considerations

Patient education is of the greatest importance. Avoiding joint abuse, weight reduction, counseling on occupation and sports-related activities, as well as appropriate exercise are necessary to preserve joint function. Physical therapy, directed at improving motion, increasing strength, and reducing pain are fundamental components of any treatment plan. Moist heat provides benefit, as does an exercise program that includes active rather than passive motion, and isometric rather than isotonic maneuvers. Medical therapy is usually initiated with salicylates or other nonsteroidal anti-inflammatory drugs (NSAIDs). Several newer modalities are discussed in the next section. Once advanced radiographically evident changes occur and pain and disability are sufficiently advanced to interfere with function and daily life, surgical intervention is often of benefit. Total joint replacement and osteotomy to restore biomechanical alignment have their principal applications to the hip and knee. Arthrodesis is useful to relieve pain and improve support in thumb OA.

Medical Therapy: Nonspecific and Targeted

NSAIDs are usually the first medications to be prescribed for OA.[96] Although the mechanism of their action was at first ascribed solely to inhibition of prostaglandin production, these agents are now known to have multiple effects. They inhibit superoxide and protease release from polymorphonuclear leukocytes and decrease aggregation of these cells.[97] These actions are of anti-inflammatory and analgesic benefit. In addition, recent studies indicate that NSAIDs have direct effects on articular cartilage. This introduces the concept of "chondrotoxic" and "chondroprotective" agents. It is based largely on in vitro and animal model studies and is predicated on the view that proteoglycan production is of benefit to cartilage and that a decrease is detrimental.

In organ cultures of normal dog knee cartilage, salicylates, fenoprofen, isoxicam, tolmetin, and ibuprofen inhibited sulfated proteoglycan synthesis; indomethacin, piroxicam, and diclofenac had no effect; and benoxaprofen and sulindac actually increased it.[98] The damaging effect of salicylates was even more marked when the knee was altered by transection of the cruciate ligament or immobilized. Analogous results were obtained when aged human cartilage was treated with salicylates or indomethacin.[99] The chondroprotective action of the newer agent, tiaprofenic acid, is attributed to its inhibition of metalloprotease-mediated proteoglycan degradation. Diclofenac and piroxicam may have similar actions.

We are in agreement with the conservative view of Doherty[100] that extrapolations from these artificial test conditions to the choice of particular NSAIDs in the management of OA is premature. They may in time prove to be valid. One well-designed clinical investigation has supported the idea that long-term use of a powerful prostaglandin synthetase inhibitor, indomethacin, accelerated progression of hip OA over that found with a less powerful agent, azapropazone.[101] The complexity of choosing particular agents is made no easier by the possibility that analgesics may permit joints to be overused and so to deteriorate more quickly.

Intra-articular steroid injections sometimes give relief in OA. Controlled clinical trials have reported short-lived benefit (up to 2 weeks), while others indicated no advantage above placebo injections.[102] A small risk of complications must be weighed: septic arthritis occurs in 0.01 to 0.001 percent of patients. A Charcot-like arthropathy, tendon rupture, and steroid crystal deposition synovitis also are infrequent occurrences. Intra-articular administration of the superoxide dismutase, orgotein, has been reported in Europe to benefit various joint diseases.[102] A recent double-blind, placebo-controlled trial in the United States supported its efficacy in OA of the knee.[103] Side effects were infrequent and confined to the skin.

Three semisynthetic complex sugar preparations (Arteparon, a polysulfated glycosaminglycan; Rumalon, a glycosaminoglycan-peptide complex; and pentosan polysulfate, SP54, a polysaccharide sulfate ester) have their advocates in several foreign countries.[104] These agents are administered by intramuscular or intra-articular injection. The proposed modes of action include broad-spectrum enzyme inhibition and perhaps augmentation of proteoglycan synthesis. Despite some favorable clinical reports abroad and experimental support in animal models of OA, these preparations have not been approved for clinical trial in the United States. Arteparon has heparinoid effects and bleeding is a potential problem.

Recent studies of S-adenosylmethionine (SAME) offer a new approach. This compound is a methyl group donor in membrane transmethylation and has multiple clinical actions: analgesic, anti-inflammatory, antidepressive, and protective to the gastrointestinal tract. SAME enhances proteoglycan production by chondrocytes cultured from human OA patients. The clinical benefit from orally administered SAME is the same as that of several NSAIDs. Its long-term efficacy and tolerability have been demonstrated over a 1- to 2-year period. The antidepressive action may be of adjunctive benefit. SAME may be prototypic of a new class of drugs to be employed in therapy of OA.[105]

Biochemical Monitoring

Detection of specific markers of articular cartilage degradation in body fluids hypothetically might be of great value for diagnosing the onset of OA and monitoring its response to treatment. Several sensitive tests for breakdown products have been developed. Serum levels of keratan sulfate[106] and urine concentration of the collagen cross-linked compound pyridinoline[107] are elevated in OA. So, too, are levels of antichondrocyte membrane and antitype II collagen antibodies.[108] Unfortunately, these changes are also found in rheumatoid and other destructive arthritides. Furthermore, articular cartilage is only a small part of the total body cartilage and derangement of other pools might contribute to these levels. Thus at present, there are no satisfactory biochemical tests for measuring the therapeutic worth of medications for degenerative joint disease.[109]

References

1. Sokoloff, L: Osteoarthritis as a remodeling process. J Rheumatol 14 (Suppl 14):7, 1987.
2. Mankin, HJ, and Treadwell, BV: Osteoarthritis: A 1987 update. Bull Rheum Dis 36:1, 1986.
3. Peyron, JG, and Altman, RD: The epidemiology of osteoarthritis. In: Moskowitz, RW et al (eds): Osteoarthritis: Diagnosis and Medical/Surgical Management. Philadelphia, WB Saunders, 1992, pp 15–37.
4. Lawrence, JS, Bremner, JM, and Bier, F: Osteoarthritis: Prevalence in the popoulation and relationship between symptoms and x-ray changes. Ann Rheum Dis 25:1, 1966.
5. Kellgren, JH, and Lawrence, JS: Radiological assessment of osteoarthritis. Ann Rheum Dis 16:494, 1957.
6. Moskowitz, RW: Osteoarthritis: A clinical overview. In: Lawrence, RC, and Shulman, LE (eds): Current topics in Rheumatology: Epidemiology of the Rheumatic diseases. New York, Gower Medical Publishing, 1984, pp 267–276.
7. Hadler, NM: Osteoarthritis as a public health problem. Clin Rheum Dis 11:175, 1985.
8. Hough, AJ, and Sokoloff, L: Pathology of osteoarthritis. In: McCarty, DJ (ed): Arthritis and Allied Conditions, ed: 11. Philadelphia, Lea & Febiger, 1989, pp 1571–1594.
9. Howell, DS, Treadwell, BV, and Trippel, SB: Etiopathogenesis of osteoarthritis. In: Moskowitz, RW et al (eds): Osteoarthritis: Diagnosis and Medical/Surgical Management. Philadelphia, WB Saunders, 1992, pp 129–146.
10. Rubin, CT, and Hausman, MR: The cellular basis of Wolff's law: Transduction of physical stimuli to skeletal adaptation. Clin Rheum Dis 14:503, 1988.
11. Mintz, G, and Fraga, A: Severe osteoarthritis of the elbow in foundry workers. Arch Environ Health 27:78, 1973.
12. Partridge, REH, and Duthie, JJR: Rheumatisim in dockers and civil servants: A comparison of heavy manual and sedentary workers. Ann Rheum Dis 27:559, 1968.
13. Lawrence, JS: Rheumatism in cotton operatives. Br J Ind Med 18:270, 1961.
14. Hadler, NM et al: Hand structure and function in an industrial setting: Influence of three patterns of stereotyped repetitive usage. Arthritis Rheum 21:210, 1978.
15. Lane, NE et al: Osteoarthritis of the hands: A comparison of handedness and hand use. J Rheumatol 16:637, 1989.
16. Radin, EL, Paul, IL, and Rose, RM: Role of mechanical factors in pathogenesis of primary osteoarthritis. Lancet i:519, 1971.
17. Burke, MJ, Fean, EC, and Wright, V: Bone and joint changes in pneumatic drillers. Ann Rheum Dis 36:276, 1977.
18. Barry, HC: Sport, exercise and arthritis. Br J Rheumatol 26:386, 1987.
19. Lane, NE et al: Long distance running, bone density, and osteoarthritis. JAMA 255:1147, 1986.

20. Anderson, JJ, and Felson, DT: Factors associated with osteoarthritis of the knee in the first National Health and Nutrition Examination Survey (HANES I): Evidence for an association with overweight, race, and physical demands of work. Am J Epidemiol 128:179, 1988.
21. Panush, RS et al: Is running associated with degenerative joint disease? JAMA 255:1152, 1986.
22. Monti, B et al: Is excessive running predictive of degenerative hip disease: Controlled study of former elite athletes. Br Med J 299:91, 1989.
23. Dequeker, J: The relationship between osteoporosis and osteoarthritis. Clin Rheum Dis 11:271, 1985.
24. van Saase, JLCM et al: Epidemiology of osteoarthritis: Zoefermeer survey. Comparison of radiological osteoarthritis in a Dutch population with that in 10 other populations. Ann Rheum Dis 48:271, 1989.
25. Moskowitz, RW: Clinical and laboratory findings in osteoarthritis. In: McCarty DJ (ed): Arthritis and Allied Conditions, ed 11. Philadelphia, Lea & Febiger, 1989, pp 1605–1630.
26. Sokoloff, L: The biology of degenerative joint disease. Chicago, University of Chicago Press, 1969.
27. Brandt, KD: Osteoarthritis. Clin Geriatr Med 4:279, 1988.
28. Tomer, Y et al: HLA antigens in patients with Heberden's nodes. Isr J Med Sci 24:24, 1988.
29. Pattrick, M et al: HLA-A, B antigens and alpha-1- antitrypsin phenotypes in nodal generalized osteoarthritis and erosive osteoarthritis. Ann Rheum Dis 48:470, 1989.
30. Ala-kokko, L et al: Single base mutation in the type II procollagen gene (COL 2 A1) as a cause of primary osteoarthritis associated with a mild chondrodysplasia. Proc Nat Acad Sci USA 87:6565, 1990.
31. Silberberg, M, and Silberberg, R: Modifying action of estrogen on the evolution of osteoarthritis in mice of different ages. Endocrinology 72:449, 1963.
32. Sokoloff, L, Varney, DA, and Scott, JF: Sex hormones, bone changes, and osteoarthritis in DBA/2JN mice. Arthritis Rheum 8:1027, 1965.
33. Rosner, IA et al: Pathologic and metabolic responses of experimental osteoarthritis to estradiol and an estradiol antagonist. Clin Orthop 171:280, 1982.
34. Felson, DT et al: Obesity and knee osteoarthritis: The Framingham study. Ann Intern Med 109:18, 1988.
35. Hochberg, MC et al: Epidemiologic associations of pain in osteoarthritis of the knee: Data from the National Health and Nutrition Examination survey and the National Health and Nutrition Examination I Epidemiologic follow-up survey. Semin Arthritis Rheum 18, 4 (Suppl 2):4, 1989.
36. Carman, WJ: Factors associated with pain and osteoarthritis in the Tecumseh Community Health study. Semin Arthritis Rheum 18, 1:4 (Suppl 2):10, 1989.
37. Davis, MA et al: Sex differences in osteoarthritis of the knee: The role of obesity. Am J Epidemiol 127:1019, 1988.
38. Felson, DT et al: The prevalence of knee osteoarthritis in the elderly: The Framingham osteoarthritis study. Arthritis Rheum 30:914, 1987.
39. van Saase, JLCM et al: Osteoarthritis and obesity in the general population: A relationship calling for an explanation. J Rheumatol 15:1152, 1988.
40. Davis, MA, Ettinger, WH, and Neuhaus, JM: The role of metabolic factors and blood pressure in the association of obesity with osteoarthritis of the knee. J Rheumatol 15:1827, 1988.
41. Hamerman, D: The biology of osteoarthritis. N Engl J Med 320:1322, 1989.
42. Maroudas, A: Glycosaminoglycan turnover in articular cartilage. Philos Trans R Soc London [Biol] 271:293, 1975.
43. Castor, CW: Regulation of connective tissue metabolism. In McCarty, DJ (ed): Arthritis and Allied Conditions, ed 11. Philadelphia, Lea & Febiger, 1989, pp 256–272.
44. Tyler, JA and Benton, HP: Synthesis of type II collagen is decreased in cartilage cultured with interleukin-1 while the rate of intracellular degradation remains unchanged. Collagen Rel Res 8:393 1988.
45. Harris, ED Jr, and McCroskery, PA: The influence of temperature and fibril stability on degradation of cartilage collagen by rheumatoid synovial collagenase. N Engl J Med 290:1, 1974.
46. Gibilisco, PA et al: Synovial fluid crystals in osteoarthritis. Arthritis Rheum 28:211, 1985.
47. Sokoloff, L, and Varma, AA: Chondrocalcinosis in surgically resected joints. Arthritis Rheum 31:750, 1988.
48. Wood, DD et al: Isolation of an interleukin-1 like factor from human joint effusions. Arthritis Rheum 26:975, 1983.
49. Pelletier, JP et al: Role of synovial membrane inflammation in cartilage matrix breakdown in the Pond-Nuki dog model of osteoarthrtis. Arthritis Rheum 28:554, 1985.
50. Alwan, WH et al: Hydroxyapatite and urate crystal induced cytokine release by macrophages. Ann Rheum Dis 48:476 1989.
51. Cooke, TDV: Pathogenetic mechanisms in polyarticular osteoarthritis. Clin Rheum Dis 11:203, 1985.
52. Altman, RD et al: Development of criteria for the classification and reporting of osteoarthritis. Arthritis Rheum 29:1039, 1986.
53. Leigh, TJ et al: Comparison of sleep in osteoarthritic patients and age and sex matched healthy controls. Ann Rheum Dis 47:40, 1988.
54. Altman, RD, and Dean, D: Introduction and overview: Pain in osteoarthritis. Semin Arthritis Rheum 18, 4 (Suppl 2):1, 1989.
55. Goddard, NJ, and Gosling, PT: Intra-articular fluid pressure and pain in osteoarthritis of the hip. J Bone Joint Surg (Br) 70:52, 1988.
56. Dey, A, Sharma, UC, and Dave, PK: Effect of high tibial osteotomy on upper tibial venous drainage: Study by intraosseous phlebography in primary osteoarthritis of knee joint. Ann Rheum Dis 48:188, 1989.

57. Meachim, G et al: An investigation of radiological, clinical, and pathological correlations in osteoarthritis of the hip. Clin Radiol 31:565, 1980.
58. Zimmerman, M: Pain mechanisms and mediators in osteoarthritis. Semin Arthirtis Rheum 18, 4 (Suppl 2): 22, 1989.
59. Lotz, M, Carson, DA, and Vaughan, JH: Substance P activation of rheumatoid synoviocytes: Neural pathway in pathogenesis of arthritis. Science 235:893, 1987.
60. Gronblad, M et al: Neuropeptides in synovium of patients with rheumatoid arthritis and osteoarthritis. J Rheumatol 15:1807, 1988.
61. Badalamente, MA, and Cherney, SB: Periosteal and vascular innervation of the human patella in degenerative joint disease. Semin Arthritis Rheum 18 (Suppl 2):61, 1989.
62. Sokoloff, L: Aging and degenerative diseases affecting cartilage. In: Hall, BK (ed): Cartilage, Vol 3. New York, Academic Press, 1983, pp 109–141.
63. Kellgren, JH, and Moore, R: Generalized osteoarthritis and Heberden's nodes. Br Med J 1:181, 1952.
64. Simkin, PA, Campbell, PM, and Larson, EB: Gout in Heberden's nodes. Arthritis Rheum 26:94, 1983.
65. McGoldrick, F, O'Brien, TM: Osteoarthritis of the hip and Heberden's nodes. Ann Rheum Dis 48:53, 1989.
66. Resnick, D, and Niwayama, G: Degenerative disease of extraspinal locations. In: Resnick, D, and Niwayama, G (eds): Diagnosis of Bone and Joint Disorders, ed 2. Philadelphia, WB Saunders, 1988, pp 1364–1479.
67. Ilardi, CF, and Sokoloff, L: Secondary osteonecrosis in osteoarthritis of the femoral head. Hum Pathol 15:79, 1984.
68. Brown, MD: The source of low back pain and sciatica. Semin Arthritis Rheum 18, 4(Suppl 2):67, 1989.
69. Resnick, D, and Niwayama G: Radiographic and pathologic features of spinal involvement in diffuse idiopathic skeletal hyperostosis (DISH). Radiology 119:559, 1976.
70. Utsinger, PD: Diffuse idiopathic skeletal hyperostosis. Clin Rheum Dis 11:325, 1985.
71. Pittsley, RA, and Yoder, FW: Skeletal toxicity associated with long term administration of 13-Cis-Retinoic Acid for refractory ichthyosis. N Engl J Med 308:1012, 1983.
72. Ehrlich, GE: Osteoarthritis beginning with inflammation. JAMA 232:157, 1975.
73. Altman, RD, and Gray, R: Inflammation in osteoarthritis. Clin Rheum Dis 11:353, 1985.
74. Shuckett, R, Russell, ML, and Gladman, DD: Atypical erosive osteoarthritis and Sjögren's syndrome. Ann Rheum Dis 45:281, 1986.
75. Sokoloff, L: Endemic forms of osteoarthritis. Clin Rheum Dis 11:187, 1985.
76. Schumacher, HR, Straka, PC, and Krikker, MA: The arthropathy of hemochromatosis: Recent studies. Ann N Y Acad Sci 526:224, 1988.
77. Sokoloff, L: Elasticity of articular cartilage: Effect of ions and viscous solutions. Science 141:1055, 1963.
78. Okazaki, I et al: Iron increases collagenase production by rabbit synovial fibroblasts. J Lab Clin Med 97:396, 1981.
79. Blake, DR et al: The importance of iron in rheumatoid disease: An hypothesis. Lancet ii:1142, 1981.
80. McCarty, DJ, and Pepe, PF: Erythrocyte neutral inorganic pyrophosphatase in pseudogout. J Lab Clin Med 79:277, 1972.
81. Bluestone, R et al: Acromegalic arthropathy. Ann Rheum Dis 30:243, 1971.
82. Johanson, NA: Endocrine arthropathies. Clin Rheum Dis 11:297, 1985.
83. Schumacher, HR, and Holdsworth, DE: Ochronotic arthropathy. I. Clinicopathologic Studies. Semin Arthritis Rheum 6:207, 1977.
84. Hunter, T, Gordon, DA, and Ogryzlo, MA: The ground pepper sign of synovial fluid: A new diagnostic feature of ochronosis. J Rheumatol 1:45, 1974.
85. Lustberg, TD, Schulman, JD, and Seegmiller, JE: Decreased binding of ^{14}C-homogentisic acid induced by ascorbic acid in connective tissues of rats with experimental alcaptonuria. Nature 228:770, 1970.
86. Golding, DN, and Walshe, JM: Arthropathy of Wilson's disease. Ann Rheum Dis 36:99, 1977.
87. Steven, MM et al: Hemophilic arthritis. Q J Med 58:181, 1986.
88. Smit, C et al: Physical condition, longevity, and social performance of Dutch hemophiliacs, 1972–85. Br Med J 298:235, 1989.
89. Greene, WB, Yankaskas, BC, and Guilford, WB: Roentgenographic classifications of hemophilic arthropathy. J Bone Joint Surg (Am) 71:237, 1989.
90. Yulish, BS et al: Hemophilic arthropathy: Assessment with MR imaging. Radiology 164:759, 1987.
91. Gregosiewicz, A, Wosko, I, and Kandzierski, G: Intraarticular bleeding in children with hemophilia: The prevention of arthropathy. J Pediatr Orthop 9:182, 1989.
92. Montane, L, McCollough, NC, and Chun-Yet Lian, E: Synovectomy of the knee for hemophilic arthropathy. J Bone Joint Surg (Am) 68:210, 1986.
93. Ellman, MH: Neuropathic joint disease (Charcot Joints). In: McCarty, DJ (ed): Arthritis and Allied Conditions, ed 11. Philadelphia, Lea & Febiger, 1989, pp 1255–1272.
94. Resnick, D: Neuroarthropathy. In: Resnick, D, and Niwayama, G (eds): Diagnosis of Bone and Joint Disorders, ed 2. Philadelphia, WB Saunders, 1988, pp 3154–3185.
95. Knight, D et al: Imaging for infection: Caution required with the Charcot joint. Eur J Nucl Med 13:523, 1988.
96. Moskowitz, RW: Primary osteoarthritis: Epidemiology, clinical aspects, and general management. Am J Med 83 (Suppl 5A):5, 1987.
97. Abramson, SB, and Weissman, G: The mechanisms of action of nonsteroidal antiinflammatory drugs. Arthritis Rheum 32:1, 1989.

98. Brandt, KD: Effects of nonsteroidal antiinflammatory drugs on chondrocyte metabolism in vitro and in vivo. Am J Med 83 (Suppl 5A):29, 1987.
99. McKenzie, LS et al: Effect of anti-inflammatory drugs on sulphated glycosaminoglycan synthesis in aged human articular cartilage. Ann Rheum Dis 35:487, 1976.
100. Doherty, M: "Chondroprotection" by non-steroidal anti-inflammatory drugs. Ann Rheum Dis 48:619, 1989.
101. Rashad, S et al: Effect of non-steroidal anti-inflammatory drugs on the course of osteoarthritis. Lancet ii:519, 1989.
102. Fife, RS, and Brandt, KD: Other approaches to therapy. In: Moskowitz, RW et al (eds): Osteoarthritis: Diagnosis and Medical/Surgical Management. Philadelphia, WB Saunders, 1992, pp 511–526.
103. McIlwain, H et al: Intra-articular orgotein in osteoarthritis of the knee: A placebo controlled efficacy, safety, and dosage comparison. Am J Med 87:295, 1989.
104. Burkhardt, D, and Ghosh, P: Laboratory evaluation of anti-arthritic drugs as potential chondroprotective agents. Semin Arthritis Rheum 17, 2 (Suppl 1):3, 1987.
105. DiPadova, C: S-Adenosylmethionine in the treatment of osteoarthritis: Review of the clinical studies. Am J Med 83 (Suppl 5A):60, 1987.
106. Thonar, EJ-MA et al: Quantification of keratan sulfate in blood as a marker of cartilage catabolism. Arthritis Rheum 28:1367, 1985.
107. Robins, SP et al: Measurement of the cross linking compound, pyridinoline, in urine as an index of collagen degradation in joint disease. Ann Rheum Dis 45:969, 1986.
108. Nemeth-Csoka, M, Paroczai, C, and Meszaros, TH: The clinical diagnostic significance of serum anti-chondrocyte membrane antibodies in osteoarthritis. Agents Actions 23:50, 1988.
109. Brandt, KD: A pessimistic view of serologic markers for diagnosis and management of osteoarthritis: Biochemical, immunologic and clinicopathologic barriers. J Rheumatol 16(Suppl 18):39, 1989.

Chapter 6
Reiter's Syndrome and Reactive Arthritis

R.D. INMAN, M.D.

Introduction

The syndrome named after Hans Reiter had its first full expression in the literature with a case report describing a Prussian lieutenant who in 1914 developed diarrhea and shortly thereafter arthritis, conjunctivitis, and urethritis.[1] There is some suggestion of earlier cases, affecting even as notable a patient as Christopher Columbus,[2] and there has been some controversy regarding the political career of Reiter himself[3] but the name appears firmly fixed in the medical literature. The original case outlining the triad of arthritis, conjunctivitis, and urethritis guided the diagnostic criteria for a long time, with fewer signs than the triad termed "incomplete Reiter's." In general most authors now accept the presence of a seronegative asymmetric arthritis plus one extra-articular feature as sufficient for the diagnosis. The latter may involve genitourinary, ocular, or mucocutaneous systems. An antecedent infection may or may not be clinically identifiable. The term *reactive arthritis* (ReA) refers to a seronegative asymmetric arthritis that follows an antecedent extra-articular infection usually within a 3- to 4-week interval. The infection may be documented by culture or implicated by history and serologic tests. The terms ReA and Reiter's syndrome (RS) are closely related and RS may be regarded as a subset of ReA, as evidenced by the appearance of both RS and ReA after a unique environmental trigger in a susceptible population. At present there is no identifiable marker in such cases to predict which disease will be restricted to joints (ReA) and which will involve other organ systems (RS).

Both RS and ReA are representative of a larger clinical diagnostic category, the seronegative spondyloarthropathies.[4] These include ankylosing spondylitis, psoriatic arthritis and the arthritis accompanying inflammatory bowel disease, as well as RS and ReA. The unifying characteristics of the spondyloarthropathies are (1) predilection for involvement of sacroiliac joints and spine; (2) oligoarticular asymmetric arthritis; (3) enthesopathy (plantar fasciitis, Achilles tendinitis, etc.); (4) absence of rheumatoid factor and autoantibodies; (5) extra-articular disease in characteristic sites (eye, heart, skin, mucous membranes); (6) male predominance; and (7) a strong association with the HLA class I antigen B27. There is one clinical subset of the spondyloarthropathies that currently falls through the net of our nomenclature. This is the young male with recurrent asymmetric arthritis and enthesitis who lacks any clue to an antecedent infection, has no extra-articular disease, and who does not meet criteria for ankylosing spondylitis. This is a relatively common syndrome in my experience. At present, such patients may be regarded as having an unclassified spondyloarthropathy but the term is unwieldy and reflects the shortcomings in our understanding of the basic pathogenesis. It has been proposed that the entire group of diseases be termed the "HLA-B27-associated diseases"[5] but there is no consensus yet. This does, however, recognize the centrality of immunogenetic susceptibility in our current understanding of this group of diseases.

Clinical Manifestations

The cardinal feature of RS and ReA is an asymmetric arthritis, typically oligoarticular and predominantly of the lower extremity. The most commonly affected joints are knees, ankles, and metatarsophalangeal joints, but upper extremity involvement does occur. Heel pain is a common feature that is quite specific[6] and reflects inflammation at tendinous insertion sites such as plantar fascia and Achilles tendon. The basis for this characteristic enthesopathy is not known. Axial involvement is reflected in back pain, although radiographic sacroiliitis occurs in the acute phase in only 28 percent of patients.[7] In followup studies radiographically evident axial changes are seen in the same percentage, but syndesmophyte formation is uncommon. When these occur they are distinguishable from classic ankylosing spondylitis by their asymmetry and nonmarginal location.

The extra-articular features of RS frequently provide the correct diagnostic clues for the clinician. When they occur independent of active joint disease, however, they may pose diagnostic problems. In such circumstances the patient may be seen by various specialists, such as a urologist for urethritis or an ophthalmologist for iritis, without a comprehensive synthesis of the different target organ manifestations. Inflammatory eye disease occurred in 59 percent of patients in one series[8] and urethritis/cervicitis in 88 percent. The latter may sometimes pose a problem in disease classification since urethritis may reflect the site of the antecedent arthritogenic infection (e.g., Chlamydia trachomatis) or may occur as a sterile inflammatory manifestation of postdysenteric RS. Symptoms of dysuria may be mild, as the penile discharge may be, and these must be inquired about directly. Circinate balanitis may appear as superficial ulcers or scaling plaques and although classically painless, they may be painful in certain patients. The oral ulcers on the hard palate or tongue are usually painless. Less common manifestations include cardiac (varying degrees of heart block, aortic insufficiency, pericarditis) and neurologic (myelopathy, cranial nerve lesions), but these are rare.

The laboratory assessment provides no diagnostic test for RS and ReA. The erythrocyte sedimentation rate is generally elevated, but not invariably, even in the setting of active inflammatory joint disease. The anemia of chronic disease may by its severity provide some clue to the duration of the inflammation. Serum immunoglobulins are generally normal, with the exception of serum IgA which can be markedly elevated. This finding is more characteristic of postdysenteric RS than postvenereal RS, and is circumstantial evidence implicating an inciting antigen crossing gut epithelial mucosal defenses.[9] This also bears an interesting relationship to elevated serum IgA levels in ankylosing spondylitis, which may in turn provide clues to the causes of that disease.[10] Immune complexes have been observed[11] but not consistently.[12] Testing for identification of the provocative infection is most rigorously performed by culture, but serologic testing may be of value on occasion. Culture of stool samples and of urethral swabs must be correctly obtained, transported, and processed for meaningful results. This is particularly true for Chlamydia trachomatis, which is an obligate intracellular pathogen. Anti-Chlamydia antibodies provide supportive evidence for a patient with postvenereal RS but are sufficiently common in the population to fall short of a diagnostic test. Anti-Yersinia antibodies, although useful in some clinical studies,[13] are of little diagnostic value in the individual case. HLA-B27 as a diagnostic test lacks sufficient sensitivity (there is a 20 percent "false-negative" rate in RS) and specificity (of the 7 percent of a normal population who are HLA-B27 positive, greater than 80 percent will probably never develop a spondyloarthropathy) to be a useful test for the clinician. Nevertheless, in atypical chronic arthritis (in which the pretest probability is higher), a positive HLA-B27 result can help to categorize the problem diagnostically.

Current Concepts of Pathogenesis

The working hypothesis for the pathogenesis of RS/ReA may be formulated as follows: (1) certain microorganisms can result in a sterile synovitis, (2) primarily in an HLA-B27-positive population, (3) following infection of the genitourinary or gastrointestinal tracts, (4) by virtue of an aberrant host immune response to the pathogen. Each of these premises has given rise to testable hypotheses in recent years and has broadened our concepts of the origins of the disease.

The arthritogenic organisms that are generally included in this list are Salmonella sp., Shigella sp., Yersinia enterocolitica, Campylobacter jejuni, and Chlamydia trachomatis.[14] A number of case reports substantiate these relationships, but it is an epidemic outbreak that has allowed a clearer definition of the arthritogenic potential of certain organisms. In a recent outbreak of Salmonella typhimurium dysentery caused by a single contaminated food source we observed that of 260 persons infected there were 19 cases of RS/ReA (7.8 percent) within 4 weeks of the onset of diarrhea.[15] These episodes constituted new onset of joint symptoms and provide strong epidemiologic evidence for a causal relationship of an enteric pathogen to arthritis. Other causes of gastrointestinal infection with secondary arthritis include parasitic infestation[16] and Clostridium difficile gut colonization,[17] but the role of HLA-B27 is undefined in these syndromes. Acute rheumatic fever in a sense fulfills the criteria for ReA,[18] with the group A streptococcus being the arthritogenic agent but generally this is not included with the ReA group, and acute rheumatic fever differs from them in its association with class II rather than class I HLA antigens.[19]

The HLA-B27-positive precondition is reflected in the 60 to 80 percent positive rate in most series of RS and ReA. In our recent studies of post-Salmonella ReA, 11 patients were typed and four were HLA-B27-positive.[15] Of the remainder all had cross-reacting group (CREG) antigens: six were HLA-B7, one was HLA-Bw60. This finding of CREG antigens in HLA-B27-negative RS had previously been observed by Arnett and colleagues.[20] The precise role that the class I antigen is playing in the pathogenesis of the disease has been one of the most provocative conundrums in current rheumatology research. The recent advances in our knowledge of the structure and function of these surface molecules have been extensive. The x-ray crystallographic structure of the molecules[21] reveals an antigen-binding groove that appears ideally suited to the function of presenting processed peptides to the T-cell receptor of an HLA-CD8-positive cytotoxic T cell. Furthermore, cloning and sequencing studies have defined those key amino acid residues that render the HLA-B27 molecule different from other class I antigens,[22] and mutagenesis experiments have identified key epitopes for the binding of anti-HLA-B27 monoclonal antibodies.[23] Theories to apply this new knowledge to the unknown mechanisms underlying the development of ReA have included molecular mimicry, which postulates that cross-reactivity of endogenous and microbial antigens plays a key role in the process. Support comes from sequence homology studies[24,25] and monoclonal antibodies,[26-28] but the identification of cross-reacting antibodies in patient sera has proved more difficult.[29,30] Several centers are actively pursuing this question. The possibility that the HLA-B27 molecule may function as a receptor for these intracellular pathogens has been raised, by analogy with human immunodeficiency virus (HIV) for the HLA-CD4 molecule,[31] but this remains unresolved. The major histocompatibility complex (MHC) region of the sixth chromosome in humans is the site of genes encoding several important immune reactants (tumor necrosis factor, complement components) and it may be that genes as yet unidentified encoding immune regulatory proteins are in strong linkage disequilibrium with the HLA class I genes but this remains at present speculative only.

The sites of the antecedent infections that are harbingers of ReA are primarily genitourinary and gastrointestinal. Whether a common mechanism, for example, microbial interaction with mucosal epithelial receptors, underlies this fact is unknown. Antecedent central nervous system infection may on occasion initiate a sterile synovitis as in the case of Neisseria meningitidis[32] or Hemophilus influenzae.[33] Chronic pulmonary infections as in cystic fibrosis may develop an ReA-like picture,[34] but in these examples the HLA relationships have not been defined.

The characteristic immune response that differentiates the HLA-B27-positive infected patient with ReA from his HLA-B27-negative counterpart with an uncomplicated course of infection has proved elusive. Serologic studies comparing Chlamydia-related RS and nonspecific urethritis have found differing reactivity to microbial antigens in these two patient groups.[35] It is of interest that one of the primary antigens recognized by the postvenereal RS sera is a 57-kd protein. Recently Morisson and colleagues[36] have determined that this component of Chlamydia trachomatis is a heat-shock protein and that it is the key antigen eliciting a cellular immune response in experimental chlamydial conjunctivitis.

A point source epidemic allows a more rigorous examination of the question of a characteristic immune response to infection. In our cohort of patients with and without ReA following infection with Salmonella typhimurium, we compared the cellular immune response to the pathogen in the two patient groups.[37] The causative pathogen was used to examine peripheral blood lymphocyte proliferation by ^{3}H-thymidine incorporation. Impairment in lymphocyte response to the antigen in the patients with ReA was demonstrated by (1) lower stimulation index, (2) lower in vitro immunoglobulin production, and (3) lower antigen-induced interleukin-2 (IL-2) production. Exogenous IL-2 when added to the proliferation assay corrected the depressed lymphocyte response in the ReA patients. The basis for this altered response has not yet been defined, although a soluble suppressor factor appears not to be the basis for the phenomenon. Because antigenicity is regarded as the degree of foreignness from self, this may indirectly relate to the notion of molecular mimicry in individuals bearing the cross-reacting host antigens. This is presently under investigation.

The fundamental mechanisms underlying the synovitis itself in ReA have not been defined. In the postjejunoileal bypass syndrome there is evidence of circulating immune complexes formed in part by enteric microbial antigens.[38] As mentioned above, immune complexes have not been consistently demonstrable in ReA.[12] There are few studies to define the immunohistopathology of the disease. The articular involvement in ReA is not adequately explained by postulating autoreactivity against HLA-B27 as the central event since the class I MHC antigens are represented on all nucleated cells in the body. On the other hand, if there is cross-reactivity between a microbial antigen and an articular antigen in the host, then inflammation restricted to the joints might be explained. A precedent for this exists in the model of adjuvant arthritis in which T-cell clones have been identified that cross-react with the peptidoglycan moiety of Mycobacterium tuberculosis and cartilage proteoglycan in the joint.[39] This hypothesis awaits formal testing in ReA.

Differential Diagnosis

The primary diagnostic challenge confronting the clinician with this group of diseases is to rule out a septic process. It is noteworthy that some of the organisms that can trigger ReA such as Yersinia and Salmonella may themselves produce a septic arthritis; therefore sterile synovial fluid on appropriate culture remains a precondition for the diagnosis of ReA. Of interest is the recent demonstration of Chlamydia antigens in the synovial membrane and synovial fluid of some patients with postvenereal RS.[40,41] Although the organism may not be recoverable on culture in such cases, the demonstration of local antigen in a sense blurs the distinction between a reactive process and a septic one.[42] The most common diagnosis to exclude in evaluating polyarthritis in a young male is gonococcal arthritis. Both gonococcal arthritis and RS may involve tenosynovitis, urethritis, conjunctivitis, and skin lesions. An attentive approach to culturing synovial fluid and extra-articular sites is necessary to rule out gonococcal arthritis. On occasion the syndromes may overlap. We have encountered three HLA-B27-positive patients with oligoarthritis who had positive urethral cultures for gonococcus. The arthritis did not respond to antibiotic therapy although the urethritis was cured. Whether such cases are attributable to a coexisting Chlamydia infection or to the fact that Neisseria gonorrhoeae may itself be a legitimate microbial trigger for RS in an immunogenetically susceptible patient has not been defined. The other common exclusion in differential diagnosis is one of the other seronegative spondyloarthropathies. Postdiarrheal arthritis may represent the rheumatic manifestation of inflammatory bowel disease, particularly if an enteric pathogen is not isolated. Such cases may necessitate gastrointestinal radiographic studies to exclude this possibility. An unusual skin rash and arthritis may represent psoriatic arthritis rather than RS and in fact the histopathology of the skin lesions are remarkably similar. Coexisting urethritis and mouth ulcers, or antecedent diarrhea would favor RS in the differential diagnosis. On some occasions, it is only the natural history and the evolution of the disease that correctly defines the diagnostic category.

Treatment

In general the newer nonsteroidal anti-inflammatory drugs (NSAIDs) are superior to aspirin in controlling the synovitis. Indomethacin and diclofenac are generally well tolerated in the young patients who constitute the majority of the disease population, but dyspepsia and gastritis may be a problem with either drug. Often high-dose, sustained therapy with a NSAID is required to make an impact on the activity of the arthritis. Intermittent intra-articular corticosteroid injections are of benefit particularly in monoarthritis or oligoarthritis. Oral steroids are rarely if ever indicated for the joint disease and it has been our observation that the acute synovitis in RS is more steroid-resistant than is rheumatoid arthritis in any event.

In a case of inflammation triggered by a microbial antigen it is rational to try to eliminate the source of that antigen. Nevertheless it has not been definitely proved by any means that antibiotic therapy alters the natural history of RS. In the case of an established positive culture (e.g., recovery of Chlamydia trachomatis from the urethra), appropriate antibiotic therapy is indicated. It is of interest to note that tetracycline may have immunoregulatory properties independent of its antimicrobial action.[43] This same question of dual mechanism is also raised for sulfasalazine, a drug being used increasingly as second-line therapy in RS patients who have a suboptimal response to NSAIDs.[44] Whether sulfasalazine works primarily as an antimicrobial agent altering gut flora or as anti-inflammatory agent is as unresolved in RS as it is in Crohn's disease.

Management of patients with chronic progressive disease is more difficult. Methotrexate has been used for several years in RS.[45-48] With the current popularity of methotrexate in treating rheumatoid arthritis there has been renewed interest in its use in RS.[49] Low-dose methotrexate (10 to 15 mg per week orally) appears to be safe and well tolerated, with the same precautionary measures as applied in the rheumatoid population. In the only controlled study using azathioprine, eight patients were entered into a 16-week crossover study.[50] Joint scores diminished during azathioprine therapy and NSAID requirements decreased. This small study suggests that azathioprine may work rapidly in RS and a larger study is warranted.

An additional issue in management is the important role of education and reassurance of the patient. Particularly in postvenereal RS, or in a case of postdysenteric RS in which balanitis and urethritis are prominent, the patient may express considerable anxiety over the genital symptoms. A thorough discussion about what is known and not known about the cause of RS should be included in the care of the patient. Some authors have recommended the use of condoms for future sexual activity once the disease has settled and if there is a chance of new exposure to sexually transmitted infections this is sound advice. For the patient who has had previous postdysenteric ReA and who inquires about foreign travel to an area of endemic intestinal pathogens, there is currently no proven role for prophylactic antimicrobial therapy and one can only exercise the logical travel precautions regarding local food and water consumption that any traveler would employ.

Prognosis

The medical literature contains a broad view on the natural history of RS, from one predicting a self-limited benign course to a disease of serious long-term morbidity. Part of this variability relates to different diagnostic criteria for study entry, different approaches to therapy, and a retrieval bias in which the patients who do well may be lost to followup while those with more severe disease are more easily identified. Csonka[51] described recurrent attacks of RS occurring over a long followup period, and Hawkes[52] reported that 40 percent of RS patients had recurrent attacks. The acute episodes lasted from 3 weeks to 5 years, and symptom-free intervals were from 3 weeks to 18 years.

Butler and co-workers[53] described 48 RS patients with a mean followup period of 6.5 years. At followup 22 percent were asymptomatic, 24 percent had recurrent minor symptoms, 24 percent had recurrent moderate symptoms, and 30 percent had recurrent major symptoms. However, even in the last groups all patients were in functional classes 1 or 2 between the flareups of disease. In contrast, the study of Fox and associates[8] described a more significant degree of long-term disability in their study of 131 RS patients at a university clinic and community health center. The mean followup period was 5.6 years. Twenty-two percent of patients had annoying symptoms, 34 percent had sustained disease activity, 16 percent had to change jobs, and 11 percent were unemployable. In this study, the presence of the HLA-B27 antigen (83 percent of patients) conferred a higher risk of sacroiliitis and uveitis. Leirisalo and associates[7] also reported the relationship between HLA-B27 and sacroiliitis, as well as more severe disease during the acute phase. A late followup (21-year interval) of 17 patients with RS was reported by Marks and Holt.[54] Five of the original group went on to develop ankylosing spondylitis, but this was unrelated to the extent of the initial peripheral arthritis. Larger joint disease (hip and shoulder) were related to the development of ankylosing spondylitis, whereas small joint destruction appeared to be a feature of RS per se.

The variable reports on the natural history of RS make it difficult not only to accurately prognosticate for an individual patient but also to determine the efficacy of any new therapeutic modalities. While the identification of HLA-B27 as the immunogenetic marker of the seronegative spondyloarthropathies allowed their segregation from other rheumatic diseases, there is still great clinical heterogeneity in the RS/ReA group of patients. A more accurate patient stratification probably awaits a better understanding of the fundamental mechanisms underlying the arthritis. As this forefront advances in the laboratory, prospective studies integrating clinical, microbiologic, and immunologic variables should be ongoing to allow a definition of optimal clinical care of these patients.

References

1. Reiter, G: Ueber eine bisher unerkannte spirochateninfektien. Dtsch Med Wochenschr 42:1535, 1916.
2. Allison, DJ: Christopher Columbus: First case of Reiter's disease in the old world? Lancet ii:1309, 1980.
3. Shafer, N: Why Reiter's disease? N Y State J Med 77:1913, 1977.
4. Arnett, FC: Seronegative spondyloarthropathies. Bull Rheum Dis 37:1, 1987.
5. Linssen, A, and Feltkamp, TEW: B27 positive diseases versus B27 negative diseases. Ann Rheum Dis 47:431, 1988.
6. Willkins, RF et al: Reiter's syndrome: Evaluation of preliminary criteria for definite disease. Bull Rheum Dis 32:31, 1982.

7. Leirisalo, M et al: Follow-up study on patients with Reiter's disease and reactive arthritis, with special reference to HLA-B27. Arthritis Rheum 25:249, 1982.
8. Fox, R et al: The chronicity of symptoms and disability in Reiter's syndrome. An analysis of 131 consecutive patients. Ann Intern Med 91:190, 1979.
9. Inman, RD, Johnston, MEA, and Klein, MH: Analysis of serum and synovial fluid IgA in Reiter's syndrome and reactive arthritis. Clin Immunol Immunopathol 43:195, 1987.
10. Inman, RD, Chiu, B, and Rajanayagam, C: Humoral immune response to Klebsiella pneumoniae in ankylosing spondylitis. Arthritis Rheum 32:S37, 1989.
11. Rosenbaum, JT et al: Presence of circulating immune complexes in Reiter's syndrome and ankylosing spondylitis. Clin Immunol Immunopathol 18:291, 1981.
12. Inman, RD, and Klein, MH: Immunological studies of serum and synovial fluid in Reiter's syndrome. Arthritis Rheum 27:85, 1984.
13. Granfors, K et al: Persistence of IgM, IgG and IgA antibodies to Yersinia in Yersinia arthritis. J Infect Dis 141:424, 1980.
14. Keat, AC: Reiter's syndrome and reactive arthritis in perspective. N Engl J Med 309:1606, 1983.
15. Inman, RD et al: Post-dysenteric reactive arthritis: A clinical and immunogenetic study following an outbreak of salmonellosis. Arthritis Rheum 31:1377, 1988.
16. Doury, P et al: Le rheumatisme de l'anguillulose. Nouv Presse Med 4:805, 1975.
17. Gertner, E, and Inman, RD: Aseptic arthritis in a man with toxic shock syndrome. Arthritis Rheum 29:910, 1986.
18. Inman, RD: Antigenic cross reactions in rheumatic fever. In: Toivanen A, Toivanen P (eds): Reactive Arthritis. Boca Raton, Fla., CRC Press, 1988, p 273.
19. Ayoub, EM et al: Association of class II human histocompatibility leukocyte antigens with rheumatic fever. J Clin Invest 77:2019, 1986.
20. Arnett, FC, Hochberg, MC, and Bias, WG: Cross-reactive HLA antigens in B27-negative Reiter's syndrome and sacroiliitis. Johns Hopkins Med J 141:193, 1977.
21. Bjorkman PJ et al: The foreign antigen binding site and T cell recognition regions of class I histocompatibility antigens. Nature 329:512, 1987.
22. Parham P et al: Nature of polymorphism in HLA-A, -B, and -C molecules. Proc Natl Acad Sci USA 85:4005, 1988.
23. El-Zaatari, F, Carter, KL, and Taurog, JD: Analysis of HLA-B27 antigenic structure by site-directed mutagenesis. Arthritis Rheum 32:S82, 1989.
24. Schwimmbeck, PL, Yu, DTY, and Oldstone, MBA: Autoantibodies to HLA-B27 in the sera of HLA-B27 patients with ankylosing spondylitis and Reiter's syndrome. J Exp Med 166:173, 1987.
25. Steiglitz, H, Fosmire, S, and Lipsky, PE: Bacterial epitopes involved in the induction of reactive arthritis. Am J Med 85:56, 1988.
26. Ogasawara, M, Kono, DH, and Yu, DTY: Mimicry of human histocompatability HLA B27 antigen by Klebsiella pneumoniae. Infect Immun 51:901, 1986.
27. Van Bohemen, CG, Grumet, FC, and Zanen, HC: Identification of HLA B27 M1 and M2 cross-reactive antigens in Klebsiella, Shigella, and Yersinia. Immunology 52:607, 1984.
28. Raybourne, RB, Bunning, VK, and Williams, KM: Reaction of anti-HLA B monoclonal antibodies with envelope proteins of Shigella species. J Immunol 140:3489, 1988.
29. Cavender, D, and Ziff, M: Anti-HLA-B27 antibodies in sera from patients with gram-negative bacterial infections. Arthritis Rheum 29:352, 1986.
30. Inman, RD, Johnston, MEA, and Falk, J: Molecular mimicry in Reiter's syndrome: Cytotoxicity and ELISA studies of HLA-microbial relationships. Immunology 58:501, 1986.
31. Sattentau, QJ, and Weiss, RA: The CD4 antigen: Physiological ligand and HIV receptor. Cell 52:631, 1988.
32. Fam, AG, Tanenbaum, J, and Stein, JL: Clinical forms of meningococcal arthritis: A study of five cases. J Rheumatol 6:567, 1979.
33. Rush, PJ et al: Arthritis associated with Hemophilus influenzae. J Pediatr 109:412, 1986.
34. Rush, PJ et al: The musculoskeletal manifestations of cystic fibrosis. Semin Arthritis Rheum 15:213, 1986.
35. Inman, RD et al: Immunochemical analysis of immune response to Chlamydia trachomatis in Reiter's syndrome and nonspecific urethritis. Clin Exp Immunol 69:246, 1987.
36. Morrison, RP, Lyng, K, and Caldwell, HD: Chlamydial disease pathogenesis: Ocular hypersensitivity elicited by a genus-specific 57-KD protein. J Exp Med 169:663, 1989.
37. Inman, RD et al: HLA Class-I related impairment in IL-2 production and lymphocyte response to microbial antigens in reactive arthritis. J Immunol 142:4256, 1989.
38. Wands, JR et al: Arthritis associated with intestinal bypass procedure for marked obesity. N Engl J Med 294:121, 1976.
39. Van Eden, W et al: Arthritis induced by a T-lymphocyte clone that responds to Mycobacterium tuberculosis and to cartilage proteoglycans. Proc Natl Acad Sci USA 82: 5117, 1985.
40. Keat, A et al: Chlamydia trachomatis and reactive arthritis: The missing link. Lancet i:72, 1987.
41. Schumacher, HR et al: Light and electron microscopic studies on the synovial membrane in Reiter's syndrome. Arthritis Rheum 31:937, 1988.
42. Inman, RD, Chiu, B, and Katz A: Immunological features of "reactive arthritis" due to Chlamydia trachomatis. Arthritis Rheum 32:S113, 1989.
43. Arsenis, C et al: Tetracyclines inhibit the synthesis and activity of neutral proteinase activities in vitro and in vivo. Arthritis Rheum 32:S319, 1989.
44. Dougados, M et al: Sulfasalazine in spondyloarthropathies. Arthritis Rheum 37:S38, 1989.

45. Farber, GA, Forshner, JG, and O'Quinn, SE: Reiter's syndrome: Treatment with methotrexate. JAMA 200:181, 1967.
46. Jefton, RL, and Duncan, WC: Treatment of Reiter's syndrome with methotrexate. Ann Intern Med 70:349, 1969.
47. Topp, JR, Fam, AG, and Hart, GD: Treatment of Reiter's syndrome with methotrexate. Can Med Assoc J 105:1168, 1971.
48. Owen, ET, and Cohen, ML: Methotrexate in Reiter's disease. Ann Rheum Dis 38:48, 1979.
49. Lally, EV, and HO, G: A review of methotrexate in Reiter's syndrome. Semin Arthritis Rheum 15:139, 1985.
50. Calin, A: A placebo controlled crossover study of azathioprine in Reiter's syndrome. Ann Rheum Dis 45:653, 1986.
51. Csonka, GW: The course of Reiter's syndrome. Br Med J 1:1088, 1958.
52. Hawkes, JG: Clinical and diagnostic features of Reiter's disease: A follow-up study of 39 patients. N Z Med J 78:347, 1973.
53. Butler, MJ et al: A follow-up study of 48 patients with Reiter's syndrome. Am J Med 67:808, 1979.
54. Marks, JS, and Holt, PLJ: The natural history of Reiter's disease—21 years of observation. Q J Med 60:685, 1986.

Chapter 7
Vasculitis

MICHAEL D. LOCKSHIN, M.D., F.A.C.P.

Introduction

Although the term *vasculitis* is common in medical parlance, the use by different disciplines of different definitions, many imprecise, causes considerable confusion. Scattered occlusion of multiple anatomically dispersed blood vessels of any size is the common denominator of all definitions. The variables of definitions include vessel size, vessel wall necrosis, demonstration of (certain types) of inflammation, and acceptance in the absence of biopsy of clinical, dermatologic, and neurologic syndromes. This chapter reviews the many definitions of vasculitis but accepts the clinical (rheumatologic) definition; focus is on differential diagnosis and treatment. Since little is known about the causes or pathogenesis of vasculitis, there is only brief mention of these aspects.

Definitions

The clinical syndromes of vasculitis are differentiable according to involved vessel size, presence of underlying disease, and time course. The major elements of classification are outlined in Table 7-1, and the definitions used by various medical disciplines in Table 7-2.

Rheumatologic Definition. The most common definition is that of clinical rheumatology.[1-5] In this definition diagnoses are made according to the presence or absence of underlying disease (for instance, polyarteritis nodosa [no accompanying disease] vs. rheumatoid vasculitis), according to vessel size (polyarteritis nodosa vs. Takayasu's arteritis), and according to time course ("allergic" vasculitis vs. polyarteritis nodosa). The rheumatologic definition of vasculitis assumes the presence of inflammation. Its

Table 7-1. Classification of Vasculitis Syndromes

Method of Differentiation	Examples
By vessel size:	
Small artery and/or vein	Leukocytoclastic vasculitis
Medium-sized artery and/or vein	Polyarteritis nodosa
Large artery	Takayasu's arteritis
Capillary	Capillary vasculitis
By presence of underlying disease:	
No underlying disease	Leukocytoclastic vasculitis
Underlying disease	
Collagen disease	Leukocytoclastic vasculitis due to Sjögren's syndrome
	Rheumatoid vasculitis
	Lupus vasculitis
Infection	Leukocytoclastic vasculitis due to endocarditis
Malignancy	Leukocytoclastic vasculitis due to lymphoma
Allergen	Allergic vasculitis
By time course:	
Abrupt, unicyclic	Allergic vasculitis
Polycyclic, relapsing	Polyarteritis nodosa
Chronic	Takayasu's arteritis

accompanying phenomena are sought: elevated erythrocyte sedimentation rate, hypergammaglobulinemia, anemia of chronic disease, and leukocytosis. Fever, malaise, myalgia, and weight loss are also common. There may be rashes that reflect the involved vessel size, and there must be evidence of end-organ damage. In this construction vasculitis is not an independent diagnosis but a syndrome description. Similarly, the rheumatologic definition implies systemic illness. Pathologic confirmation is not obligatory but is often useful. *Vessel wall necrosis*

Table 7-2. Definitions of Vasculitis by Different Specialty Groups

Group	Primary criteria	Comments
Rheumatology	Systemic illness Inflammation present End-organ damage present	Syndrome description rather than diagnosis; primary causes must be sought
Pathology	Vessel wall necrosis (endothelial cell necrosis) (disruption of internal elastic membrane)	Inflammation not required End-organ damage not required Differential diagnosis depends on specific pathology features
Radiology	Angiography: tapering, narrowing, constriction and/or dilatation of arteries (not explained by atherosclerosis or other known vascular abnormality) CT or MRI: multiple areas consistent with infarction MRI: perivascular inflammation	Abnormalities can be mimicked by spasm Nonsystemic diagnoses fullfill criteria Abnormalities can be mimicked by nonvascular disease, e.g., demyelination
Neurology	Mononeuritis multiplex CT or MRI abnormality as above Severe symmetric peripheral neuropathy Nonatherosclerotic, nonembolic multiple stroke syndrome Rapidly progressive cerebral vascular disease	After exclusion of other known causes Systemic illness not necessarily implied Inflammation not necessarily implied Separate syndrome
Dermatology	Various forms of palpable purpura or atypical urticaria (livedo reticularis)	Systemic illness not necessarily implied

and *inflammatory (usually polymorphonuclear leukocyte) response* is present. Noninflammatory vascular injury or occlusion would not satisfy this definition, nor would angiographic or other radiologic demonstration of vascular abnormality if the accompanying clinical phenomena were not simultaneously present.

At the margins of the definition, patients with collagen diseases frequently develop small vessel vascular changes in periungual areas, at the finger pads, over the extensor surfaces, of the small joints, and on the palms. Although these lesions have diagnostic importance, represent forms of vascular abnormality, and are often casually referred to by clinicians as vasculitis, these lesions fall within the definitions of the specific collagen disease and are not considered in the discussion of vasculitis.

Pathologic Definition. A pathologist's use of the term vasculitis differs from that of the clinical rheumatologist.[6-8] By light, immuno-, and electron-microscopy, *vascular necrosis* is the predominant characteristic sought by pathologists. Usually identified by fibrinoid change within the muscular arterial wall or by disruption of the muscular arterial wall or by disruption of the arterial internal elastic membrane, the criterion for necrosis may also be satisfied by isolated evidence of endothelial cell or venous injury. Infiltration of inflammatory cells within and through the arterial wall is commonly present but not obligatory. End-organ ischemia or infarction is also not obligatory. Perivascular inflammation without vascular necrosis, common in the collagen diseases, does not fulfill the pathologist's definition of vasculitis. The noninflammatory vascular injuries of scleroderma, renal crisis or malignant hypertension fulfill many pathologists' definitions of vasculitis. Severe inflammatory sites, and some malignances, often have inflammatory vascular necrosis in the immediate area of the lesion. Pathologically present, vasculitis in this setting does not imply systemic disease.

The size of the involved vessel and the simultaneity of lesions (if many are found) permit the pathologist to suggest clinical classifications, for instance to distinguish polyarteritis nodosa from allergic vasculitis, and to make fine distinctions based on the presence or absence of venous abnormalities; types of inflammatory cells; presence or absence of immunoglobulins, fibrin, and complement; and evidence of utilization of complement.

The pathologist's definitions are often based on autopsy rather than biopsy material; the distinctions taught in medical school are seldom achievable with the small amounts from limited areas of materials available to the treating physician. The most important lesson for the clinican is to accept a pathology report of vasculitis as a description, not a diagnosis, and to place it in context with other information available.

Radiologic Definition. Radiologists diagnose as vasculitis angiographic abnormalities of blood vessels that have no alternative explanations.[9-17] These abnormalities include *alternating areas of constriction and dilatation (aneurysms), and multiple unexplained cutoffs.* Radiologists impute neither systemic illness nor inflammation to the visualized abnormality. In angiography, *vascular spasm* induced by drugs, by local infection or tumor, or by processes such as migraine may suggest vasculitis. In computed tomography (CT) scans, *multiple areas of infarction* caused by thrombi, as in the antiphospholipid antibody syndrome, may also suggest vasculitis, as may scattered high intensity signals in magnetic resonance imaging (MRI).

Neurologic Definition. The neurologic definition[18,19] of vasculitis depends in part on interpretation (with radiologists) of head and spinal cord CT and MRI scans and in part on the clinical appearance without other explanation of vascular occlusions (usually stroke), *mononeuritis multiplex,* or *severe peripheral neuropathy.* As with the definitions offered by other disciplines, the definition offered by neurology does not necessarily imply systemic illness or inflammation.

Syndromes

The clinical syndromes recognized by rheumatologists are listed in Table 7-3.

Small Vessel Vasculitis (Leukocytoclastic Vasculitis)

Leukocytoclastic vasculitis occurs either as an isolated phenomenon or as a symptom or complication of another disease. Leukocytoclastic vasculitis is recognized by a clinically variable rash. The lesions of leukocytoclastic vasculitis are raised and hemorrhagic: "palpable purpura" (Fig. 7-1). The size and appearance of lesions varies among patients (a few millimeters to more than a centimeter) but is rather constant for an individual patient. The lesions frequently have necrotic centers. Clusters of lesions may ulcerate widely leaving only an ankle or other ulcer as a diagnostic clue. Lesions in patients with Wegener's granulomatosis tend to have more heaped

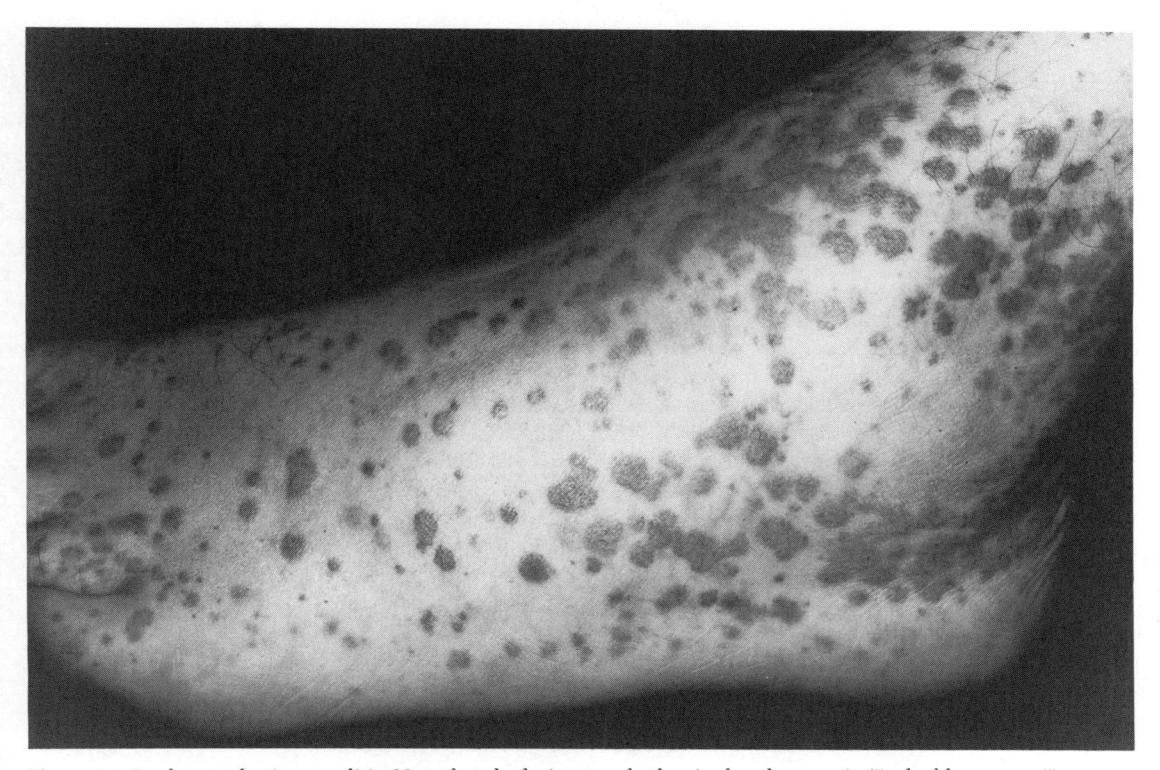

Figure 7-1. Leukocytoclastic vasculitis. Note that the lesions are both raised and purpuric ("palpable purpura").

Table 7-3. Forms of Vasculitis

Vessel Size	Diagnosis	Underlying Disease	Course
Small artery and/or vein	Leukocytoclastic vasculitis	None	Polycyclic
		Sjögren's syndrome	Polycyclic or chronic
		Systemic lupus erythematosus	Polycyclic
		Rheumatoid arthritis	Polycyclic
		Wegener's granulomatosis	Polycyclic
		Infection	Unicyclic
		Malignancy	Unicyclic
		Allergic	Unicyclic
		Henoch-Schönlein	Polycyclic
		Cryoglobulinemia	Polycyclic
Small arteriole and/or venule	Periungual telangiectasia	Systemic lupus erythematosus	Chronic
		Scleroderma	Chronic
		Dermatomyositis	Chronic
Medium-sized artery and/or vein	Polyarteritis nodosa	Rheumatoid arthritis	Chronic
		Systemic lupus erythematosus	Unicyclic or chronic
		Wegener's granulomatosis	Polycyclic or chronic
		Dermatomyositis	Chronic
		Hepatitis B infection	Unicyclic or chronic
		Allergic	Unicyclic
		None (PAN)	Unicyclic, polycyclic or chronic
		None (cutaneous PAN)	Polycyclic
	Isolated cranial arteritis	None	Unicyclic
Large artery	Takayasu's arteritis	—	Chronic
	Giant cell arteritis	—	Polycyclic or chronic
	Syphilis	Syphilis	Unicyclic
	Tuberculosis	Tuberculosis	Unicyclic
	Polychondritis	Relapsing polychondritis	Chronic
Capillary	Capillary vasculitis	—	Chronic

PAN = polyarteritis nodosa.

up bases than do lesions in patients with other diagnoses. The rash is neither painful nor pruritic. It appears in crops over the lower legs and feet. Less commonly, but characteristically, it appears over the anterior knee and extensor aspect of the elbow, and occasionally on the dorsum of the hands overlying the metacarpophalangeal joints. The reasons for this distribution are unknown. In some diseases the distribution of lesions has diagnostic importance: patients with systemic lupus erythematosus frequently have lesions over the elbows; those with Henoch-Schönlein purpura frequently have lesions on the buttocks. The lesions are clinically very distinct from the much larger, painful, highly erythematous and nonulcerating lesions of erythema nodosum. Urticaria, atypical in the large size of the hive, its duration over many hours to days, and its relative absence of pruritus, is a less common manifestation of leukocytoclastic vasculitis. The lesions of leukocytoclastic vasculitis commonly leave scars when they heal.[20–22]

Although in the majority of patients involvement is limited to the skin and subcutaneous tissue, limited visceral involvement may occur. Three extracutaneous organ systems are affected: peripheral nerves, small intestine, and kidney.[23] The presence of leukocytoclastic vasculitis does not exclude the simultaneous presence of other forms of vasculitis, but this is uncommon.

Without Associated Collagen Disease. Isolated leukocytoclastic vasculitis occurs predominantly in young women, recurs episodically over years, causes little visceral disease, and eventually disappears, leaving chronically scarred, often ulcerated, legs. During episodes patients have fatigue and malaise. The erythrocyte sedimentation rate may be elevated. Urinalysis is usually normal, as are the fluorescent antinuclear antibody test and tests for specific antinuclear and cytoplasmic antibodies. A chronic, slowly progressive glomerulonephritis may occur. Intestinal perforation due to involvement of the small bowel is rare and is a late phenomenon. Once underlying named collagen disease has been initially excluded, patients with isolated leukocytoclastic vasculitis do not progress to develop another collagen disease.

With Associated Collagen Disease. Leukocytoclastic vasculitis occurs by definition in patients with Henoch-Schönlein purpura, commonly occurs in patients with Sjögren's syndrome and with IgG-IgM cryoglobulinemia, and occasionally occurs in patients with rheumatoid arthritis, Wegener's granulomatosis, and systemic lupus erythematosus. Microscopic ("capillary") vasculitis may be a variant of Wegener's granulomatosis limited to the kidneys. (In both of these latter diseases antineutrophil cytoplasmic antibody is present). In each of the above diseases a characteristic clinical pattern is the main criterion for differentiating the disease from nonspecific leukocytoclastic vasculitis. In Henoch-Schönlein purpura, gastrointestinal and renal involvement are the rule. A relapsing course with eventual remission occurs in most cases, but lethal intestinal perforation or renal failure may occur. Hypertension is uncommon. The disease is most common in children; the apparent rarity in older age groups may simply reflect a preference of physicians' caring for older patients to use a more general terminology when neither the biopsy nor the clinical course is definitive. Childhood Henoch-Schönlein purpura may occur after a defined viral infection; in adult leukocytoclastic vasculitis, infections have also been triggers in some circumstances. In patients with cryoglobulinemia an indolent but progressive glomerulonephritis, manifested by microscopic hematuria and quantitatively small amounts of proteinuria, may over years lead to renal failure.

Glomerulonephritis, intestinal perforation, and severe peripheral neuropathy are uncommon complications of leukocytoclastic vasculitis. In the majority of patients, if the rash does not ulcerate it is seldom more than a cosmetic nuisance; overall prognosis is good, but recurrent periods of malaise, fatigue, arthralgia, and rash are the rule.

With Other Diseases. Leukocytoclastic vasculitis probably represents an (allergic) immunologic response to an extrinsic antigen. Leukocytoclastic vasculitis therefore is often the first symptom of systemic infection.[24-26] Commonly encountered infections in the United States that cause leukocytoclastic vasculitis include chronic bacteremias such as infectious endocarditis and chronic meningococcemia or gonococcemia. Nonbacterial infections may also cause leukocytoclastic vasculitis. Examples include a variety of viral infections, including hepatitis B, tuberculosis, atypical mycobacterial infection, and leprosy. The visual appearance of leukocytoclastic vasculitis associated with infection does not differ from that associated with collagen disease, but detailed clinical history and laboratory evaluation suggests the former diagnosis. There is less of a tendency of infection-associated leukocytoclastic vasculitis to remit; high fevers, seldom present in isolated leukocytoclastic vasculitis, profound illness, weight loss, and rapid clinical deterioration are all clues to infection. Immunizations and defined allergens have also on occasion triggered leukocytoclastic vasculitis.[27,28,29]

When there is known exposure to an allergen, when the illness is sudden in onset and appears to have peaked within a single time point, it is appropriate to attribute leukocytoclastic vasculitis to an allergic exposure. This form of leukocytoclastic vasculitis is occasionally catastrophic. Acute renal failure and extensive infarction of skin and other viscera occur. There is high mortality. If recovery occurs, end-organ damage (renal insufficiency, amputation) limits activity, but there is no recurrence of disease.

Another form of "allergic" exposure is leukocytoclastic vasculitis secondary to malignancy. Leukemias and lymphomas are most commonly reported, but any form of malignancy is possible. Occasionally leukocytoclastic vasculitis occurs with no apparent other cause in midpregnancy. Whether this represents coincidence or a specific patient's response to pregnancy, such as has been suggested for erythema nodosum gravidarum, is unknown.

Differential Diagnosis

Leukocytoclastic vasculitis is differentiated from other diseases by the appearance and distribution of the rash. Small infarctive lesions resembling leukocytoclastic vasculitis also occur in septicemia and in bacteremias with Neisseria, Pseudomonas, Streptococcus pneumoniae, and some staphylococci. Patients with these infections tend to be sicker than patients with leukocytoclastic vasculitis, and to have high fevers and other signs of sepsis. Systemic nonbacterial infections such as disseminated zoster or rickettsial disease (Rocky Mountain spotted fever) may also cause confusion. Small vessel embolization may also occur from cholesterol, fat, amniotic fluid, and fragmenting emboli from intracardiac myxomas. Simultaneous clinical events usually make distinction of the first three circumstances easy. Petechial hemorrhage due to thrombocytopenia, thrombasthenia, or vascular fragility (scurvy) should also be easily distinguishable. Similarly, erythema nodosum, pustular psoriasis, lichen planus, and Kaposi's sarcoma can be distinguished by inspection alone.

In the pseudohive presentation of leukocytoclastic vasculitis, if clinical circumstances do not permit distinction, skin biopsy may be necessary for diagnosis. Skin biopsy may also be useful in hyperacute (allergic) vasculitis and for unexplained ulcers. Skin biopsy is otherwise seldom necessary to diagnose "palpable purpura."

Differential diagnosis among the causes for leukocytoclastic vasculitis requires consideration of the possibilities listed above. Tests for antinuclear antibody, urinalysis, tests for cryoglobulins, clinical examination for associated collagen or infectious disease, and, on occasion, blood culture for bacteria is usually appropriate in the initial evaluation of a patient with a new diagnosis of leukocytoclastic vasculitis.

Pathology

The lesions of leukocytoclastic vasculitis occur in the precapillary or postcapillary vascular bed; the former tend to have leukocytic infiltrates and are associated with hypocomplementemia.[8] The latter have lymphocytic infiltrates and are not associated with hypocomplementemia. As expected, immunopathologic evidence for vessel-bound immunoglobulin and complement is present.[30-35] However, knowledge of these data seldom helps in the differential diagnosis or management of individual patients. Rare patients with leukocytoclastic vasculitis have concomitant complement deficiencies.[36,37]

Treatment

The best treatment is elimination of the primary cause, when one can be found. When there is no identified primary cause, or when symptomatic treatment is necessary, nonsteroidal anti-inflammatory drugs, antimalarial drugs, colchicine, and corticosteroid drugs should be chosen according to the perceived seriousness and chronicity of the problem.[38,39] Corticosteroid preparations, however, have disappointing effectiveness for all but the malaise and myalgia of the syndrome. Even at high doses they seldom completely control the vasculitis. On occasion experimental therapies such as apheresis have been tried. In most cases neither the systemic involvement nor the time course justify immunosuppressive agents such as cyclophosphamide.

Medium Vessel Vasculitis

Polyarteritis nodosa is the prototype of medium-sized vessel vasculitis. Except for tempo of illness and minor differences of organ predilection, medium-sized vessel vasculitis occurring in patients with systemic lupus erythematosus, rheumatoid arthritis, or other collagen disease does not differ from that occurring in the absence of collagen disease. The pathology in all cases is that of necrosis occurring throughout the entire vessel wall, frequently in a spotty fashion, with intense inflammatory infiltrate, healing with scarring, and always disruption of the internal elastic membrane (Fig. 7-2). This type of vasculitis may produce angiographically visible alternating constrictions and aneuryms.

Without Associated Collagen Disease. There are several variants of polyarteritis nodosa. The most common variant has abrupt onset, with severe myalgia, weight loss, fever, hypertension, and, often, catastrophic interruption of blood supply, resulting in bowel, extremity, or cardiac infarction.[40-45] Mononeuritis multiplex or cutaneous signs of vasculitis are often clues to the diagnosis. A less common variant has a multiyear antecedent history of allergy, including asthma and prominent eosinophilia followed by abrupt multisystem polyarteritis nodosa (Churg-Strauss type). A third form is that of an indolent rather than abrupt, remitting and recurring illness with prominence of cutaneous ulcers and mononeuritis multiplex. A fourth type is frequently called cutaneous polyarteritis nodosa.[45] Patients with this form have nodular and ulcerating skin disease, more evident in the lower extremities, and symptomatic peripheral neuropathy, but rarely have visceral disease. The first three types most commonly occur in middle-aged men; the fourth is more common in young women, but all types occur in both sexes at all ages. Not discussed here is a primarily pediatric disorder consisting of lymphatic hyperplasia, rash, mucositis, and predominantly coronary necrotizing vasculitis (Kawasaki disease, mucocutaneous lymph node syndrome).

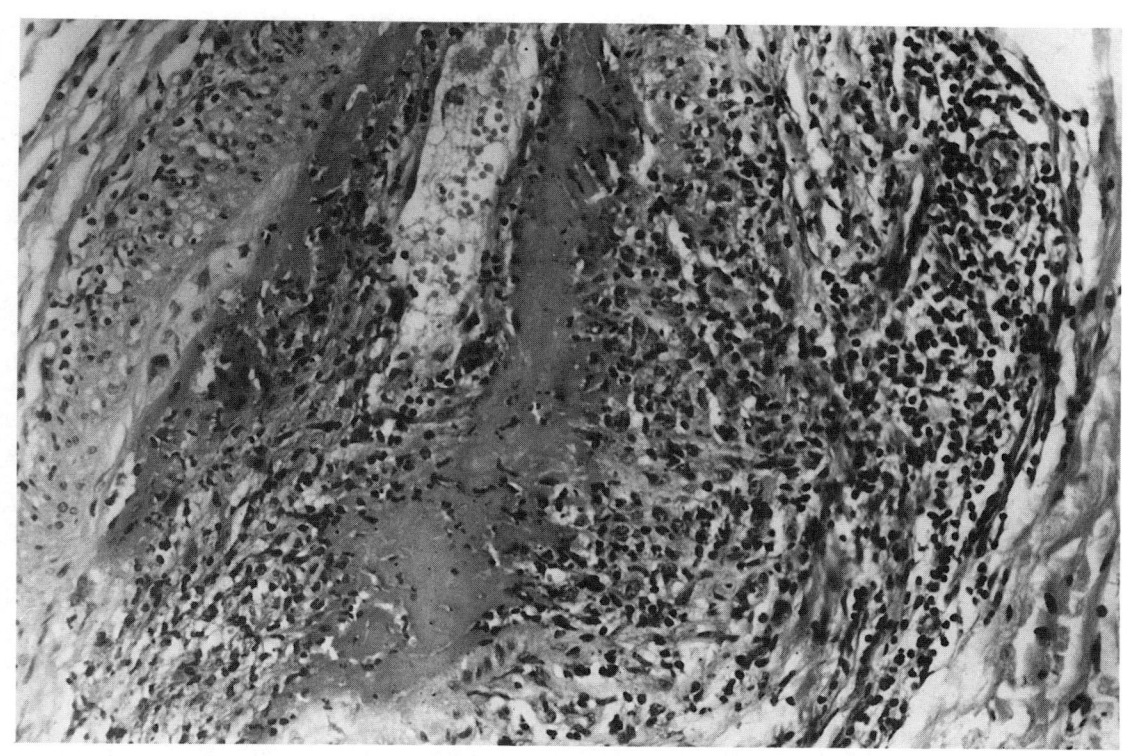

Figure 7-2. Necrotizing vasculitis of the polyarteritis type. There is vessel wall necrosis and through-and-through infiltration with polymorphonuclear leukocytes.

Multiorgan ischemic events are a sine qua non for the diagnosis of systemic necrotizing vasculitis. These include (in order of clinical frequency) renovascular hypertension, mononeuritis multiplex, cutaneous, digital or extremity gangrene, bowel gangrene, stroke, and cardiac infarction. In polyarteritis nodosa the erythrocyte sedimentation rate is usually elevated; leukocytosis is usually present. Other laboratory tests, including antinuclear antibody, complement, and immune complex measurements add very little diagnostic information.

A minority of patients with polyarteritis nodosa has had antecedent infection with the hepatitis B virus (antibody to hepatitis B surface antigen).[46-51] In some studies the date of the exposure to hepatitis virus was known. Polyarteritis nodosa occurred within approximately 3 months of the infection. Other infections have also been implicated in the occurrence of polyarteritis nodosa,[52-55] as has illicit use of street drugs,[56] allergy, and immunization.[57-58] Animal models implicating infection, diet, hypertension, and other phenomena have also suggested pathogeneses for polyarteritis nodosa.[59-63] Occasional patients with malignancy, most notably hairy cell leukemia, have polyarteritis nodosa.[64,65] The vasculitis of hepatitis B infection is most commonly abrupt and unicyclic, but all forms of vasculitis, including leukocytoclastic vasculitis, have occurred. These triggers imply that all polyarteritis nodosa represents a host reaction to an extrinsic agent. Regardless of the trigger, the clinical presentation of the vasculitis does not differ.

With Associated Collagen Disease. When polyarteritis nodosa complicates another rheumatic disease it is, by convention, referred to by the name of the original diagnosis: lupus vasculitis, rheumatoid vasculitis, etc.[66-68] These forms of vasculitis often differ from idiopathic polyarteritis nodosa in tempo and organ system involvement, but the pathology is indistinguishable. Rheumatoid vasculitis tends to be the indolent type producing leg ulcers, but may cause digital gangrene or bowel infarction; unlike spontaneous polyarteritis nodosa it rarely involves the renal vessels or kidneys. Lupus vasculitis is often catastrophic, progressing rapidly to multiorgan infarction. Dermatomyositis vasculitis occurs in children much more than in adults; bowel infarction is common. Although vasculitis is an integral part of

Wegener's granulomatosis, the pulmonary infiltrates and glomerulonephritis dominate the clinical picture.

Pathology

Pathologic demonstration of necrotizing vasculitis is confirmatory, not diagnostic. Necrotizing vasculitis occurs in the vicinity of intense (septic or neoplastic) inflammation and occasionally without obvious explanation in an apparently otherwise healthy person. The isolated finding of vascular necrosis around a recently removed gall bladder or appendix is *not* sufficient reason to make a diagnosis of polyarteritis nodosa. Conversely, a negative biopsy result does not exclude the diagnosis. Muscle biopsy of the deltoid, gastrocnemius, or quadriceps in a patient in whom there is clinical suspicion of systemic necrotizing vasculitis identifies the diagnosis in over two thirds of patients. Except for an occasional inflamed nodule, there is little merit to directing biopsies to epididymis or sural nerve; the latter in particular often results in nonhealing biopsy sites (if done distally) or unpleasant symptomatic anesthesia or dysesthesia (if done proximally). Biopsy is preferable as a first diagnostic step because it may demonstrate an unsuspected myxoma, tumor, cholesterol, or septic embolus.

Detailed studies of both the antigen and the host have not revealed the mechanism by which polyarteritis nodosa occurred, nor have these studies indicated why a minute fraction of persons infected with hepatitis B develop vasculitis. Circulating immune complexes, complement-mediated defects in phagocytosis, viral cytotoxicity, and other mechanisms have been suggested,[69–77] but none has been definitively accepted. Moreover, after vasculitis has remitted, serologic evidence of hepatitis B infection persists with no apparent change in circulating immune reactants.[77]

Differential Diagnosis

Differential diagnosis of medium-sized vessel vasculitis depends first on clinical pattern recognition, second on documentation of a consistent pathologic or radiographic finding, and third on reasonable exclusion of alternative diagnoses.

Since the clinical events of polyarteritis nodosa reflect vascular occlusion, other causes of vascular occlusion must be excluded. These alternative diagnoses include atherosclerotic emboli, septic emboli, fragmenting myxoma, and a variety of rare arteriopathies.[78,79] Transient hypotension, with inadequate perfusion of areas with poor vascular supply (because of atherosclerosis or congenital abnormality) can cause a clinical appearance similar to that of a necrotizing vasculitis, as can intense vasospasm seen in ergotism or other drug-induced vascular spastic states. Diabetes and heavy metal intoxications can cause mononeuritis multiplex. Noninflammatory thromboses occur in the primary antiphospholipid antibody syndrome, in protein C, protein S, and antithrombin III deficiencies, and in thrombotic thrombocytopenic purpura. The absence of inflammatory symptoms usually suffices to exclude vasulitis.

Angiographic demonstration of aneurysms, constrictions, or occlusions is an alternative, indirect method of diagnosis (Figs. 7-3 and 7-4). Although these findings can occasionally be diagnostic, most often they are subtle and potentially misleading. Vascular spasm, emboli, atherosclerosis, and, occasionally, fibromuscular dysplasia can cause confusion. Angiography is useful as the first diagnostic test if renovascular hypertension, bowel ischemia, or intraabdominal hemorrhage is the initial presentation.

Treatment

There is no consensus about treatment for non-life-threatening forms of polyarteritis nodosa. Rare patients with indolent, remitting, polycyclic disease improve spontaneously with no treatment. Many patients with unicyclic disease have recovered with high-dose (60 mg prednisone per day) oral corticosteroid, given for 4 to 8 weeks, then tapered and discontinued. In my experience the majority of patients who do not have a lethal complication (such as bowel or cardiac infarction) when first seen respond to this therapy alone. Those with life-threatening complications, those who have not responded within 3 weeks to corticosteroid, and those with recurrent, polycyclic disease usually respond to cyclophosphamide, 100 to 150 mg per day (dose adjusted to keep leukocyte count above 3000 per mm^3). Other immunosuppressive agents, such as azathioprine, tend to be less effective. A septic complication such as bowel infarction with peritoneal contamination importantly restricts therapy options and is usually lethal.[80–83]

Patients who survive the initial illness frequently have residua; permanent neuropathy (foot drop or wrist drop), hypertension, renal insufficiency, or vascular insufficiency of an extremity are common.[47]

Large Vessel Vasculitis

There are two forms of large vessel vasculitis, usually distinguishable clinically but not pathologically.

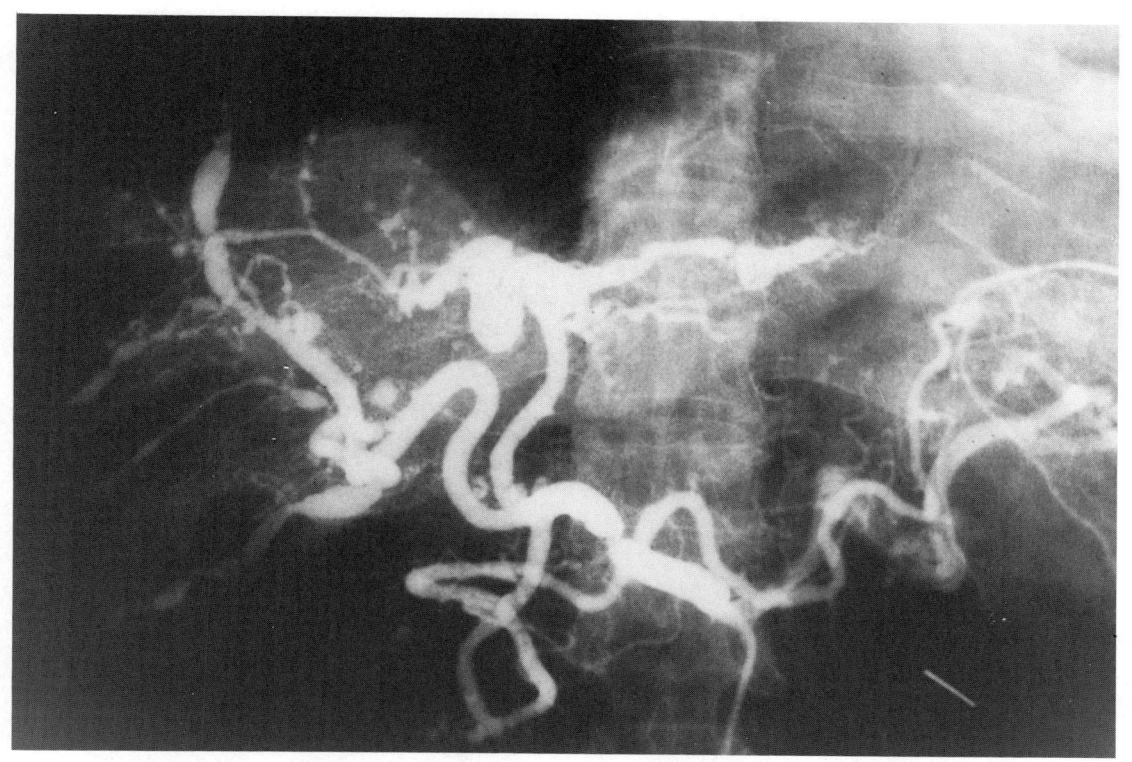

Figure 7-3. Celiac arteriogram of a patient with polyarteritis nodosa. Note the alternating constrictions and dilated areas, particularly in the hepatic circulation (left side of photograph).

Takayasu's arteritis is a disease primarily of young women, that causes inflammation most often of the aorta and brachiocephalic vessels; giant cell or temporal arteritis affects the elderly and attacks the cranial vessels. In occasional patients of intermediate age a clear distinction between diagnoses may not be possible.

Takayasu's Arteritis

Takayasu's arteritis has two major clinical presentations. The most common is that of symptoms related to local arterial constriction or dilatation, including absent pulses (with or without claudication), asymptomatic bruit, cerebrovascular ischemic symptoms, renovascular hypertension, or aortic insufficiency. Patients with these findings usually do not have systemic symptoms or elevated erythrocyte sedimentation rates. The alternative presentation is that of a systemic collagen disease; symptoms include fever, malaise, arthralgia, weight loss, anemia, mild leukocytosis, and an elevated erythrocyte sedimentation rate. In these patients careful physical examination demonstrates arterial tenderness, bruit, or occlusion. An important proportion of patients with Takayasu's arteritis have evidence for antecedent tuberculosis.[84]

Differential Diagnosis. The differential diagnosis for those patients presenting with symptoms related to local arterial disease is that of vascular occlusion, aortic dissection, atherosclerosis, embolus, congenital abnormality, and fibromuscular dysplasia. Arteriography, or possibly magnetic resonance imaging, is almost always indicated; both distinguish among the alternatives. Syphilitic aortitis and relapsing polychondritis are also rarely encountered and are usually diagnosed by other organ involvement or by direct biopsy. For patients presenting with systemic collagen disease symptoms, all of the collagen diseases and many infectious illnesses must be considered; differential diagnosis depends on targeting and visualization of a suspect arterial system (Fig. 7-5). Rarely is arterial biopsy necessary. If done, it shows intense inflammation with giant cells, thick onion-skinned vessels, and striking perivascular scarring. Because of the degree of scarring, rupture or dissection of an involved vessel is rare. Investigation for

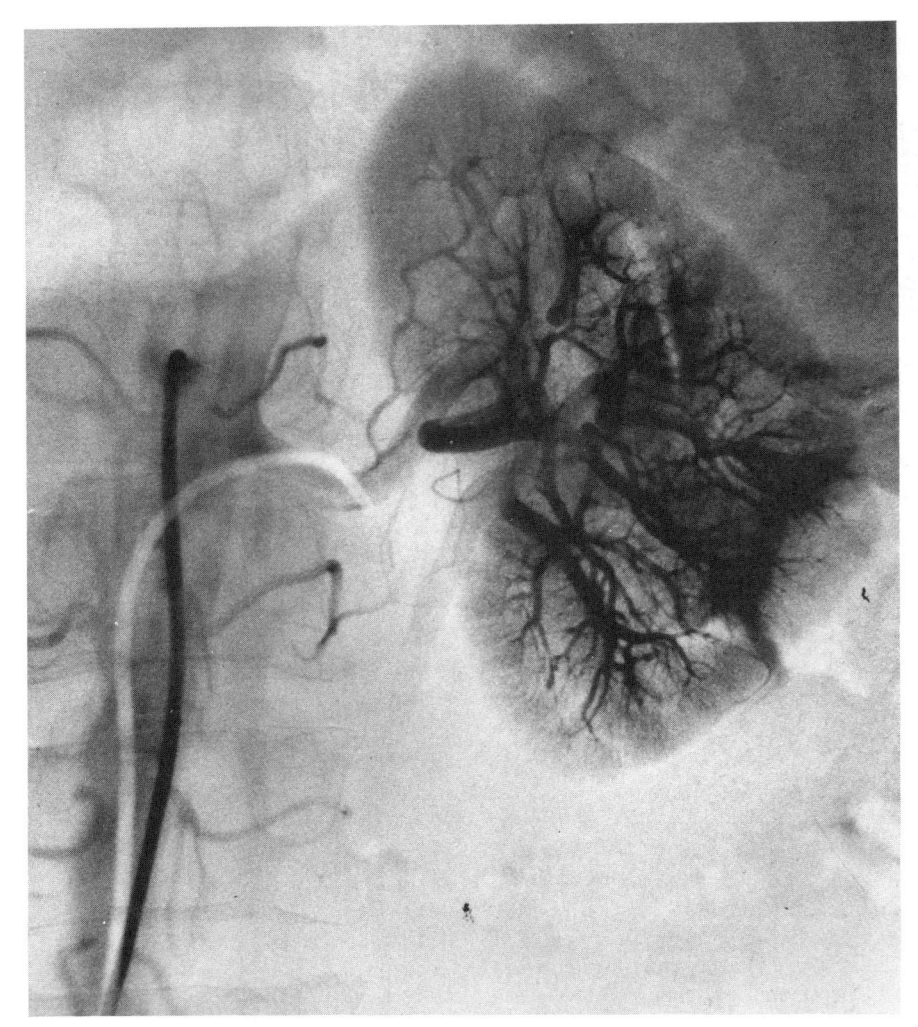

Figure 7-4. Renal arteriogram of another patient with polyarteritis nodosa. This appearance is more typical than that of Figure 3, and is much more subtle. There are small aneurysms visible in the lower pole, in the clear space above the center of the lower pole, and at approximately 2 o'clock in the upper pole.

coexistent tuberculosis is appropriate in all patients with a confirmed diagnosis of Takayasu's arteritis.

Treatment. Patients without signs of inflammation do not need anti-inflammatory treatment, nor is anticoagulation helpful. When indicated, surgical bypass of stenotic areas or replacement of ectatically insufficient aortic valves is possible. For patients with systemic symptoms, corticosteroid therapy improves sense of well-being, reduces pain of tender arteries, and lowers the erythrocyte sedimentation rate. It is controversial whether stenotic arteries will reopen or further occlusions be prevented. The rare patient who does not respond to corticosteroid alone may have the disease controlled if azathioprine or cyclophosphamide is added; it is seldom possible to discontinue this therapy once it is started.[85,87]

Giant Cell Arteritis

Giant cell, temporal, or cranial arteritis also may present with either local or systemic symptoms. Local symptoms may include a swollen, tender, red temporal artery, headache, diplopia, or sudden visual loss.[86-91] The systemic presentation of temporal arteritis includes abrupt, severe shoulder and hip

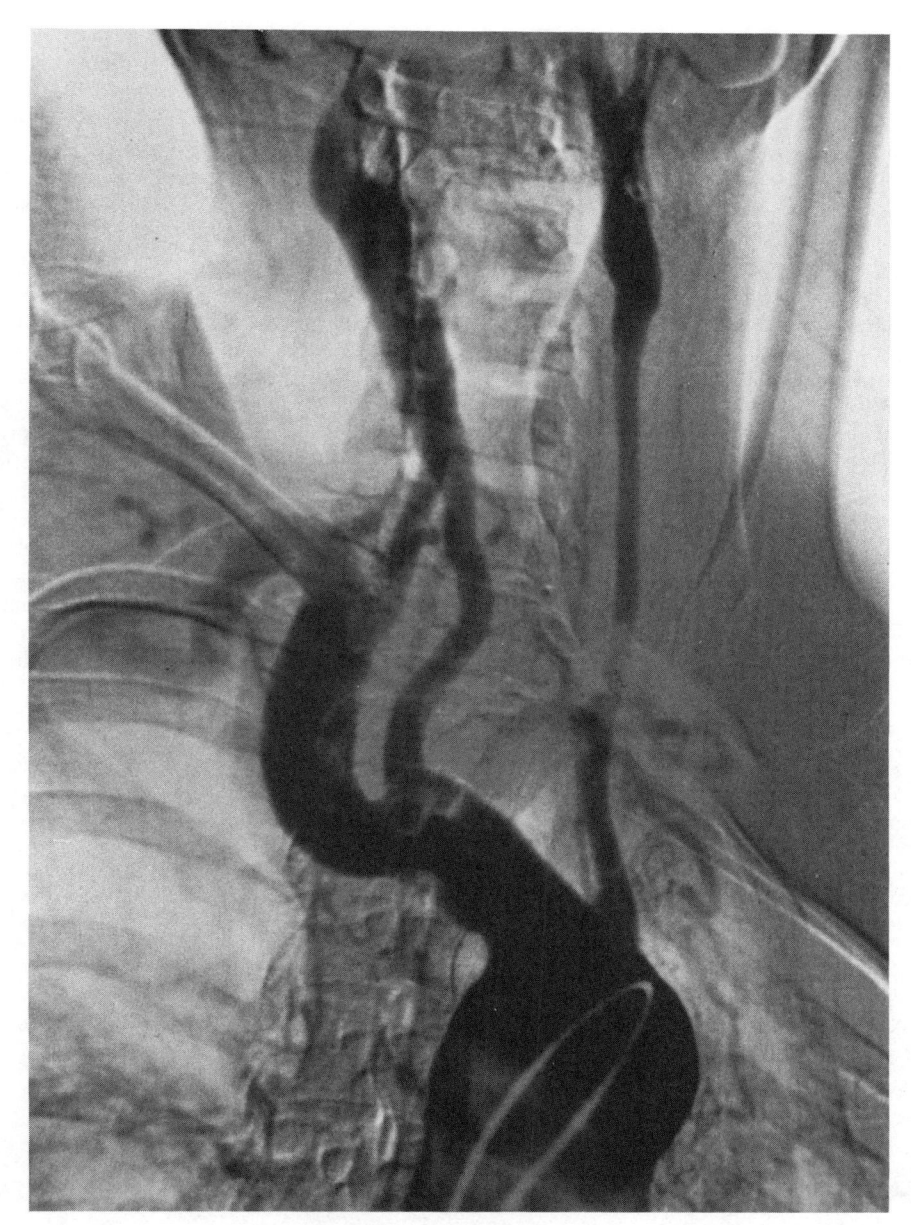

Figure 7-5. Aortic arch arteriogram of a patient with Takayasu's arteritis. There is ectasia of the ascending aortic arch, complete blockage of the left subclavian artery, partial blockage of the right subclavian, and extensive involvement of both carotids.

girdle aching with restricted motion but (early) with little weakness (polymyalgia rheumatica), fever, weight loss, anemia, and other symptoms. Blindness usually occurs with very little warning, that warning being transient diplopia or amaurosis fugax.

The erythrocyte sedimentation rate is almost always very high; serum alkaline phosphatase is also frequently abnormal, and normochromic, normocytic anemia is common. Biopsy of the affected artery, or, if none is palpated, of the anterior (frontal) branch of the temporal artery, is frequently diagnostic, but a negative biopsy finding does not exclude the diagnosis. Microscopic pathology demonstrates necrosis and through-and-through inflammation of the artery; giant cells are present. The microscopic appearance is similar to that of Takayasu's arteritis.[92-96]

Differential Diagnosis. Giant cell arteritis is rare before age 50. In those patients in whom the diagnosis is considered possible, the swollen tender artery has very few alternative explanations; polyarteritis nodosa and, rarely, an infection or tumor may mimic the superficial findings. If the presenting symptoms are vaso-occlusive, the more common atherosclerosis or embolism must be considered, especially if the expected laboratory abnormalities are not present.

In patients presenting with fever, anemia, weight loss, or other systemic symptoms, the differential diagnosis includes a large number of diseases. In these cases temporal artery biopsy should be done even if there are no subjective or objective abnormalities suggesting abnormality of the selected artery. A positive biopsy result is sufficient evidence presumptively to exclude alternative diagnoses and to initiate a therapy trial.

An occasional elderly patient develops unilateral pulselessness; polymyalgia rheumatica may be present; angiography shows occlusive disease of the brachiocephalic vessels (Fig. 7-6). It is convention to refer to this as giant cell arteritis of the aorta and great vessels, but there is no known way to distinguish this syndrome from that of Takayasu's arteritis occurring in the elderly.[97-99]

Treatment. Temporal arteritis usually responds quickly to moderate- or high-dose corticosteroid therapy (30 to 60 mg prednisone per day). Patients with *any* visual symptoms should be treated instantaneously; parenteral corticosteroid, given the moment the diagnosis is suspected, is appropriate, since blindless, once it occurs, is usually irreversible. Standard doses of corticosteroid (300 mg hydrocortisone per day or 48 mg methylprednisolone per day in divided doses) suffice to reduce inflammation. There is no published documentaion that "pulses" of 1000 mg methylprednisolone accomplish anything more.

It is necessary to maintain moderate- to high-dose corticosteroid therapy for several (4 to 6) weeks

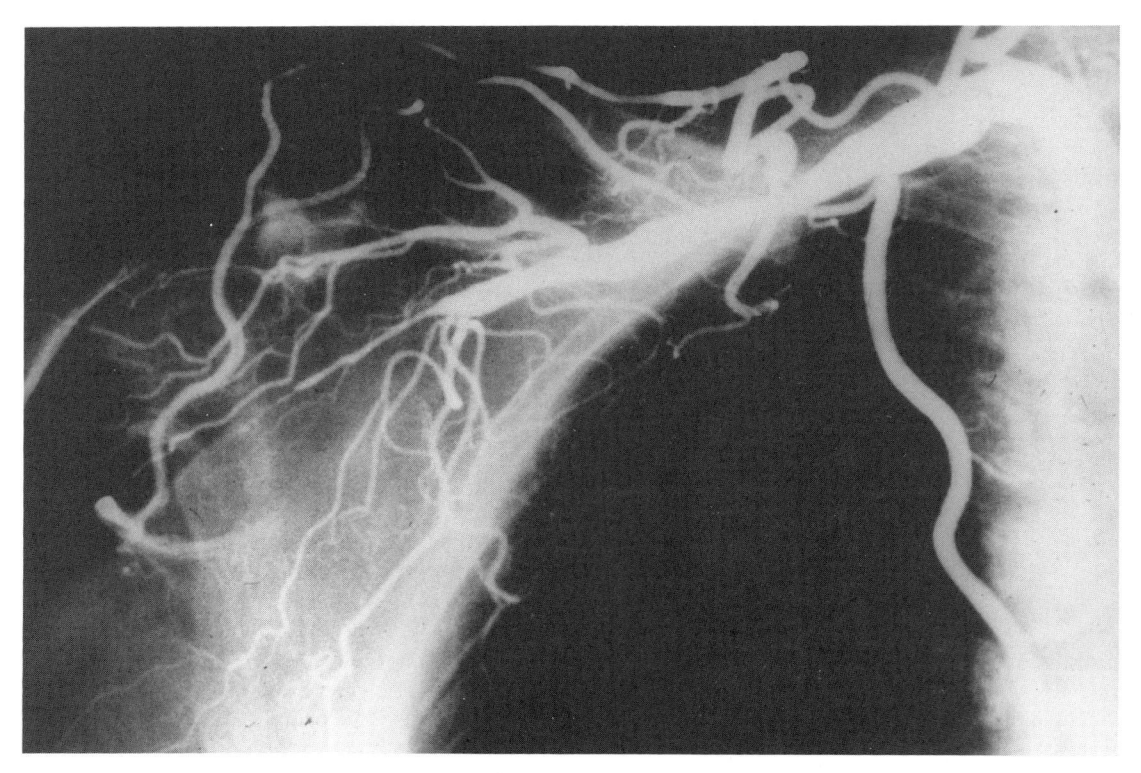

Figure 7-6. Aortic arch arteriogram of an elderly patient presenting with polymyalgia rheumatica and pulselessness. There is extensive involvement of the subclavian artery. This patient could equally well be diagnosed as having giant cell arteritis of the great vessels or Takayasu's arteritis occurring in the elderly.

before tapering is initiated.[100] Recurrence of disease is possible.[101] To monitor tapering, it is helpful to follow the erythrocyte sedimentation rate (ESR). A rising ESR, however, may signify intercurrent infection, such as diverticulitis. The toxicity of corticosteroid is high in this age group. Infections, osteoporotic fractures, diabetes, and hypertension occur easily. Approximately half of affected patients can discontinue corticosteroid therapy within 6 months to 1 year. In those who cannot, the physician must weigh the risk of corticosteroid toxicity against that of recurrent disease. Patients whose ESRs remain below 50 mm per hour (Westergren method) are not at high risk for disease recurrence; it is my practice not to increase maintenance therapy for ESR fluctuations in this range. Although often prescribed for patients needing prolonged or high-dose corticosteroid therapy, immunosuppressive agents such as azathioprine or cyclophosphamide are not of proven value in this illness.

Isolated Cranial Vasculitis

A rare, devastating condition known as isolated cranial vasculitis or granulomatous vasculitis of the central nervous system appears to be a localized disease.[102,103] Presenting symptoms are rapidly progressive vascular insufficiency of (usually posterior) intracranial circulation. The cerebrospinal fluid, but not the peripheral blood, shows evidence of inflammation. Angiography demonstrates diffuse intracranial vascular abnormalities. Leptomeningeal biopsy, usually required for diagnosis, demonstrates necrotizing vasculitis. Differential diagnosis includes chronic infectious or neoplastic meningitis and herpetic encephalitis. The cause is unknown. Corticosteroid therapy is usually ineffective; cyclophosphamide may be useful. Blindness often occurs early, and fatal outcome is common.

References

1. Lockshin, MD: Vasculitis. Bull N Y Acad Med 55:867, 1979.
2. Christian, CL, and Sergent, JS: Vasculitis syndromes: Clinical and experimental models. Am J Med 61:385, 1976.
3. Fauci AS: Vasculitis: New insights amid old enigmas. Am J Med 67: 916, 1970.
4. Fan, PT et al: A clinical approach to systemic vasculitis. Semin Arthritis Rheum 9: 248, 1980.
5. Fauci, AS, Haynes, BF, and Katz, P: The spectrum of vasculitis. Ann Intern Med 89: 660, 1978.
6. Zeek, PM: Periarteritis nodosa: A critical review. Am J Clin Pathol 22: 777, 1952.
7. Zeek, PM: Periarteritis nodosa and other forms of necrotizing angiitis N Engl J Med 248: 764, 1953.
8. Soter, NA et al: Two distinct cellular patterns in cutaneous necrotizing angiitis. J Invest Dermatol 66: 344, 1976.
9. Fisher, RG: Renal artery aneurysms in polyarteritis nodosa: A multiepisodic phenomenon. Am J Roentgenol 136: 983, 1981.
10. Bron, KM, Strott, CA, and Shapiro, AP: The diagnostic value of angiographic observations in polyarteritis nodosa. Arch Intern Med 116: 450, 1965.
11. Travers, RL et al: Polyarteritis nodosa: A clinical and angiographic analysis of 17 cases. Semin Arthritis Rheum 8: 184, 1979.
12. d'Izarn JJ et al: Arteriography in polyarteritis nodosa: 15 cases. J Radiol Electrol 57: 505, 1976.
13. Bron, KM, and Gajaraj, A: Demonstration of hepatic aneurysms in polyarteritis nodosa by arteriography. N Engl J Med 282: 1024, 1970.
14. Leonhardt, ETG, Jakobson J, and Ringqvist, CTA: Angiographic and clinicophysiologic investigation of a case of polyarteritis nodosa. Am J Med 53: 242, 1972.
15. Vallat M et al: Periarterite noueuse a manifestation hepato-vesiculaire mortelle: Aspects arteriographiques. Sem Hôp Paris 53: 1953, 1977.
16. Fisher RG et al: Polyarteritis nodosa and hepatitis-B surface antigen: Role of angiography in diagnosis. Am J Roentgenol 129: 77, 1977.
17. Lemieux, G et al: Importance de l'angiographie renal dans le diagnostic de la polyarterite noueuse. Union Med Can 102: 1064, 1973.
18. Moore, PM, and Fauci, AS: Neurologic manifestations of systemic vasculitis. Am J Med 71: 517, 1981.
19. Moore, PM, and Cupps, TR: Neurological complications of vasculitis. Ann Neurol 14: 155, 1983.
20. Cupps, TR, Springer, RM, and Fauci, AS: Chronic, recurrent small-vessel cutaneous vasculitis. JAMA 247: 1994, 1982.
21. Sibbald, RG, Roberts, JT, and Rosenthal, D: Cutaneous vasculitis. Can Med Assoc J 118: 142, 1978.
22. Gilliam, JN, and Smiley, JD: Cutaneous necrotizing vasculitis and related disorders. Ann Allergy 37: 328, 1976.
23. Lopez, LR et al: Gastrointestinal involvement in leukocytoclastic vaculitis and polyarteritis nodosa. J Rheumatol 7: 677, 1980.
24. Heumann, HAM et al: Hepatitis B surface antigen deposition in the blood vessel walls of urticarial lesions in acute hepatitis B. Br J Dermatol 104: 383. 1981.
25. Gower RG et al: Small vessel vasculitis caused by hepatitis B virus immune complexes. J Allergy Clin Immunol 62: 222, 1978.
26. Phinney, PR et al: Necrotizing vasculitis in a case of disseminated neonatal herpes simplex infection. Arch Pathol Lab Med 106: 64, 1982.

27. Blumberg, S, Bienfang, D, and Kantrowitz, FG: A possible association between influenza vaccination and small-vessel vasculitis. Arch Intern Med 140: 847, 1980.
28. Mullick, FG et al: Drug related vasculitis. Hum Pathol 10: 313, 1979.
29. Perrillo, RP, Tedesco, FJ, and Wise, L: The role of additives in allergic vasculitis during intavenous hyperalimentation. Digest Dis 20: 1191, 1975.
30. Soter, NA, Austen, KF, and Gigli, I: The complement system in necrotizing angiitis of the skin: Analysis of complement activities in serum of patients with concomitant collagen-disease. J Invest Dermatol 63: 219, 1974.
31. Mackel, SE, Tappeniner, G, and Brumfield, H: Circulating immune complexes in cutaneous vasculitis. J Clin Invest 64: 1652, 1979.
32. Ullman, S et al: Deposits of immunoglobulins and complement in the dermoepidermal junction of patients with anaphylactoid purpura. Acta Derm Venereol 55: 359, 1975.
33. Kauffmann, RH et al: Circulating and tissue-bound immune complexes in allergic vasculitis: Relationship between immunogloblin class and clinical features. Clin Exp Immunol 41: 459, 1980.
34. Kammer, GM, Soter, NA, and Schur, PH: Circulating immune complexes in patients with necrotizing vasculitis. Clin Immunol Immunopathol 15: 658, 1980.
35. Monroe EW et al: Vasculitis in chronic urticaria: An immunopathologic study. J Invest Dermatol 76: 103, 1981.
36. Marder RJ et al: Clq deficiency associated with urticarial-like lesions and cutaneous vasculitis. Am J Med 61: 560, 1976.
37. Moorthy, AV, and Pringle, D: Urticaria, vasculitis, hypocomplementemia, and immune-complex glomerulonephritis. Arch Pathol Lab Med 106: 68, 1982.
38. Schroeter AL et al: Livedo vasculitis (the vasculitis of atrophie blanche). Arch Dermatol 111: 188, 1975.
39. Hazen, PG, and Michel, B: Management of necrotizing vasculitis with colchicine. Arch Dermatol 115: 1303, 1979.
40. Frohnert, PP, and Sheps, SG: Long-term follow-up study of periarteritis nodosa. Am J Med 43: 8, 1967.
41. Stockigt, JR, Topliss, DJ, and Hewett, MJ: High-renin hypertension in necrotizing vasculitis. New Engl J Med 300: 1218, 1979.
42. Lejonc JL et al: Hypertension in systemic necrotizing vasculitis. Ann Intern Med 93: 149, 1980.
43. White, RH, and Schambelan, M: Hypertension and angiographic findings in necrotizing vasculitis. Ann Intern Med 94: 410, 1981.
44. Robins, JM, and Bookstein, JJ: Regressing aneurysms in periarteritis nodosa. Radiology 104: 39, 1972.
45. Diaz-Lopez, JL, and Winkelmann, RK: Cutaneous periarteritis nodosa. Arch Dermatol 110: 407, 1974.
46. Gocke, D et al: Association between polyarteritis and Australia antigen. Lancet ii: 1149, 1970.
47. Sergent J et al: Vasculitis with hepatitis B antigenemia: Long-term observation in 9 patients. Medicine (Baltimore) 55: 1, 1976.
48. Trepo, CJ, and Thivolet, J: Hepatitis associated antigen and periarteritis nodosa (PAN). Vox Sang 19: 410, 1970.
49. Trepo, CJ, and Thivolet, K: Antigene australien, hepatite a virus et periarterite noueuse. Presse Med 78: 1575, 1970.
50. McMahon, BJ et al: Vasculitis in eskimos living in an area hyperendemic for hepatitis B. JAMA 244: 2180, 1980.
51. Walsh JC: Mononeuritis multiplex complicating the post-perfusion syndrome. Australas Ann Med 17: 327, 1968.
52. Sergent, JS, and Christian, CL: Necrotizing vasculitis after acute serous otitis media. Ann Intern Med 81: 195, 1974.
53. Hoffman, GS, and Franck, WA: Infectious mononucleosis, autoimmunity, and vasculitis. JAMA 241: 2735, 1979.
54. Doherty, M, and Bradfield, JWB: Polyarteritis nodosa associated with acute cytomegalovirus infection. Ann Rheum Dis 40: 419, 1981.
55. Frayha, RA: Trichinosis-related polyarteritis nodosa. Am J Med 71: 307, 1981.
56. Citron BP et al: Necrotizing angiitis associated with drug abuse. New Engl J Med 283: 1003, 1970.
57. Bishop, WB, Carlton, RF, and Sanders, LL: Diffuse vasculitis and death after hyperimmunization with pertussis vaccine. New Engl J Med 274: 616, 1966.
58. Phanuphak, P, and Kohler, PF: Onset of polyarteritis nodosa during allergic hyposensitization treatment. Am J Med 68: 479, 1980.
59. Elling, F: Nutritionally induced necrotizing glomerulonephritis and polyarteritis nodosa in pigs. Acta Pathol Microbiol Scand 87: 387, 1979.
60. Nordstoga, K, and Westbye, KR: Polyarteritis nodosa associated with nosematosis in blue foxes. Acta Pathol Microbiol Scand 84: 291, 1976.
61. Porter, DD, Larsen, AE, and Porter, HG: The pathogenesis of aleutian disease of mink. Am J Pathol 71: 331, 1973.
62. Mullink, JWMA: Polyarteritis in mice due to spontaneous hypertension. J Comp Pathol 89: 99, 1979.
63. Svendsen, UG: Thymus dependency of periarteritis nodosa in DOCA and salt treated mice. Acta Pathol Microbiol Scand 62: 30, 1974.
64. Gerber, MA et al: Periarteritis nodosa, australia antigen and lymphatic leukemia. New Engl J Med 286: 14, 1972.
65. Goedert, JJ et al: Polyarteritis nodosa, hairy cell leukemia and splenosis. Am J Med 71: 323, 1981.
66. Lakhanpal, S, Conn, DL, and Lie, JT: Clinical and prognostic significance of vasculitis as an early manifestation of connective tissue syndromes. Ann Intern Med 101: 743, 1984.
67. Gladstein, GS et al: Gangrene of a foot secondary to systemic lupus erythematosus with large vessel vasculitis. J Rheumatol 6: 549, 1979.

68. Scott, DGIM, Bacon, PA, and Tribe, CR: Systemic rheumatoid vasculitis: A clinical and laboratory study of 50 cases. Medicine (Baltimore) 60: 288, 1981.
69. Michalak, T: Immune complexes of hepatitis B surface antigen in the pathogenesis of periarteritis nodosa. Am J Pathol 90: 619, 1978.
70. Prince, AM: Role of immune complexes involving SH antigen in pathogenesis of chronic active hepatitis and polyarteritis nodosa. Lancet i: 1309, 1971.
71. Hurst, NP, and Nuke, G: Evidence for defect of complement-mediated phagocytosis by monocytes from patients with rheumatoid arthritis and cutaneous vasculitis. Br Med J 282: 2081, 1981.
72. Ronco, P et al: Immunopathological studies of polyarteritis nodosa and Wegener's granulomatosis: A report of 43 patients with 51 renal biopsies. Q J Med 52: 212, 1983.
73. Trepo CG et al: The role of circulating hepatits b antigen/antibody immune complexes in the pathogenesis of vascular and hepatic manifestations in polyarteritis nodosa. J Clin Pathol 27: 863, 1974.
74. Prince, AM, and Trepo, C: Role of immune complexes involving SH antigen in pathogenesis of chronic active hepatitis and polyarteritis nodosa. Lancet i: 1309, 1971.
75. Scott, DGI et al: Precipitating antibodies to nuclear antigens in systemic vasculitis. Clin Exp Immunol 56: 601, 1984.
76. Fye, KH et al: Immune complexes in hepatitis B antigen-associated polyarteritis nodosa: Detection by antibody-dependent cell-mediated cytotoxicity and the Raji cell. Am J Med 62: 783, 1977.
77. Korbet, SM, Schwartz, MM, and Lewis, EJ: Immune complex deposition and coronary vasculitis in systemic lupus erythematosus. Am J Med 77: 141, 1984.
78. Leonhardt, ETG, and Kullenberg, KP-G: Bilateral atrial myxomas with multiple arterial aneurysms—a syndrome mimicking polyarteritis nodosa. Am J Med 62: 792, 1977.
79. Strole, WE, Clark, WH, and Isselbacher, KJ: Progressive arterial occlusive disease (Kohlmeier-Degos). New Engl J Med 276: 195, 1967.
80. Cohen, RK, Conn, DL, and Ilstrup, DM: Clinical features, prognosis, and response to treatment in polyarteritis. Mayo Clin Proc 55: 146, 1980.
81. Fauci, AS, Doppman, JL, and Wolff, S: Cyclophosphamide-induced remissions in advanced polyarteritis nodosa. Am J Med 64: 890, 1978.
82. Scott, DGI, and Bacon, PA: Intravenous cyclophosphamide plus methylprednisolone in treatment of systemic rheumatoid vasculitis. Am J Med 76: 377, 1984.
83. Leib, ES, Restivo, C, and Paulus, HE: Immunosuppressive and corticosteroid therapy of polyarteritis nodosa. Am J Med 67: 941, 1979.
84. Fiessinger J-N et al: Maladie de Horton et maladie de Takayasu: Criteres anatomopathologiques. Nouv Presse Med 7: 639, 1978.
85. Shelhamer JH et al: Takayasu's arteritis and its therapy. Ann Intern Med 103: 121, 1985.
86. Healey, LA: Giant cell arteritis. Ann Intern Med 88: 709, 1978.
87. Kyle, V, and Hazleman, BL: Polymyalgia rheumatica/giant cell arteritis. Clin Exp Rheumatol 1: 171, 1983.
88. Hailton, CR, Shelley, WM, and Tumulty, PA: Giant cell arteritis: Including temporal arteritis and polymyalgia rheumatica. Medicine (Baltimore) 50: 1, 1971.
89. Hauser, WA et al: Temporal arteritis in Rochester, Minnesota, 1951 to 1967. Mayo Clin Proc 46: 597, 1971.
90. Wilske, KR, and Healey, LA: Polymyalgia rheumatica. Ann Intern Med 66: 77, 1967.
91. Lockshin, MD: Diplopia as early sign of temporal arteritis. Arthritis Rheum 13: 419, 1970.
92. Parker F et al: Light and electron microscopic studies on human temporal arteries with special reference to alterations related to senescence, atherosclerosis and giant cell arteritis. Am J Pathol 79: 57, 1975.
93. Waaler, E, Tonder, O, and Milde, E-J: Immunological and histological studies of temporal arteries from patients with temporal arteritis and/or polymyalgia rheumatica. Acta Pathol Microbiol Scand 84: 55, 1976.
94. Hamrin, B, Jonsson, N, and Hellsten, S: "Polymyalgia arteritica": Further clinical and histopathological studies with a report of six autopsy cases. Ann Rheum Dis 27: 397, 1968.
95. Liang, GC, Simkin, PA, and Mannik, M: Immunoglobulins in temporal arteries. Ann Intern Med 81:19, 1974.
96. Bonnetblanc, JM et al: Immunofluorescence in temporal arteritis. New Engl J Med 298: 458, 1978.
97. Lie, JT: Disseminated visceral giant cell arteritis. Am J Clin Pathol 69: 299, 1978.
98. Pollock, M, Blennerhassett, JB, and Clarke, AM: Giant cell arteritis and the subclavian steal syndrome. Neurology 23: 653, 1973.
99. Hunder, CG, Ward, LE, and Burbank, MK: Giant-cell arteritis producing an aortic arch syndrome. Ann Intern Med 66: 578, 1967.
100. Blumberg, S et al: Recurrence of temporal arteritis. JAMA 244: 1713, 1980.
101. Beevers, DG, Harpur, JE, and Turk, KAD: Giant cell arteritis—the need for prolonged treatment. J Chron Dis 26: 571, 1973.
102. Zappia RJ et al: Progressive intracranial arterial occlusion syndrome. Arch Ophthalmol 86: 455, 1971.
103. Diliberti, JH: Granulomatous vasculiltis. N Engl J Med 306: 1365, 1982.

Chapter 8
Crystal-Induced Inflammatory Joint Disease

THEODORE FIELDS, M.D.
LAWRENCE RYAN, M.D.

Introduction

Acute, intermittent attacks of inflammatory arthritis are often caused by crystals. Sodium urate, calcium pyrophosphate, and basic calcium phosphate (especially hydroxyapatite) are the crystals most commonly involved. There are distinct similarities in the pathophysiology of the inflammation caused by each of these crystal types. There are also many similarities in the treatment modalities available for management of the acute inflammatory episodes that result. The development of effective prophylactic regimens for gout has dramatically altered the natural history of severe gout in the present era. Effective acute and chronic therapies often allow successful control of crystal-induced inflammation.

Pathophysiology

This chapter considers pathogenetic mechanisms involved in articular crystal-induced diseases, focusing on the more common monosodium urate monohydrate (MSU), calcium pyrophosphate dihydrate (CPPD), and basic calcium phosphate (BCP) crystals. The latter grouping includes hydroxyapatite with partial carbonate substitution and octacalcium phosphate. Rare or less pathogenetically significant crystals such as cholesterol, liquid lipid, and calcium oxalate are covered briefly. Factors affecting crystal formation, biologic impact of crystals, and modulators of crystal-induced effects are addressed.

Crystal Formation

CPPD, BCP, and MSU crystals form from ionic species in a matrix, usually cartilage or periarticular tissue. Simple fluid phase crystal formation is probably rare outside the test tube. Crystallogenesis in tissue is determined by the interaction of three factors: cation concentration, anion concentration, and matrix components, both organic and inorganic (Table 8-1).

In CPPD deposition the role of matrix changes, particularly of cartilage proteoglycan abnormalities, has been examined. The matrix surrounding mature crystal deposits is abnormal. In familial cases depletion of mucinlike oligosaccharides antedating crystal formation has been described in articular cartilage from three kindreds.[1] Other evidence for abnormal proteoglycan in CPPD deposits comes from the observations of Ishikawa and co-workers[2] that glycosaminoglycan-rich cells appear in areas of early CPPD deposition. They hypothesize that inorganic pyrophosphate (PPi) produced during disordered glycosaminoglycan synthesis accumulates in these safranin O–staining cells. Intracellular PPi is released when these cells are disrupted and then participates in matrix mineralization. Abnormal accumulation of chloroform- and methanol-soluble lipid

Table 8-1. Clinical Factors Affecting Crystal Formation

	Crystal Type		
	MSU	CPPD	BCP
Matrix	Favors degenerated	Favors degenerated ?Vesicles ↑ Lipid ↑ "Red cells" ↓ Mg, ? ↑ Fe (hemochromatosis)	Favors degenerated ?Vesicles
Cation	Unknown	↑ Systemic with parathyroid ↑ Articular in degenerated cartilage	↑ Calcium phosphate product in renal failure
Anion	Systemic urate	↑ Local PPi (hypophosphatasia), ↓ Mg (overproduction)	Unknown

deposits detected by Sudan III staining are also apparent in cartilage near CPPD deposits, suggesting yet a third organic matrix anomaly. Early deposits are geographically unrelated to matrix vesicles and are not aligned along collagen fibers, although they are adjacent to collagen fibers. In vitro studies suggest, however, that collagen may play a role in crystallization. In aqueous solution CPPD crystals do not form at physiologic ionic concentrations and at physiologic pH. However, when precipitation studies are performed in collagen gels, typical triclinic and monoclinic crystals form at pH 7.5 and at physiologic calcium and PPi levels.[3] Theoretically proteoglycans could serve as a sink for the cation in CPPD crystals or as an inhibitor of crystallization. Proteoglycans inhibit formation of apatite. Moreover, both the sulfate and carboxylate moieties on proteoglycans suppress CPPD precipitation from aqueous solution. Clinically CPPD deposits are common in degenerated cartilages, and hypothetically matrix degeneration favors crystal deposition by depletion of inhibitory molecules or exposure of nucleating sites. Preferential anatomic distribution of CPPD in fibrocartilage, as opposed to hyaline cartilage, may be related to the presence of type I collagen in fibrocartilage or the lesser concentrations of inhibitory glycosaminoglycans. Inorganic matrix factors such as pH, concentrations of other ions, and water content may have a bearing on CPPD accumulation. For example, iron, inorganic phosphate, and acid pH all inhibit calcification. However, the primary inorganic considerations are PPi and calcium.

Systemically elevated calcium concentrations appear to play a role in CPPD deposits associated with hyperparathyroidism. Even there the role is suspect, since the radiographic calcification does not resolve after surgical correction of the systemic hypercalcemia. So-called normocalcemic hyperparathyroidism has been reported in association with CPPD, again suggesting that hypercalcemia is not solely responsible for production of hyperparathyroidism-associated CPPD deposition disease.

Local ionic calcium concentrations have not been measured in adult articular cartilage matrix, but degenerated cartilage contains more total calcium than normal cartilage.[4] Much of this may be intracellular, crystalline, or chelated, and thus unimportant in the formation of extracellular ionic crystals. However, there is strong evidence for abnormally elevated local (articular) PPi accumulation contributing to CPPD deposition.[5]

Disordered PPi metabolism may be expressed phenotypically in CPPD-containing cartilage. Elevated levels of joint fluid PPi are seen in osteoarthritis and CPPD deposition disease. The source is likely to be cartilage, since concentrations in the joint are regularly higher than in plasma, the downgradient implying local production; and since cartilage is the only joint tissue that spontaneously elaborates extracellular PPi when cultured in defined media.[6] This scheme would conveniently place the site of PPi production proximate to the site of crystal formation, the smallest and presumably earliest crystals appearing in cartilage adjacent to chondrocytes. The mechanism by which PPi escapes cells to participate in crystal formation is uncertain. One hypothesis suggests that PPi, a byproduct of multiple synthetic reactions, may be coexported from the cell with newly synthesized matrix components. Cytosolic synthetic reactions generate PPi, which is efficiently hydrolyzed by an abundant neutral magnesium-dependent pyrophosphatase. Portions of macromolecules destined for export, such as collagen or proteoglycan, are synthesized in the Golgi apparatus or endoplasmic reticulum with PPi. In these sites PPi is protected from the cytosolic pyrophosphatase and is available for coexport with the matrix coproduct. Evidence against this construct is provided by reports that inhibition of sulfated glycosaminoglycan synthesis and export has little or no effect on PPi extrusion by cartilage.[7] Conversely, ascorbate stimulation of collagen synthesis is accompanied by a substantial increase in chondrocyte PPi elaboration into the media bathing cartilage, indicating a potential cosecretion pathway involving PPi and collagen.

Alternatively, the PPi which participates in extracellular crystal formation may not be an intracellular product. Adenosine triphosphate (ATP) is released by damaged cells. In degenerated cartilage ATP from chondrocytes interacts with nucleoside triphosphate pyrophosphohydrolase (NTPPPH). This enzyme generates PPi and adenosine monophosphate (AMP) in an energetically favorable hydrolysis. Importantly, it is an ectoenzyme on chondrocytes where it can generate matrix PPi.[8] In addition, excess enzyme activity has been described in extracts of chondrocalcinotic cartilage and in synovial fluid containing CPPD (and sometimes BCP) crystals.[5,9] This ectoenzyme is found in active form on many cells and raised levels are described on skin-derived fibroblasts of some patients with sporadic, but not with the familial type of, chondrocalcinosis.[10]

Unlike true gout, in which the plasma levels of the pertinent anion are elevated, PPi concentration is not high in the plasma of most patients with CPPD deposits, the exception being the few with hypophosphatasia. Support for an underlying systemic abnormality in PPi metabolism derives from observations indicating that nonarticular cultured cells, including lymphoblasts and skin-derived fibroblasts from patients with CPPD deposition disease, contain more PPi than do control cells from patients with primary osteoarthritis.[10] In unusual circumstances systemically high PPi concentrations may produce crystals. CPPD deposits occur frequently in patients with adult hypophosphatasia, a deficiency of alkaline phosphatase isoenzyme. Since PPi is a substrate for alkaline phosphatase at physiologic pH, PPi might be expected to accumulate in extracellular fluids. Such elevations in the plasma and urine of these patients has been observed. Decreased serum magnesium levels due to renal wasting seems to predispose to CPPD deposition. This predisposition likely accounts for the association of CPPD deposition with Bartter's syndrome, in which hypomagnesemia is common. The etiopathogenesis of the association is unclear, but may be multifactorial. First, magnesium is a necessary cofactor for hydrolysis of PPi by alkaline phosphatase and some pyrophosphatases. Hypomagnesemia, therefore, might result in deficient PPi hydrolysis. Second, magnesium directly affects CPPD solubility, causing dissolution of crystals as dramatically demonstrated by attempted therapeutic joint lavage with magnesium, which resulted in partial crystal dissolution and initiation of an acute pseudogout attack. Oral magnesium supplementation has been advocated as a treatment for CPPD deposits, but therapeutic efficacy has not been established. Overall, circumstantial evidence favors aberrant PPi metabolism as a contributing factor in crystallization, but a single specific error has not been identified. Perhaps the situation is analogous to gout, in which many causes of hyperuricemia lead to the common final precipitation of MSU crystals.

Monosodium Urate

Monosodium urate (MSU) crystals result from hyperuricemia. The other MSU constituents, water and sodium, are abundant and are not limiting factors. Most often renal urate retention causes the hyperuricemia, but a host of reasons for urate overproduction are known. Overproducers and undersecretors are conveniently separated by determination of the urate secretion in a 24-hour urine specimen. A value of greater than 800 mg per day on a standard diet (or 600 mg per 24 hours in a reliable and compliant patient on a low-purine diet) indicates overproduction. This differentiation also assists diagnostically and in deciding which hypouricemic agent is most suitable for a given patient. Cautious interpretation is demanded by a host of influences on the urinary determination including diet, medications, methodology, and completeness of collection.

Whatever the cause of hyperuricemia, at 37°C MSU crystals form in physiologic solutions when the urate concentration exceeds 6.5 mg per dl. Local factors may increase urate concentrations beyond systemic (plasma) levels. For example, Simkin and co-workers describe faster clearance of water from joints compared with urate.[11] Thus, dependent joints, such as the first metatarsophalangeal, may accumulate water and urate while the person is upright and while the joint is traumatized during waking hours. At night preferential resorption of water could result in local hyperuricemia, favoring crystal formation or growth of preexisting crystals. This scheme fits well with the observation that attacks of podagra frequently begin at night. The solubility product of MSU is temperature-dependent, and precipitates form at concentrations as low as 4.5 mg/dl at 4°C. This may explain characteristic deposition in cooler acral joints. Lastly, matrix abnormalities may influence MSU precipitation. A number of older women with chronic hyperuricemia due to hypertension and thiazide treatment have developed gout in Heberden's nodes. Loss of proteoglycans, which normally inhibit crystal deposition, may potentiate it at this site.

Basic Calcium Phosphate

Factors affecting BCP precipitation are uncertain. However, BCP crystals regularly occur in joint fluids containing excess NTPPPH and PPi.[5] Both NTPPPH and PPi are necessary for matrix vesicle–induced apatite mineralization. Morphologic observation of juxtaposition of BCP crystals and matrix vesicles, particularly near the tidemark in degenerative cartilage, supports a causal link, but BCP is often seen at a distance from matrix vesicles. Other factors promoting BCP crystal formation include loss of inhibitory proteoglycans from cartilage matrix, excess ATP substrate for matrix vesicles in BCP-containing fluids, and release of BCP from subchondral bone or osteophytes. The calcium content of osteoarthritic cartilage is also high compared with normal cartilage, but it is not known how much is ionic and available to participate in crystal formation.

Crystal Release

Once formed, crystals must reach the synovium or synovial space to engender most biologic responses, particularly acute inflammation. Three general mechanisms appear to be involved in crystal release: abrupt changes in crystal size, trauma, and matrix degradation.[12] When crystals rapidly enlarge they can break through the matrix, gaining access to the synovial space. Similarly, if partially dissolved, they may be released from their matrix. Rapid change in urate levels, such as at the onset of hypouricemic treatment, may initiate attacks of gout. For this reason prophylactic colchicine is prescribed. Similarly, rapid lowering of the serum calcium is a well-recognized precipitant of acute pseudogout. Many persons who have hyperparathyroidism and radiographic evidence of chondrocalcinosis experience acute pseudogout attacks in the postoperative period following parathyroidectomy. Another mode of transit into the synovial space is by microfracture of the cartilage-containing crystals. Thus trauma may antedate acute attacks. Enzymatic release of crystals due to matrix digestion, a phenomenon termed enzymatic strip-mining, could cause acute flareups of disease. This can be especially confusing when bacterial infection leads to enzymatic crystal shedding. Multiple published examples of the concurrence of gout or pseudogout with septic arthritis should alert the clinician to the possibility of overlooking joint sepsis in inflamed joints containing crystals (Table 8-2).

Inflammation

Once out of avascular tissues, crystals are exposed to several cell types and fluid phase mediators that can engender inflammation.[13] Synovial lining cells phagocytose all three types of crystals. Subsequently release of interleukin-1 (IL-1), tumor necrosis factor-alpha (TNF-alpha), and PGE_2 promote inflammation and tissue damage. Neutrophils are the prime movers of the phlogistic response. When animals are depleted of neutrophils the response to MSU crystals is markedly attenuated.[14] Following phagocytosis neutrophils release leukotrienes, lysosomal proteases, and chemotactic factors, promoting local injury and recruitment of more inflammatory cells. Activated oxygen species are detectable. Once ingested, MSU crystals are lytic to phagolysosomes, resulting in cell death and reentry of the intracellular crystal into the synovial fluid. Some crystals are dissolved while in the phagolysosome. Intracellular dissolution and/or release of crystal has been termed "crystal traffic" to emphasize the concept of a dynamic path from release of crystals into the joint until their eventual clearance. Other possible cellular effectors include platelets, which are found in inflamed joints and contain proinflammatory peptides, proteolytic enzymes, and mitogenic factors. Fluid phase reactants may be directly generated by crystals. Monosodium urate crystals activate complement by both the classic and alternative pathways in vitro.[13] Hageman factor is activated, leading to generation of kinins. Lastly, substance P released from sensory nerves potentially augments inflammation by effecting increased vascular permeability,

Table 8-2. Modes of Crystal Shedding

Altered size	MSU release at onset of hypouricemic therapy as crystals shrink; CPPD release from cartilage after parathyroidectomy
"Strip-mining"	Release of crystals by enzymatic dissolution of the matrix in which they are embedded, for example, released by neutrophil and bacterial enzymes during joint sepsis
Trauma	Release by microfracture of cartilage or trauma to periarticular deposits

while activating synovial lining and mast cells. Immunoglobulins coating crystals modify the inflammatory response by stimulating phagocytosis and superoxide production by neutrophils.

Attacks of crystal-induced inflammation are self-limited. Many factors contribute to cessation. Certainly crystals are solubilized and cleared from the joint, as embodied in the concept of crystal traffic.[15] However, numerous crystals are often seen in fluids from joints in which the inflammatory process is waning, and "joint milk" laden with MSU has been aspirated from noninflamed joints. Inhibition of phlogistic properties has been extensively studied in gout. Factors such as urate concentration, crystal size, and hyaluronic acid affect the inflammatory response. Incubation of MSU crystals with normal serum inhibits phlogistic properties. The primary factor is apolipoprotein. Terkeltaub and colleagues[16] have shown that high molecular weight apolipoprotein, normally excluded from the synovial space, enters through inflamed synovial membrane, coats crystals, and inhibits further inflammation. Neutrophil cytolysis is also inhibited. Apolipoprotein binding is inhibited by glycosaminoglycans in the synovial fluid. Other factors, such as attachment of cytolytic cell fragments to crystals, may also interfere with crystal-cell interactions. Inhibitors of hydroxyapatite-induced inflammation have also been described.[17] In a system analogous to the interaction of lipoprotein and MSU crystals, an apatite binding protein, alpha$_2$-HS glycoprotein, coats hydroxyapatite crystals and blunts superoxide release by polymorphonuclear white cells exposed to the coated MSU crystals.

Other Crystals

Calcium oxalate monohydrate and dihydrate crystals have been identified in inflamed joints. All affected patients have had chronic renal insufficiency and were on either peritoneal dialysis or hemodialysis. Most have been receiving ascorbic acid supplementation, ascorbate being metabolized to oxalate in mammals. Thus the hyperoxaluria produced by renal retention is magnified by vitamin C–induced overproduction. Extracellular fluids are supersaturated with respect to oxalate at concentrations of 50 nM.[18] This level occurs in virtually all patients with serum creatinine concentrations higher than 9 mg/dl. Like MSU crystals, oxalate often deposits in Heberden's nodes, suggesting a role for matrix abnormalities and/or lower acral temperature on deposition.[19] Episodic inflammation in oxalate crystal–containing joints is in keeping with observed inflammatory reaction after injection of these crystals into canine joints.[20] Beware that artifactual calcium oxalate crystals form when synovial fluid is introduced into collection tubes containing sodium oxalate anticoagulant.

Cholesterol crystals occur in many chronically inflamed joints and bursae, especially in association with rheumatoid arthritis. The source of the crystals may be excess cellular synthesis or breakdown of cellular membranes. No causal relationship between cholesterol crystals and joint inflammation or damage has been established in human arthritis.

Liquid lipid crystals are brightly birefringent spherules with a Maltese cross appearance. They have been described typically in acutely inflamed joints or bursae in which inflammation is often preceded by trauma.[21] The source of the constituent lipids is indeterminate, but derivation from cell membrane is likely. Synthetic liposomes, prepared from phosphatidylcholine, x-diacetyl phosphate and cholesterol then injected into rabbit knees, had the Maltese cross appearance and provoked an acute inflammatory response.[22] Mediators of this inflammation have not yet been characterized.

Gout

Clinical Manifestations and Diagnosis

Gout is a relatively common disorder, involving especially middle-aged men and, to a lesser extent, postmenopausal women. Gout is a disorder defined by the metabolic consequences of hyperuricemia and tissue deposition of urate.

Preliminary diagnostic criteria for gout have been established (Table 8-3). The presence of either criterion A or criterion B is sufficient to make the diagnosis; both involve microscopic identification of urate crystals using polarized light microscopy (Fig. 8-1). Since the treatment of gout often involves lifelong medication, making a definitive diagnosis is of great importance. Therefore, crystal identification is highly recommended whenever possible. Attacks of gout occur most commonly in the lower extremities, especially at the first metatarsophalangeal (MTP) joint, but great caution must be taken in assuming that an arthritic episode at the first MTP joint is necessarily due to gout. Conditions such as pseudogout (see later section), hydroxyapatite deposition disease,[23] rheumatoid arthritis, osteoarthritis, and Reiter's syndrome are among other conditions that can involve this joint. At times the diagnosis of gout needs to be made in a patient who is not having an acute attack. In these cases it has been shown that urate crystals can be identified even in asymptomatic MTP[24] and knee joints.[25] It is important to examine joint fluid within hours of aspiration, since crystals may become more difficult to recognize, and artifactual crystals may form.[26]

If six of the twelve clinical, laboratory, and x-ray criteria are present, a diagnosis of gout is made, but crystal identification is always preferable. The important aspects of gouty arthritis are brought out by these criteria. Note that response to colchicine was not listed as a diagnostic factor, since the response is not thought to be sufficiently specific. Gout attacks tend to reach their peak of clinically evident inflammation quickly, certainly within 24 hours, and may often present with extensive enlarging areas of erythema that may be suggestive of cellulitis. The skin may even desquamate afterward. Early in the gouty process there is often only one joint involved, especially the first MTP or a tarsal joint. Not uncommonly a contiguous joint becomes involved shortly (Fig. 8-2).

Over time tophi may form, representing large local depositions of urate. They form especially at the helix of the ear, around the olecranon bursa, along the Achilles tendon, and on the ulnar forearm. Those patients with tophi are much more likely to have associated joint abnormalities, such as subcortical cysts, and subsequent joint damage. Tophi tend to be firmer in consistency than the subcutaneous nodules that may be seen in rheumatoid arthritis and lupus.

Kidney stones are an important complication of gout and of hyperuricemia. The presence of urate kidney stones suggests that the patient is an overproducer of uric acid, with high lelvels of urinary urate.

Late in the course of gout some patients develop a chronic polyarticular arthritis. Absence of symmetry, typical x-ray changes, and crystal indentification help to separate this condition from other chronic arthropathies.

Only a very small percentage of patients with gout have identifiable enzyme defects leading to hyperuricemia. Most patients with idiopathic gout have hyperuricemia on the basis of decreased excretion of uric acid. A large number of factors may either cause gout or worsen already present gout by virtue of increasing serum uric acid concentrations. These factors may work by increasing uric acid production, for example, obesity and excessive alcohol consumption[27]; other factors decrease excretion of urate, including renal vascular disease, the use of diuretics, lead nephropathy,[28] and cyclosporine.[29]

Treatment

The vast majority of patients with gout can be helped with medications that are presently available. Acute attacks can be controlled, and, when indicated, prophylactic therapy is quite effective. Treatments used for acute inflammatory episodes must be clearly distinguished from those used in chronic prophylaxis. Drugs used to lower the serum uric acid concentration are of no value in the treatment of acute gout, and may actually worsen an acute episode. Patient education begins with instruction on the chronic nature of the condition. Alcohol use needs to be limited, and purine restriction, although of somewhat limited value, needs to be discussed (see prophylaxis of acute gout later in the chapter). Keeping fluid intake at 2L daily can help prevent kidney stones. The patient should be advised to avoid low-dose aspirin, less than 2 g per day, which can decrease urate excretion.

Acute Gout

Treatment should be started as soon as an acute attack of gout is diagnosed. The more prolonged the delay before treatment starts, the longer treatment

Table 8-3. Diagnostic Criteria for Gout

Diagnosis Made by:
A. Characteristic urate crystals documented in joint fluid or
B. Tophus documented to have urate crystals or
C. In some cases the presence of six out of the following 12 clinical, laboratory and x-ray criteria (note that criterion on A or B are preferable):
  1. More than one acute arthritis attack
  2. Maximal inflammation within 24 hours
  3. Episode of monoarticular arthritis
  4. Joint redness
  5. First metatarsophalangeal (MTP) joint swelling or pain
  6. Unilateral MTP joint inflammation
  7. Unilateral tarsal joint inflammation
  8. Possible tophus
  9. Hyperuricemia
  10. Asymmetric swelling in a joint on x-ray study
  11. X-ray study showing subcortical cysts without erosion
  12. Negative bacterial culture of joint fluid during an attack

Adapted with permission of the American College of Rheumatology from Wallace, SL, et al: Preliminary criteria for the diagnosis of primary gout. Arthritis Rheum 20:895, 1977.

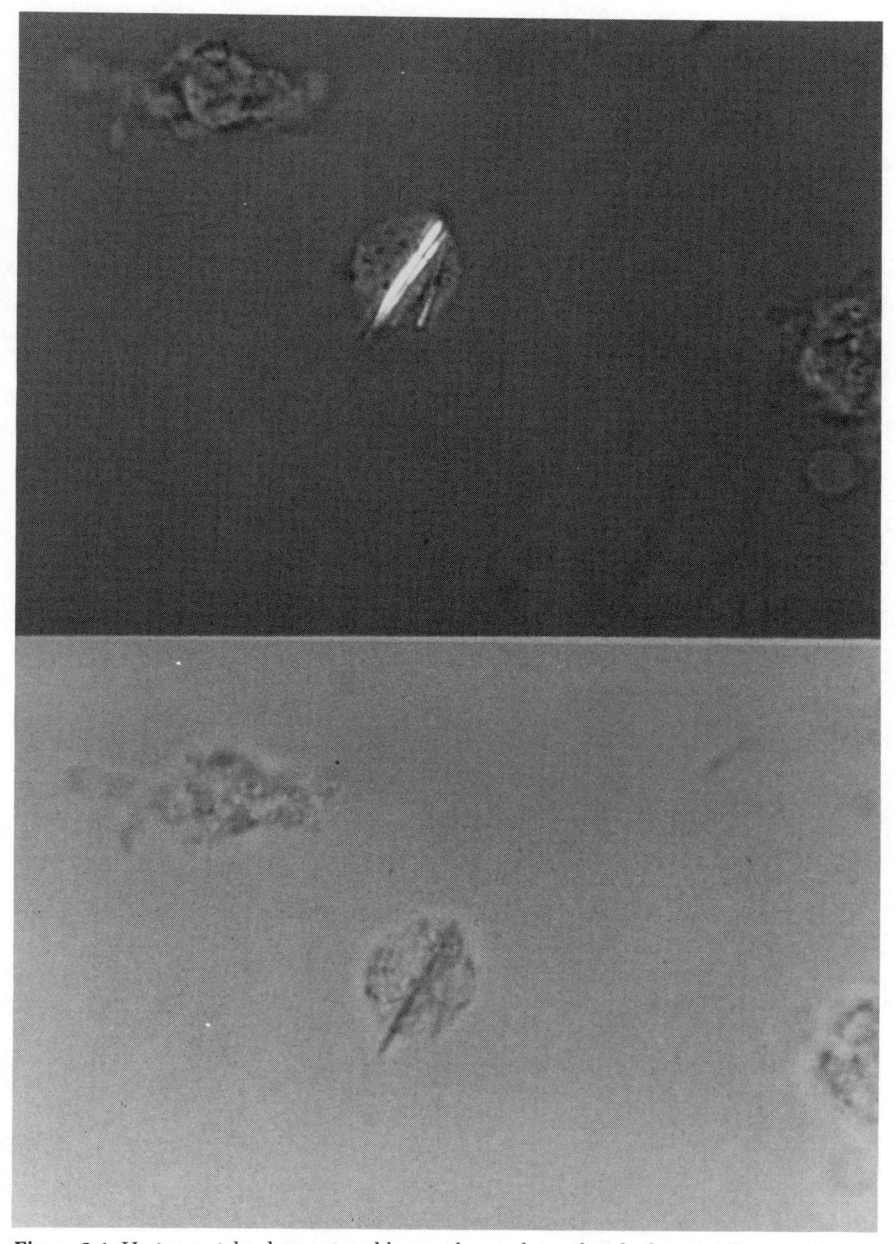

Figure 8-1. Urate crystals phagocytosed by a polymorphonuclear leukocyte. The crystals are much more easily seen in the top photograph, using compensated polarized light, than in the bottom photograph, using ordinary light. (From the 1981 Revised Clinical Slide Collection. Used with permission of the American College of Rheumatology.)

generally takes to become effective. Putting the involved joint at rest is also important to prevent delay in response.

Nonsteroidal anti-inflammatory drugs (NSAIDs) are the medications of choice for acute gout. Patients should have a NSAID available at home, to start at the first sign of an attack. A large number of NSAIDs have been shown to work when given in their anti-inflammatory doses,[30] for example, indomethacin 50 mg t.i.d., naproxen 500 mg b.i.d., or sulindac 200

142 RHEUMATIC DISORDERS IN CLINICAL PRACTICE

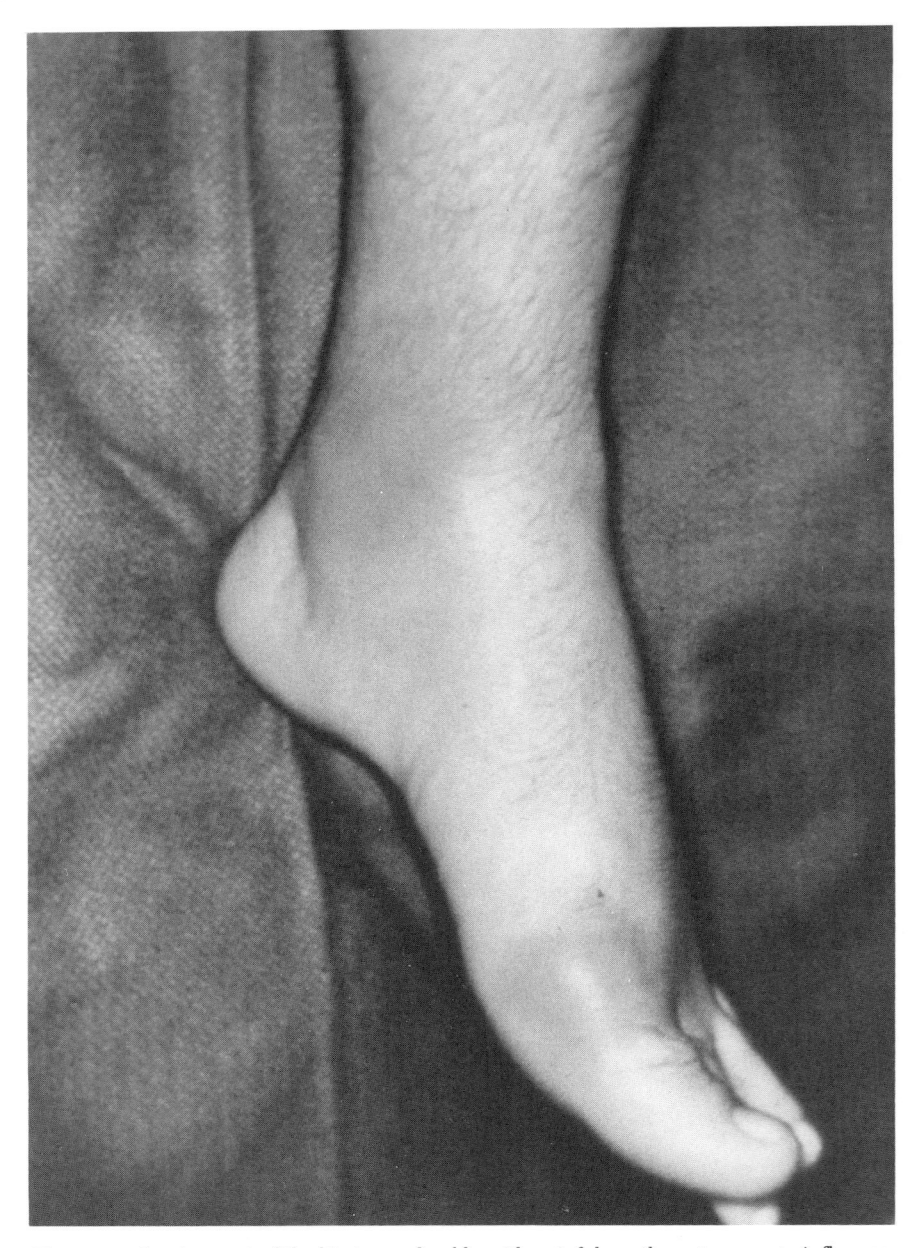

Figure 8-2. Involvement of the big toe and ankle with painful, erythematous gouty inflammation. (From the 1981 Revised Clinical Slide Collection. Used with permission of the American College of Rheumatology.)

mg b.i.d. A nonsteroidal anti-inflammatory drug should be continued for 24 hours after the acute attack is completely resolved, and then tapered to discontinuation over the following 2 days. Phenylbutazone, once used fairly widely for gout, is now generally avoided because of the risk of bone marrow toxicity. Indomethacin has been used commonly for gout for many years, and most patients can tolerate it for the short periods needed to treat an acute gout attack. However, headache and dizziness, especially in the elderly, may limit its use, and gastrointestinal side effects may be a problem with this medication, as with all of the other NSAIDs. Patients with impaired renal function, congestive heart failure, ulcerative colitis, and active peptic ulcer disease may also pose problems. (See Appendix 3-2 on p. 60, for review of side effects of NSAIDs.)

Oral colchicine is sometimes helpful in acute gout, if started very early after the attack has begun. When started early, relatively low oral doses may be needed, given at 0.6 mg every hour for no more than 6 hours. When given later in an attack of gout, the amount of colchicine required to abort the attack frequently causes significant gastrointestinal upset and diarrhea before full resolution of the attack has been achieved. This makes oral colchicine very frequently impractical in the treatment of acute gout. Intravenous colchicine avoids the gastrointestinal side effects of oral colchicine, but brings its own set of problems. It is especially helpful in patients with contraindications to NSAIDs, such as active peptic ulcer disease, congestive heart failure and alcoholism, or when oral intake is contraindicated, for example, after surgery. In patients with renal or hepatic dysfunction the risk of intravenous colchicine increases considerably. The drug is irritating to the skin, and can cause significant skin damage if it extravasates. It is advised that not more than a 2-mg total dose be given to the elderly, and not more than a 4-mg total dose to anyone. Therapy is started with 1.5 to 2 mg intravenously, followed by 0.5-mg additional doses at 8-hour intervals. Ideally, patients with hepatic or renal dysfunction should not receive intravenous colchicine at all.[31] After intravenous colchicine administration, oral colchicine should be avoided for at least 1 week. Care must be taken to avoid dosage errors with intravenous colchicine, since significantly higher doses, for example, 1 g instead of 1 mg, can be fatal. It is important that each dose of intravenous colchicine be separately ordered, and the patient fully reevaluated before receiving any additional dose.

When a single joint is involved, in a patient who cannot tolerate NSAIDs, a local steroid injection can be very helpful. Rebound syndromes after such injections may be more related to local reactions to the injected steroid crystals than to failure to control the attack of gout. In patients who cannot tolerate either NSAIDs or colchicine, and who have polyarticular involvement, systemic steroid or adrenocorticotropic hormone (ACTH) therapy may be helpful. Prednisone has been used at doses of 20 to 40 mg per day for 1 to 3 days, with subsequent rapid tapering. Intramuscular ACTH has been given at 40 to 80 IU every 6 to 12 hours for up to 3 days, with gradual tapering. In the past, rebound flares of arthritis have been reported, limiting the use of systemic steroids or ACTH. A recent report suggested that a single intramuscular dose of ACTH was effective, without significant rebound problems.[32]

Medical therapies aimed at lowering serum uric acid concentrations should be kept completely separate from treatment of an acute attack of gout. If a uric acid–lowering medication is being used, and an acute attack occurs, this medication should be continued. An exception might be made if the uric acid–lowering agent has just been started, and may actually have caused the acute attack, in which case the uric acid–lowering agent may be stopped. If uric acid–lowering treatment has not yet been started, it should not be started for several weeks after an acute attack.

Prophylaxis

Gout attacks can be effectively prevented with prophylactic medication. Strict guidelines, however, should be followed in terms of which patients get treated, and the adverse effects and drug interactions of these prophylactic agents should be carefully considered. The importance of making a definite diagnosis of gout is crucial here, since patients treated with these medications will essentially be on them for a lifetime.

Before starting a long-term urate-lowering agent, several factors should be considered. The patient's present medications should be reviewed, to see if any of them could be elevating uric acid levels. Many diuretics raise serum uric acid levels, as can low-dose salicylates. The patient should be advised to markedly limit alcohol consumption, and advised that gradual weight loss is helpful; "crash" diets may worsen the situation and even precipitate acute attacks. It is still worthwhile to advise patients to avoid high purine foods, such as liver, sardines, meat gravies, and anchovies; even though purine restriction in the diet may only reduce serum urate by approximately 1 mg/dl, such dietary restriction can also reduce urinary excretion of urate by 200 to 400 mg per day. Patients should be advised to keep urine volumes high by drinking 3 to 4 quarts of fluid per day, to help reduce the risk of urate kidney stones. Patients with a history of urate kidney stones or patients with gout and very high urinary uric acid excretion are treated with allopurinol. Those who cannot take allopurinol or who continue to pass urate stones can be treated with urine alkalinization using potassium citrate (Polycitra) 20 ml q.i.d. or acetazolamide 500 mg h.s.

Colchicine Prophylaxis. Because of adverse effects associated with antihyperuricemic therapy, many patients are started only on colchicine prophylaxis in the absence of any specific indication for antihyperuricemic drugs. Because NSAIDs are very effective in treating gout attacks, a patient is often not started on prophylactic therapy after a single gout attack. After a second gout attack, many rheumatologists begin colchicine therapy, again in the absence of specific indications for antihyperuricemic drugs (see next section).

Colchicine prophylaxis is started at 0.6 mg q.d. or b.i.d. The efficacy of colchicine prophylaxis[33] has stood the test of time. Some patients started on twice-daily colchicine develop diarrhea, but may tolerate once-daily therapy. Twelve patients were recently reported who developed a neuropathy and myopathy following prophylactic use of colchicine.[34] The myopathy was associated with elevated serum levels of creatine phosphokinase, and reversed upon colchicine discontinuation. All of the patients in this reported group had decreased renal function; at this point it is difficult to extrapolate the significance of these findings to the overall population taking colchicine prophylactially.

The dose of colchicine should be modified in several clinical settings: Patients with creatinine clearances of less than 60 ml per minute should receive 0.6 mg q.d., and those with a creatinine clearance less than 30 ml per minute, 0.6 mg every other day. Dose reduction is also appropriate in patients with hepatic dysfunction. Great caution and reduced dosage are required in patients with reduced bone marrow reserve, due to the risk of colchicine-induced cytopenias.

Uricosuric Prophylaxis. In patients with recurrent gout attacks in spite of colchicine prophylaxis, chronic uricosuric therapy may be indicated, assuming that none of the indications for allopurinol therapy are met (see next section). Such patients should have less than 800 mg per 24-hour urate excretion, and a creatinine clearance greater than 80 ml per minute (since uricosuric agents are not very effective with decreased renal function). There should be no history of kidney stone, since increased urinary urate concentrations could cause further stones to form. There should be no evidence of tophi, since the dissolution of tophi can lead to very high urinary uric acid and renal stones. Some authorities think that uricosuric therapy should be used only in patients under age 60, due to decreased renal function with age.

Uricosuric agents prevent renal tubular reabsorption of urate, and can be quite effective.[35] Since sodium urate saturates extracellular fluid at a concentration of 6.4 mg/dl, the goal is to keep serum uric acid below 6 mg/dl.

Probenecid is generally considered the uricosuric drug of choice. Toxicity is similar with probenecid and sulfinpyrazone, although sulfinpyrazone has been, on rare occasions, associated with bone marrow suppression, and may have more gastrointestinal toxicity than probenecid. With either of these medications it is important to maintain urine volumes greater than 2 L per 24 hours to reduce the risk of renal stones. Both drugs cause skin rashes in 2 to 4 percent of patients. Sulfinpyrazone is slightly more potent than probenecid, and may be more successful in patients with mild degrees of renal insufficiency. With both drugs, salicylates at low doses antagonize the uricosuric effect. With either drug it is advisable to start colchicine 3 days before the uricosuric agent is started, and to continue the colchicine for 6 additional months. This helps prevent the gouty flareups that may occur on the initiation of therapy with serum urate–lowering agents.

Probenecid is started at a dose of 250 mg b.i.d. for a week, then 500 mg b.i.d. to t.i.d. The dose can be increased subsequently, depending on the uric acid response; the urate level should be checked weekly, with dose adjustment, until the uric acid is at or below 6 mg/dl. The dosage of probenecid is generally not raised above 2000 mg per day. Sulfinpyrazone is used at a dose of 50 mg b.i.d. for a week, then adjusted upward toward 100 mg t.i.d. to q.i.d., based on weekly checks of serum urate concentration.

Probenecid causes increased plasma levels of penicillin, indomethacin, and methotrexate. Sulfinpyrazone may potentiate the effects of sulfa-containing medications such as sulfamethoxazole and sulfonylurea hypoglycemics.

Allopurinol Prophylaxis. In patients who meet specific criteria, allopurinol is effective and generally well tolerated. However, because of occasional very severe toxicity, the use of this medication must be limited to only those patients who meet such criteria (Table 8-4).

When serum urate concentration is kept at 6 mg/dl or less, allopurinol is effective in markedly decreasing the incidence of gouty attacks.[36] Allopurinol inhibits xanthine oxidase, allowing xanthine and hypoxanthine to increase in concentration in the blood, and then to be excreted in the urine. Xanthine stone formation is rare, since hypoxanthine and xanthine are more soluble than uric acid.

The presence of tophi is included on the list of indications for allopurinol therapy for two reasons: patients with tophi are much more likely to go on to destructive joint disease, and the marked uric acid shifts related to dissolving tophi might significantly

Table 8-4. Indications for Allopurinol Therapy

Gout episodes refractory to colchicine prophylaxis in a patient with creatinine clearance less than 60 ml/min (and therefore not a candidate for uricosuric therapy).

Hyperuricemia with kidney stones (uric acid or calcium-containing) or urate excretion greater than 800 to 1000 mg/24 hours, associated with gouty arthritis.

Failure of uricosuric agents to bring uric acid level to 6.0 mg/dl or less in a patient with colchicine-refractory gouty arthritis.

Allergy to or intolerance of uricosuric agents in a patient with colchicine-refractory gouty arthritis.

Tophi in a patient with gouty arthritis.

As prophylaxis against acute urate nephropathy in patients on cancer chemotherapy.

---

increase the risk of kidney stone formation in patients on uricosuric therapy. Concerns about kidney stones also are the rationale for the use of allopurinol in patients with significantly elevated urinary uric acid levels.

An "allopurinol hypersensitivity syndrome" has been described, including erythematous, desquamative skin rash, fever, hepatitis, eosinophilia, and worsening of renal function.[37] The severity of this syndrome requires that special attention be given to meeting appropriate criteria before the institution of allopurinol therapy.[38] Because of the severity of some cases of allopurinol hypersensitivity, allopurinol is generally not restarted if stopped due to the development of a rash. Most severe reactions to allopurinol occur within 3 months of beginning this medication.

Allopurinol has been reported, in rare cases, to cause bone marrow suppression, and has been reported to increase the incidence of bone marrow suppression with cyclophosphamide. In patients on azathioprine or 6-mercaptopurine one third to one fourth of the usual dose should be used when the patient is taking allopurinol. The risk of side effects from allopurinol may be increased in patients taking thiazide diuretics. There is an increased risk of rash due to ampicillin in patients on allopurinol.

In patients requiring xanthine oxidase inhibition, but apparently allergic to allopurinol, oxypurinol can sometimes be tolerated.[39] Oxypurinol is an active metabolite of allopurinol, and has a 12- to 17-hour half-life. This medication is available from the manufacturer on an investigational basis. Some patients develop the same side effects on oxypurinol as on allopurinol.[40] Occasionally in very severe, refractory cases, a combination of allopurinol and probenecid can be used, at the usual doses of each.

Allopurinol is started at a dose of 100 mg daily for a week, then increased by 100 mg weekly until a dose of 300 mg daily is reached. Some patients need as much as 600 to 800 mg per day. Colchicine prophylaxis should be started 3 days before, and continued until 6 months after starting allopurinol. The allopurinol therapy should be lifelong. The dosage should be decreased in patients with renal insufficiency, and in patients without any significant kidney function a dose of 100 mg every 3 days is suggested. Most patients with renal insufficiency and hyperuricemia, however, do not require treatment with allopurinol (see later section on treatment of asymptomatic hyperuricemia).

When starting allopurinol the serum uric acid concentration should be checked in 3 weeks, and then every 3 months, adjusting the dose as needed. Renal and hepatic function should be checked 3 weeks after starting therapy, and then every 6 months. Allopurinol can be taken with meals to increase gastrointestinal tolerance, and 2 L of fluid daily should be taken to help prevent xanthine renal stones.

Chronic Gout

If tophi get infected or interfere with joint function, surgical removal is sometimes indicated. In patients with gout and renal disease, in whom the pathogenesis of the renal dysfunction is not clear, an ethylenediaminetetraacetic acid (EDTA) lead-mobilization test should be considered to uncover occult lead intoxication. In patients with polyarticular chronic gout, physical therapy is important to maintain joint function.

Treatment of Asymptomatic Hyperuricemia

Asymptomatic hyperuricemia is defined as elevated serum uric acid concentration without evidence of gouty arthritis or tophi, or a history of uric acid stones. The chief argument in favor of treatment of asymptomatic hyperuricemia has been the concept of gradual renal deterioration secondary to damage from uric acid. Several studies, however, have shown convincingly that there is no direct relationship between the level of serum uric acid and the degree of renal dysfunction.[41,42] These studies suggest that renal dysfunction, more common in gouty than nongouty patients, is actually associated with hypertension, renal vascular disease, and diabetes mellitus, which also tend to accompany gout. When these other factors were statistically accounted for, serum uric acid concentration alone was not significantly correlated with renal deterioration. Levels of serum urate greater than 13 mg per dl may be associated with future development of azotemia,[41] and therefore those patients with urate levels over 13 mg per dl might be considered for prophylactic therapy. Likewise, those patients with significant urate excretion, greater than 1000 mg per 24 hours, might be considered for prophylactic treatment to avoid kidney stones. Most patients with asymptomatic hyperuricemia never develop gouty episodes. Patients with asymptomatic hyperuricemia related to diuretics are best treated by eliminating the diuretics if possible. In view of the above considerations, a conservative approach is generally recommended for asymptomatic hyperuricemia[43]; most such patients require no treatment at all.

Gout and Cyclosporine

Patients receiving cyclosporine after organ transplantation are an especially complex group to treat. Cyclosporine increases serum urate concentration[29] because it acts to decrease renal function. The gout in these patients may be polyarticular and tophaceous, and allopurinol therapy would seen appropriate. However, allopurinol must be given with great caution in this group of patients. Many of these patients are taking azathioprine, which is metabolized by xanthine oxidase. The addition of allopurinol, which is a potent xanthine oxidase inhibitor, requires a reduction in azathioprine dose (see earlier discussion). In renal transplant patients, who often have reduced creatinine clearance, a reduced dose of allopurinol is required.[44]

Pseudogout

Clinical Manifestations and Diagnosis

Pseudogout refers to the inflammatory joint disease that occurs secondary to the deposition of calcium pyrophosphate dihydrate (CPPD) crystals. The arthritic process may occur as acute pseudogout, or may mimic rheumatoid arthritis or osteoarthritis. Diagnostic criteria have been established for the diagnosis of CPPD crystal deposition disease (Table 8-5). As in gout, specific identification of the crystal involved is the key to diagnosis. Seeing calcifications on an x-ray film is not sufficient for diagnosis, since many patients have such calcifications and remain asymptomatic (Fig. 8-3). Especially important among

Table 8-5. Criteria for the Diagnosis of CPPD Crystal Deposition Disease

Criteria

1. CPPD crystals documented in fluid obtained by joint aspiration or biopsy, by chemical analysis, or x-ray diffraction.
2A. Calcium pyrophosphate crystals seen on polarized light microscopy, with no or weakly positive birefringence.
2B. Typical calcification on x-ray studies.
3A. Acute arthritis, involving especially the knees or other large joints.
3B. Chronic arthritis, especially involving the knees, hips, wrists, elbows, shoulders, and metacarpophalangeal (MCP) joints, especially if acute exacerbations and remissions are present.

Definite diagnosis can be made if: criterion 1 or 2A is present.
Probable diagnosis can be made if: criterion 2B is present.
Possible diagnosis can be made if: criterion 3A or 3B is present.
Criteria 3A and 3B are suggestive only.

The following features can help separate pseudogout from osteoarthritis:
Uncommon site, such as wrist, MCP, elbow, or shoulder involvement.
Joint space narrowing especially localized to the radiocarpal or patellofemoral joints.
Subchondral cyst formation.
Severe degeneration, with subchondral bony collapse and fragmentation.
Tendon calcifications.

Adapted with permission of the Arthritis Foundation from McCarty DJ: Calcium pyrophosphate dihydrate crystal deposition disease. In: Schumacher, HR, Jr (ed): Primer on the Rheumatic Diseases, ed 9. Atlanta, Arthritis Foundation, 1988, p 209.

the clinical features that might suggest pseudogout is the distribution of joint involvement. As opposed to the distribution in patients with idiopathic osteoarthritis, joints such as the wrists, metacarpophalangeal joints, elbows, and shoulders are often involved in pseudogout. Certain x-ray abnormalities, such as patellofemoral joint space narrowing, suggest pseudogout.[45] The presence of certain other conditions makes pseudogout statistically more likely, for example, hyperparathyroidism and hemochromatosis, although treatment of these metabolic conditions often fails to stop the occurrence of episodes of pseudogout.[46] The knee joint is the single most common joint location for pseudogout. Polyarticular, symmetric involvement, which resembles rheumatoid arthritis, ultimately develops in about 5 percent of cases.

The diagnosis of pseudogout is most commonly confirmed by noting weakly positive birefringent

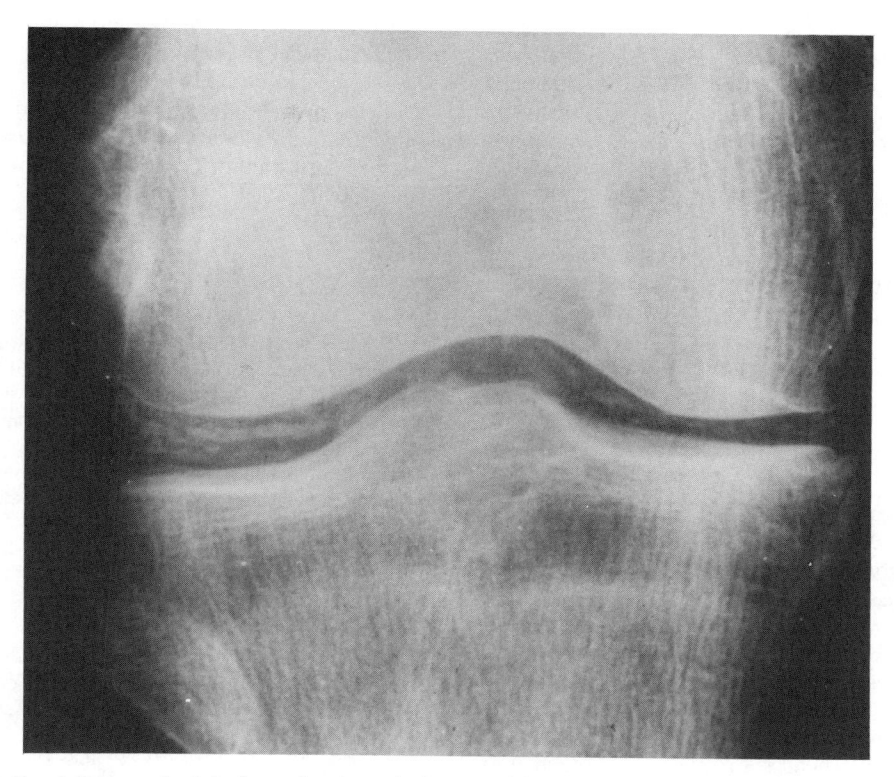

Figure 8-3. X-ray photograph of the knee showing calcification of the menisci and articular cartilage in chondrocalcinosis. Patients with such x-ray study results may or may not be symptomatic with pseudogout. (From the 1981 Revised Clinical Slide Collection. Used with permission of the American College of Rheumatology.)

crystals in inflammatory joint fluid. Crystal identification is especially important in view of the fact that gout and pseudogout may coexist in the same patient. Pseudogout, like gout, may coexist with septic arthritis, and it is therefore important to culture any joint fluid obtained when pseudogout is a consideration. Familial forms of CPPD deposition disease are rare. A Czechoslovakian series revealed an unusual tendency to periostotic calcification of the spine.[47]

Treatment

Joint aspiration, when possible, is particularly helpful in the diagnosis and management of acute pseudogout. Septic arthritis and coexistent gouty arthritis can be ruled out. The simple removal of inflammatory joint fluid can sometimes be sufficient to resolve an acute attack. Local steroid injection, such as with methylprednisolone acetate, 1 ml of a 40 mg per ml suspension, is often helpful in monoarticular attacks. The involved joint should be immobilized. Nonsteroidal anti-inflammatory drugs are generally used, for example, indomethacin 50 mg t.i.d. or naproxen 500 mg b.i.d. Intravenous colchicine is as effective in pseudogout as it is in gout. In patients who cannot tolerate NSAIDs, for example, those with acute peptic ulcer disease, congestive heart failure, or significant edema, intravenous colchicine may be a reasonable alternative. A single dose of 2 mg given intravenously in 15 ml of nonbacteriostatic normal saline injected over a 5-minute period may be sufficient.

Prophylaxis

The long-term prevention of recurrent pseudogout attacks is much less successful than it is with gouty arthritis. In gouty arthritis, chronically lowering the serum uric acid concentration may gradually reduce the amount of urate deposited in tissue. There is no way to similarly decrease tissue deposition of CPPD. Associated conditions, such as hyperparathyroidism, hemochromatosis, and gouty arthritis should be sought. Detection and treatment of these associated conditions, however, is unlikely to alter the course of pseudogout. A recent study suggested that oral colchicine prophylaxis, 0.6 to 1.2 mg per day, may help prevent attacks of pseudogout, similar to the effect of oral colchicine in gout. This study requires confirmation, since it reported on only ten patients followed for 1 year.[48]

Basic Calcium Phosphate–Related Joint Inflammation

Hydroxyapatite crystals are the most common form of basic calcium phosphate (BCP) crystals to cause joint inflammation. In general the diagnosis of hydroxyapatite crystal deposition disease must be made clinically, since the crystals can be seen with electron-microscopy, but not with routine polarizing microscopy. Shiny nonbirefringent lumps may be seen with light microscopy, but are often difficult to identify definitively.

There are three clinical syndromes that have been associated with the deposition of hydroxyapatite and other BCP crystals: acute calcific periarthritis; acute hydroxyapatite arthritis; and chronic hydroxyapatite arthropathy, such as the Milwaukee shoulder.[49] Calcific periarthritis occurs in acute self-limited episodes; calcium deposits may be documented on x-ray film, especially in the region of the shoulder. Multiple areas around joints and tendons may be calcified in some cases, especially in patients with chronic renal failure. Chronic hydroxyapatite arthropathy is typified by the Milwaukee shoulder, a condition especially of older women, leading to joint destruction and loss of motion. Inflammation of the first MTP joint secondary to hydroxyapatite deposition may be easily misdiagnosed as gout. This syndrome, associated with transient soft tissue calcifications of the first MTP joint, has been recently described as occurring especially in premenopausal women.[50]

Treatment

Intermittent attacks of calcific periarthritis, such as at the shoulder or first MTP joint, frequently respond to NSAIDs. Needle aspiration of the areas of inflammation is often helpful, and local steroid injection is frequently added. In some cases surgical removal of large calcific deposits is required. Hydroxyapatite-induced inflammation has been reported to respond to colchicine,[51] but some have reported an erratic response to this medication. Local application of physical therapy modalities is often useful.

Treatment of the Milwaukee shoulder is generally difficult. In some cases a conservative approach has been helpful, including NSAIDs, multiple shoulder aspirations, and shoulder rest. Before joint collapse occurs, anterior acromioplasty has been used. Once collapse occurs, total shoulder replacement has been an alternative.[52]

References

1. Bjelle, A: Cartilage matrix in hereditary pyrophosphate arthropathy. J Rheumatol 8:959, 1981.
2. Ishikawa, K et al: A histological study of calcium pyrophosphate dihydrate crystal-deposition disease. J Bone Joint Surg (Am) 71:875, 1989.
3. Mandel, NS et al: Calcium pyrophosphate crystal deposition: An in vitro study using a gelatin matrix. Arthritis Rheum 27:789, 1984.
4. Pritzker, KP, Chateauvert, JM, and Grynpas, MD: Osteoarthritic cartilage contains increased calcium, magnesium, and phosphorus. J Rheumatol 14:806, 1987.
5. Rachow, JW et al: Synovial fluid inorganic pyrophosphate concentration and nucleotide pyrophosphohydrolase activity in basic calcium phosphate deposition arthropathy and Milwaukee shoulder syndrome. Arthritis Rheum 31:408, 1988.
6. Howell, DS et al: Extrusion of pyrophosphate into extracellular media by osteoarthritic cartilage incubates. J Clin Invest 56:1473, 1975.
7. Prins, AP et al: Inorganic pyrophosphate release by rabbit articular chondrocytes in vitro. Arthritis Rheum 29:1485, 1986.
8. Ryan, LM et al: Cartilage nucleoside triphosphate (NTP) pyrophosphohydrolase. I. Identification as an ecto-enzyme. Arthritis Rheum 27:404, 1984.
9. Tenenbaum, J et al: Comparison of phosphohydrolase activities from articular cartilage in calcium pyrophosphate deposition disease and primary osteoarthritis. Arthritis Rheum 24:492, 1981.
10. Ryan, LM et al: Pyrophosphohydrolase activity and inorganic pyrophosphate content of cultured human skin fibroblasts: Elevated levels in some patients with calcium pyrophosphate dihydrate deposition disease. J Clin Invest 77:1689, 1986.
11. Simkin, PA: The pathogensis of podagra. Ann Intern Med 86:230, 1977.
12. McCarty, DJ: Calcium pyrophosphate dihydrate crystal deposition disease—1975. Arthritis Rheum 19:275, 1976.
13. Terkeltaub, RA, and Ginsberg, MH: The inflammatory reaction to crystals. Rheum Dis Clin North Am 14:353, 1988.
14. Phelps, P, and McCarty, DJ: Crystal-induced inflammation in canine joints. II. Importance of polymorphonuclear leukocytes. J Exp Med 124:150, 1966.
15. Halverson, PB, and McCarty, DJ: Basic calcium phosphate (apatite, octacalcium phosphate, tricalcium

phosphate) crystal deposition diseases. In: McCarty, DJ (ed): Arthritis and Allied Conditions, ed 11. Philadelphia, Lea Febiger, 1989, pp 1737–1755.
16. Terkeltaub, R et al: Apolipoprotein B mediates the capacity of low density lipoprotein to suppress neutrophil stimulation by particulates. J Biol Chem 261:15662, 1986.
17. Terkeltaub, RA et al: Serum and plasma inhibit neutrophil stimulation by hydroxyapatite crystals: Evidence that serum α 2-HS glycoprotein is a potent and specific crystal-bound inhibitor. Arthritis Rheum 31:1081, 1988.
18. Worcester, EM et al: Evidence that serum calcium oxalate supersaturation is a consequence of oxalate retention in patients with chronic renal failure. J Clin Invest 77:1888, 1986.
19. Reginato, AJ et al: Arthropathy and cutaneous calcinosis in hemodialysis oxalosis. Arthritis Rheum 29:1387, 1986.
20. Faires, JS, and McCarty, DJ: Acute arthritis in man and dog after intrasynovial injection of sodium urate crystals. Lancet ii:682, 1962.
21. Gardner, GC, and Terkeltaub, RA: Acute monoarthritis associated with intracellular positively birefringent Maltese cross appearing spherules. J Rheumatol 16:394, 1989.
22. Choi, SJ et al: Liposome-induced synovitis in rabbits. Arthritis Rheum 29:889, 1986.
23. Fam, AG, and Rubinstein, J: Hydroxyapatite pseudopodagra: A syndrome of young women. Arthritis Rheum 32:741, 1989.
24. Weinberger, A, Schumacher, HR, and Agudelo, CA: Urate crystals in asymptomatic metatarsophalangeal joints. Ann Intern Med 91:56, 1979.
25. Bomalski, JS, Lluberas, G, and Schumacher, HR Jr: Monosodium urate crystals in the knee joints of patients with asymptomatic nontophaceous gout. Arthritis Rheum 29:1480, 1986.
26. Kerolus, G, Clayburne, G, and Schumacher, HR Jr. Is it mandatory to examine synovial fluids promptly after arthrocentesis? Arthritis Rheum 32:271, 1989.
27. Faller, J, and Fox, IH: Ethanol-induced hyperuricemia: Evidence for increased urate production by activation of adenine nucleotide turnover. New Engl J Med 307:1598, 1982.
28. Batuman, VB et al: The role of lead in gout nephropathy. New Engl J Med 304:520, 1981.
29. Lin H et al: Cyclosporine-induced hyperuricemia and gout. New Engl J Med 321:387, 1989.
30. Wallace, SL, and Singer, JZ: Therapy in gout. Rheum Dis Clin North Am 14: 441, 1988.
31. Wallace, SL, and Singer, JZ: Systemic toxicity associated with the intravenous administration of colchicine: Guidelines for use (review article). J Rheumatol 15:495, 1988.
32. Axelrod, D, and Preston, S: Comparison of adrenocorticotropic hormone with oral indomethacin in the treatment of acute gout. Arthritis Rheum 31:803, 1988.
33. Yu, TF, and Gutman, AB: Efficacy of colchicine prophylaxis: Prevention of recurrent gouty arthritis over a mean period of five years in 208 gouty subjects. Ann Intern Med 55:179, 1961.
34. Kuncl, RW et al: Colchicine myopathy and neuropathy. New Engl J Med 316:1562, 1987.
35. Thompson, GR et al: Long-term uricosuric therapy in gout. Arthritis Rheum 5:384, 1962.
36. Delbarre, F et al: Treatment of gout with allopurinol: A study of 106 cases. Ann Rheum Dis 25:625, 1966.
37. Hande, AR, Noone, RM, and Stone, WJ: Severe allopurinol hypersensitivity: Description and guidelines for prevention with renal insufficiency. Am J Med 76:47, 1984.
38. Singer, JZ, and Wallace, SL: The allopurinol hypersensitivity syndrome: Unnecessary morbidity and mortality. Arthritis Rheum 29:82, 1986.
39. Puig JG et al: Plasma oxypurinol concentration in a patient with allopurinol hypersensitivity. J Rheumatol 16:842, 1989.
40. Lockard O et al: Allergic reaction to allopurinol with cross-reactivity to oxypurinol. Ann Intern Med 85:333, 1976.
41. Fessel, WJ: Renal outcomes of gout and hyperuricemia. Am J Med 67:74, 1979.
42. Campion, EW, Glynn, RJ, and DeLabry, LO: Asymptomatic hyperuricemia: Risks and consequences in the normative aging study. Am J Med 82:421, 1987.
43. Liang, MH, and Fries, JF: Asymptomatic hyperuricemia: The case for conservative management. Ann Intern Med 88:666, 1978.
44. Kahl, LE, Thompson, ME, and Griffith, BP: Gout in the heart transplant recipient: Physiologic puzzle and therapeutic challenge. Am J Med 87:289, 1989.
45. Dieppe, PA et al: Pyrophosphate arthropathy: A clinical and radiographic study of 105 cases. Ann Rheum Dis 41:371, 1982.
46. Alexander, GM et al: Pyrophosphate arthropathy: A study of metabolic association and laboratory data. Ann Rheum Dis 41:377, 1982.
47. Zitnan, D, and Sitaj, S: Natural course of articular chondrocalcinosis. Arthritis Rheum 19:363, 1976.
48. Alvarellos, A, and Spilberg, I: Colchicine prophylaxis in pseudogout. J Rheumatol 13:804, 1986.
49. Fam, AG et al: Apatite associated arthropathy: A clinical study of 14 cases and of two patients with calcific bursitis. J Rheumatol 6:461, 1979.
50. Fam, AG, and Rubinstein, J: Hydroxyapatite pseudopodagra: A syndrome of young women. Arthritis Rheum 32:741, 1989.
51. Schumacher, HR et al: Arthritis associated with apatite crystals. Ann Intern Med 87:411, 1977.
52. McCarty, DJ: Basic calcium phosphate crystal deposition diseases. In: McCarty, DJ (ed): Arthritis and Allied Conditions, ed 10. Philadelphia, Lea & Febiger, 1985, p 1560.

Chapter 9
Systemic Lupus Erythematosus

ROBERT P. KIMBERLY, M.D.

Introduction

Systemic lupus erythematosus (SLE) is a systemic, multiorgan, autoimmune disease characterized by humoral and cellular immunologic abnormalities. Although initially described as a cutaneous disease, the systemic nature of SLE was recognized in the 1870s by Moriz Kaposi. Subsequently patients with polymorphic skin lesions and other clinical manifestations including lymphadenopathy, arthritis, pleuritis, nephritis, and altered mental function were described. The recognition of SLE as a distinct, clinical disease entity gradually expanded from an initial cluster of clinical manifestations to include pathologic findings such as glomerulonephritis with "wire loop" lesions, "onion skin" lesions in the spleen, and nonbacterial verrucous endocarditis. Starting with the discovery of the lupus erythematosus (LE) cell phenomenon, clinical investigators recognized the presence of autoantibodies and immune system abnormalities reflecting an autoimmune disease process. The use of increasingly sensitive laboratory tests for the autoantibodies associated with SLE has enlarged the spectrum of disease to include new clinical associations, such as anticardiolipin antibody related thrombosis, and more mild forms of disease expression. This evolution of our recognition of SLE as a disease entity forms the basis for the definition of systemic lupus: a multisystem disease with a spectrum of clinical manifestations, a range of characteristic pathologic findings, and a series of immunologic abnormalities including an array of autoantibodies.

Etiology

The etiology of SLE remains unknown, and the multiplicity of factors contributing to the development of disease suggests that a single etiologic agent is unlikely to be found. The spectrum of disease manifestations most probably reflects an interplay between external environmentally derived stimuli and host characteristics. Factors that contribute to the pathogenesis of disease or lead to clinical exacerbations do not necessarily reflect the primary etiology of SLE. Infectious agents including viruses, drugs, and toxins continue to draw speculative interest as the causal agent(s). For example, using molecular biologic techniques, investigators are seeking protein sequence homologies between autoantigens and viral proteins as well as the presence of cross-reactive antibodies. However, compelling evidence identifying the causal agent for SLE is currently unavailable.

Among important environmental influences, exposure to ultraviolet radiation can activate cutaneous and, at times, systemic disease. Intercurrent viral infections and psychosocial stress may also contribute to disease exacerbations. Some medications, such as procainamide and hydralazine, can lead to a lupuslike syndrome. However, drug-induced lupus differs significantly from idiopathic SLE and these agents are not known to activate spontaneous SLE.

Certain biologic characteristics of patients appear to be predisposing factors for the development of disease but are not themselves causal. For example, women are much more likely to have lupus than men. On a population basis, black and Native

American groups have a higher prevalence of lupus than do whites. Several kinds of genetic markers—including the class II MHC molecules, HLA-DR2 and HLA-DR3, and deficiencies of the complement components C2 or C4 or the presence of the C4A null allele—are associated with SLE. Other inherited properties of the immune system may also contribute. However, none of these host characteristics are obligatory for disease expression.

Epidemiology

Ethnic background influences the risk for development of SLE. Among females the incidence is two to three per 100,000 for whites and seven to eight per 100,000 for blacks. Prevalence figures vary between one and ten per 10,000 in the general population but may be as much as 100 times higher in family members of SLE patients. The prevalence of SLE in black and Native American groups is higher than in whites. The peak age of onset is from the second to the fourth decades of life. In adults the ratio of female to male cases is approximately 8 to 10:1. This female predominance is less striking before menarche and after menopause. Within these groups the female to male sex ratio approximates 2 to 3:1.

Epidemiologic analysis has underscored the genetic predisposition to the development of SLE. The high prevalence of disease among patients' family members, the high concordance for clinical disease between monozygotic twins, the associations between SLE and complement deficiencies and the associations between SLE and certain HLA phenotypes, all suggest a multigene hypothesis for the inheritance of SLE. Within this context, female sex hormones have a significant influence on disease expression.

Pathogenesis

The mechanism linking this clinically manifest genetic susceptibility with specific HLA-DR molecules and other disease-associated markers are currently speculative. However, the central theme in SLE is the occurrence of an abnormal immune responsiveness directed, at least in part, against the host. The abnormalities include B-cell hyperactivity with increased antibody production, immune complex formation with tissue deposition and injury, as well as T-cell regulatory dysfunction and monocyte/macrophage abnormalities.

Genes of the major histocompatibility complex have been a major investigative focus since they participate in the regulation of immune responsiveness. Accordingly, one hypothesis ("determinant selection") suggests that certain MHC molecules will bind critical antigens more efficiently and mediate immune hyperresponsiveness leading to autoimmunity. Among white patients, the most significant associations occur with HLA-DR2 and HLA-DR3. Subsets of each of these DR groupings will likely emerge with even stronger associations, but it is important to recognize that the strength of a given histocompatibility association may vary with ethnicity. A corollary of this approach is that the occurrence of several different MHC molecular "susceptibility" configurations indicates the possibility that any given structural determinant might confer a specific immunologic reactivity and thereby a given pattern of clinical disease expression. A suggestive link between a heritable marker and disease expression is seen with subacute cutaneous lupus erythematosus, which is clearly associated with HLA-DR3 and with antibodies to the cytoplasmic ribonucleoprotein Ro. However, with the information currently available, it is difficult to conclude that tight linkages between specific heritable factors and specific disease manifestations exist.

Other genes, including some on chromosome 6 within the MHC region and some other chromosomes, are also associated with susceptibility to SLE. The class III gene cluster, situated between MHC class I and class II, includes several complement system components. Congenital deficiencies of C2 and C4 are associated with SLE in many different populations. Complement system components play an important role in opsonization for immune clearance, immune solubilization, and effector system activation. Absence of C2 or C4, components of the classic complement pathway, might create a significant functional defect predisposing to enhanced immune complex deposition or to altered ligand-receptor interactions between opsonized particles and effector cells. An interesting recent finding is that the gene for tumor necrosis factor maps to the same region. Although its role is currently undefined, the prospect of genetically linked cytokine production is intriguing. Among genes located on other chromosomes, the gene encoding for the receptor binding the complement receptor type I (CR1) may encode for a polymorphism associated with SLE. Certain immunoglobulin G heavy chain polymorphisms (Gm allotypes) may also contribute to disease susceptibility.

In the assessment of the overall immunologic reactivity of SLE, certain characteristics of the immune response are clear. B-cell hyperactivity with polyclonal hypergammaglobulinemia, a spectrum of autoantibodies and circulating antigen-antibody immune complexes, is a prominent feature of SLE (Table 9-1). Autoantibodies may lead to discrete clinical consequences that result from the antigen specificity of that antibody. For example, antilymphocyte antibodies lead to lymphopenia, and antierythrocyte antibodies may lead to a hemolytic anemia. In contrast, the pathophysiologic consequences of circulating autoantibodies targeting specific components of the cell's intracellular machinery are not understood. At times a clinical association may exist such as that between congenital heart block and antibodies to Ro/SS-A, or between lupus psychosis and antibodies recognizing ribosomal P proteins. More often, however, such precise clinical correlations between disease manifestations and autoantibody specificity cannot be discerned.

Autoantibodies may also participate in the pathogenesis of disease through important "antigen-nonspecific" mechanisms. Circulating immune complexes can influence the modulation of immunoregulatory networks through cell surface complement and Fc receptors, and they can be deposited directly in tissues with consequent inflammation and tissue injury. Much evidence supports an important role for immune complexes in SLE. Circulating complexes of various types can be detected in most patients, especially during disease activity. Deposits of immunoglobulins and complement are found at the dermal-epidermal junction in skin biopsies, in the renal glomeruli of patients with nephritis, and in regions of vascular inflammation.

Table 9-1. Autoantibodies in Systemic Lupus Erythematosus

Autoantibody Designation	Incidence (%)	Molecular Target	Comments
anti-dsDNA	80	Double-stranded DNA	Reasonable specificity for SLE; often associated with clinical activity
anti-ssDNA	70	Single-stranded DNA	
antihistone	60	Histones, histone complexes	Common in drug-induced lupus
anti-Ku	10	Nonhistone DNA binding protein	More common in Orientals
anti-Sm	30	Proteins associated with U1-U6 RNAs	Specific (not sensitive) for SLE
anti-RNP	40	Proteins associated with U1 RNA	High titers associated with MCTD-like disease
anti-Ro(SS-A)	30	Proteins complexed with Y1-Y5 RNAs	Associated with SCLE, congenital heart block, neonatal lupus, Sjögren's syndrome, C2 deficiency
anti-La(SS-B)	10	Proteins complexed with RNA PolIII	Low risk for nephritis in SLE
anti-P	15	Ribosomal P protein	Associated with psychosis
anti-U1-RNA	Rare	U1-RNA	
anti-PCNA/cyclin	5	Protein associated with DNA polymerase δ	
anti-Hsp90	50	Heat shock protein, 90 kd	
anti-Hsp73	40	Heat shock protein, 73 kd	
antilamins	Rare	Nuclear lamin proteins	
anti-topo isomerase	Rare	Chromosomal protein	
anticardiolipin	50	Phospholipids	Associated with thrombosis, thrombocytopenia, and fetal loss; often found with lupus anticoagulant and false (+) VDRL
Antierythrocyte	50	Cell surface antigens	Associated with hemolytic anemia
Antilymphocytes	70	Cell surface antigens	Associated with lymphopenia
Antiplatelet		Cell surface antigens	Associated with thrombocytopenia
Antineuronal	70	Cell surface antigens	Associated with diffuse CNS disease

Several different factors may influence how an immune complex is handled. Physical size and complement-fixing ability are probably the most important determinants of immediate handling by the mononuclear phagocyte system that itself may vary in terms of efficiency for receptor-mediated handling of an immune complex load. The net electric charge, the immunoglobulin class, the IgG isotype, and Gm allotype of the immune complex components may also contribute significantly to the accumulation of tissue deposits over time. Local formation of immune complexes may occur.

T lymphocytes influence the production of antibody by B cells and serve as effector cells. Overall B-cell activity is the result of a balance of intrinsic B-cell properties, stimulation of antibody synthesis provided by T helper cells, and suppression of antibody production by T suppressor cells. Altered T suppressor cell activity in SLE patients is commonly found but is not a uniformly predictable finding. T helper cell activity is neither consistently elevated nor decreased. The net effect, however, is B-cell hyperactivity with increased antibody production. Less clear is the role for altered effector T cells in the pathogenesis of SLE. Differences in natural killing, specific cytotoxicity, and antibody-dependent cellular cytotoxicity in SLE patients can be demonstrated in comparison with normal subjects, but the role of these differences in relation to disease pathogenesis is unclear.

Monocytes/macrophages play an important role not only as sources of soluble, antigen-nonspecific immune mediators, such as interleukin-1 and interferons, but also as phagocytes responsible for the clearance of immune complexes. Measures of decreased receptor-mediated clearance correlate with renal disease and its activity. Concurrent determination of both receptor-mediated mononuclear phagocyte system function and the characteristics of the immune complexes in the patient would likely lead to even more precise associations. Interestingly, mononuclear phagocyte system clearance and several different assays of cellular immune function or cytokine production show subtle differences in some normal subjects with the HLA phenotypes (DR2 and/or DR3) associated with SLE. These observations suggest that several heritable differences in immune function may contribute to a lupus diathesis.

Clinical Spectrum of Disease

The diagnosis of systemic lupus erythematosus rests on the recognition of a cluster of clinical findings with supportive laboratory tests. Although some findings—such as a characteristic malar rash or discoid skin lesions, high titers of antibodies to double-stranded DNA or antibodies to the Sm antigen—in the context of a systemic illness are more suggestive than others, no one finding or test in isolation makes the diagnosis. Given the broad spectrum of clinical manifestations and disease, 11 criteria for the identification and classification of patients as having SLE have been proposed by the American Rheumatism Association (Table 9-2). The presence of any four or more of these criteria at any point in time constitutes an adequate basis for the diagnosis. Eight of these criteria are based on a careful history and physical examination. Standard laboratory studies including urinalysis and complete blood count supply additional information. Only two criteria require more sophisticated laboratory testing. A positive antinuclear antibody test, in the absence of medications associated with drug-induced lupus, is highly sensitive and often used as the first immunologic laboratory screening test. The presence of other immunologic abnormalities is reflected in a positive LE preparation, anti-DNA antibody, anti-Sm antibody, or a false-positive serologic test for syphilis. All of these findings may not be present simultaneously, and early in the course of disease a definitive diagnosis may not be possible. Because features of the disease may develop over time, a patient may carry a different diagnosis, such as idiopathic thrombocytopenic purpura, early in the course of the illness, and then evolve a more multisystem disorder characteristic of SLE. While many SLE patients recurrently manifest a similar pattern of disease manifestations during disease flareups (e.g., polyarthritis, fever, serositis, and skin lesions), others may present with organ system involvement not previously characteristic of that patient's disease. Thus, longitudinal assessment may play an important role in the evaluation and diagnosis of patients with lupus and other autoimmune diseases.

Constitutional Manifestations

Constitutional signs and symptoms commonly include fever, which is a sign of active SLE. Fever secondary to infection must, of course, be excluded, especially in patients treated with corticosteroids or immunosuppressive agents. Acute severe SLE may be accompanied by fever above 40°C, but sustained fever above 39.5°C is uncommon. Fatigue, anorexia, nausea, and weight loss may also be prominent manifestations of active, systemic disease.

Table 9-2. 1982 Revised Criteria for the Classification of Systemic Lupus Erythematosus

Criterion	Definition
1. Malar rash	Fixed erythema, flat or raised, over the malar eminences
2. Discoid rash	Erythematous raised patches with adherent keratotic scaling and follicular plugging
3. Photosensitivity	Skin rash as a result of unusual reaction to sunlight
4. Oral ulcers	Oral or nasopharyngeal ulceration, usually painless
5. Arthritis	Nonerosive arthritis involving two or more peripheral joints and characterized by tenderness, swelling, or effusion
6. Serositis	Pleuritis (pleuritic pain, pleural friction rub or effusion) or pericarditis (ECG changes or pericardial friction rub or effusion)
7. Renal disorder	Persistent proteinuria (>0.5 g/day) or cellular casts
8. Neurologic disorder	Seizures or psychosis without other explanation
9. Hematologic disorder	Hemolytic anemia, or leukopenia ($<4,000/mm^3$), or lymphopenia ($<1,500/mm^3$), or thrombocytopenia ($<100,000/mm^3$)
10. Immunologic disorder	Positive LE cell preparation, or anti-DNA antibodies, or anti-Sm antibodies, or false-positive serologic test for syphilis
11. Antinuclear antibody	Abnormal titer of antinuclear antibody

Cutaneous Manifestations

Cutaneous findings are very common in SLE. Acute cutaneous lupus occurs most commonly as facial erythema in a malar or butterfly distribution involving the bridge of the nose and the cheeks. It may also occur as more extensive erythema involving the arms and trunk, primarily in sun-exposed areas. The erythema of acute cutaneous lupus is often exacerbated by exposure to ultraviolet light. Widespread morbilliform or bullous eruptions are uncommon. Subacute cutaneous lupus erythematosus (SCLE) is characterized by superficial, nonscarring papulosquamous or annular lesions of the trunk with a widespread and symmetric distribution. SCLE does not usually involve the medial aspects of the arms and the lower extremities. The skin lesions of chronic cutaneous (discoid) lupus are erythematous, raised, scaling patches usually found on the head and scalp. They may demonstrate follicular plugging, atrophic central scarring, depigmentation, and telangiectasia. Unlike SCLE lesions which may become confluent, discoid lesions are more individually discrete. Disease-related, but nonspecific, skin lesions include shallow painless ulcers found primarily on the hard palate, and on the nasal septum. Frontal or patchy alopecia occurs in about half of patients. Dermal vascular lesions including vasculitis, chronic ulcers, telangiectasias, and livedo reticularis also occur. Urticaria, pigmentary changes, and fingertip ulcerations accompanying Raynaud's phenomenon can be seen in lupus patients.

Musculoskeletal Manifestations

Systemic lupus erythematosus often leads to articular, muscular, and skeletal findings. Nearly all patients experience arthralgias and myalgias. The arthritis of lupus presents classically as nonerosive, nondeforming polyarthritis with symmetric involvement of the proximal interphalangeal joints, metacarpophalangeal joints, wrists, and knees, ankles and feet. Periarticular soft tissue swelling and tenosynovitis are frequent accompaniments to lupus arthritis, and persistent tenosynovitis may lead to tendon rupture. Reducible joint deformities (the so-called Jaccoud's arthropathy including swan-neck deformities and ulnar deviation) result from capsular laxity, not from pannus formation and bony destruction. Rarely, overlap disorders may occur in which patients with a characteristic clinical presentation of SLE may develop the erosive joint disease of rheumatoid arthritis. In SLE, radiologic evaluation often shows periarticular demineralization, and occasional acral sclerosis. Muscle weakness is common in SLE patients, and may reflect general malaise, subclinical myopathy, or overt, inflammatory myositis. Electromyographic abnormalities occur more frequently than elevations in creatine kinase; muscle biopsy may show myositis with inflammatory cells or a vacuolar myopathy. Muscle weakness may also reflect a drug side effect (corticosteroid- or antimalarial-induced myopathy). The primary skeletal findings in SLE patients are avascular necrosis of bone, and osteoporosis. Although weight-bearing joints are frequently affected by avascular necrosis, the bone of any peripheral joint can be involved, and lead to overt symptoms. Although more common in patients treated with glucocorticoids, avascular necrosis can occur without prior steroid treatment. The decreased bone mass of osteoporosis results from glucocorticoid therapy.

Hematologic Manifestations

Both blood clotting mechanisms and the cellular elements of blood can be affected by SLE. The most common clotting abnormality, the lupus anticoagulant, is evidenced by a mild prolongation of the prothrombin time, and a more significant prolongation of the partial thromboplastin time. The lupus anticoagulant interferes with the binding of phospholipid in the prothrombin activator complex (a complex of Ca^{++}, factors Xa, V, and phospholipid). In the absence of other coagulation deficiencies (e.g., thrombocytopenia), it is associated with thrombosis rather than with bleeding, and invasive procedures such as surgery can be performed without correction of the laboratory abnormality. The lupus anticoagulant is also associated with anticardiolipin antibodies, and a false-positive serologic test for syphilis (VDRL). These various antiphospholipid antibodies may be seen in association with arterial and/or venous thromboses, stroke or other cerebrovascular disorders, or fetal death. Rarely, antibodies to individual clotting factors (II, VIII, IX) occur, and cause a bleeding diathesis that may respond to glucocorticoids.

Although more than half of patients may have a positive Coombs' test at some point in time, autoimmune hemolytic anemia occurs in only abut 10 percent of cases. Anemia of chronic disease is common, and may vary with disease activity. Leukopenia is found in about half of patients, and usually reflects a reduction in lymphocytes. Granulocytopenia may also occur. The leukopenia in SLE is not usually associated with recurrent infections, and does not, by itself, obligate treatment with glucocorticoids. Thrombocytopenia is usually not profound with platelets counts remaining above 80 to 100,000 cells per mm^3, but more severe thrombocytopenia may occur and require steroid treatment.

Renal Manifestations

In lupus nephritis the full spectrum of glomerular pathologic lesions (mesangial, membranous, proliferative, and membranoproliferative) as well as interstitial abnormalities are seen. More severe and extensive lesions have a greater likelihood of progression to renal insufficiency, as do lesions with significant fibrosis and sclerotic glomeruli. Patients with limited disease on biopsy usually maintain good renal function although histologic transitions can occur. In general, an active urinary sediment with leukocytes, erythrocytes, and hyaline, granular, and/or cellular casts signifies active inflammatory disease that may respond to therapy. Patients with persistently active sediments, and with high levels of anti–double-stranded DNA antibodies and hypocomplementemia, are most likely to have active and progressive nephritis, although "clinically silent" membranoproliferative nephritis has been reported. Patients with deteriorating renal function and active urinary sediments require vigorous therapy, whereas those with static renal insufficiency of a significant degree are much less likely to benefit from such an approach. Renal biopsy may be useful in defining the extent of renal involvement, determining the degree of active disease, and assessing prognosis. This information may be useful in formulating a therapeutic plan. For example, a physician may be more aggressive with the institution of high-dose oral or pulse steroid or intravenous cyclophosphamide when a renal biopsy demonstrates an active, inflammatory process involving the glomeruli and/or interstitium (a high activity index) than he or she would if the renal lesion is predominantly that of scarring (a high chronicity index).

Nervous System Manifestations

The most common central nervous system (CNS) manifestations are seizures and psychiatric dysfunction that may range up to overt psychosis. Seizure may occur as single isolated events or as recurrent episodes; in either case, metabolic abnormalities must be evaluated and corrected since metabolic derangements often underlie CNS events in SLE. Direct parenchymal involvement is becoming increasingly apparent with magnetic resonance imaging (MRI) technology. This involvement may lead to organic brain syndrome, both extrapyramidal and cerebellar dysfunction, optic neuritis, aseptic meningitis, as well as tissue infarcts and subarachnoid hemorrhage. Headaches, which may resemble migraine and respond to corticosteroid therapy, occur frequently. Peripheral nervous system involvement incudes cranial nerve palsies, transverse myelitis, and sensory or sensorimotor neuropathies. Both depression and anxiety may occur; they often represent a reaction to chronic disease but may also result from glucocorticoid therapy ("steroid psychosis"). In the clinical assessment of neurologic disease, the physical examination plays a central role. With focal findings, radionuclide scans, computed tomography (CT) scans, MRI, and angiograms may assist in defining the anatomic lesion(s). With nonfocal findings, these tests may show only nonspecific cortical atrophy (often associated with chronic corticosteroid use) with sulcal and ventricular enlargement. Cerebrospinal fluid (CSF) examination shows an elevated protein level, often with an increased mononuclear cell count, in about half of patients. The CSF is most important in evaluating the possibility of infection. Electroencephalography may show both diffuse slowing and focal abnormalities and may be useful in evaluating a single and perhaps isolated seizure. It is important to note that while SLE patients may develop the above-mentioned disease-related neurologic problems, the physician must be aware that the problem may be related to non-SLE causes (e.g., stroke due to hypertension; depression or psychosis due to corticosteroids; or altered mental status due to metabolic causes such as electrolyte imbalance, hypoxemia, or infection).

Cardiovascular Manifestations

Cardiovascular involvement in SLE includes inflammatory disease of vessels, heart and serosal surfaces, accelerated atherosclerosis, and peripheral thrombosis. Pericarditis is the most common manifestation. Echocardiographically demonstrable effusions are more common than symptomatic disease. Tamponade rarely occurs. Infectious pericarditis (e.g., tuberculous or bacterial) must always be considered, especially in patients on immunosuppressive therapy. Myocardial disease secondary to muscle inflammation or small vessel involvement can cause conduction abnormalities. Verrucous endocarditis (Libman-Sacks endocarditis) seldom leads to clinically important valvular lesions or embolic complications, but the lesions can become secondarily infected and lead to infectious endocarditis. Peripheral vascular manifestations include small vessel vasculitis, phlebothrombosis with or without thrombophlebitis, and, rarely, gangrene. Raynaud's phenomenon occurs in approximately one fourth of patients. Accelerated atherosclerosis with early myocardial infarction and myocardiopathy is increasingly recognized as a cause of significant morbidity in lupus patients, and is probably related to a combination of steroid therapy, hyperlipidemia, and immune complex–related intimal damage.

Pulmonary Manifestations

Pleuritis is the most common pulmonary finding in SLE. Pleural effusions occur in about half of patients, whereas pleuritic pain is reported somewhat more frequently. Abnormal pulmonary function tests with both restrictive and obstructive deficits occur more frequently than radiographically evident interstitial fibrosis. Acute "lupus pneumonitis," a diagnosis of exclusion, may be limited to only patchy infiltrates and platelike atelectasis on chest x-ray studies, or it may be extensive. Acute pulmonary insufficiency with intrapulmonary hemorrhage is infrequent.

Gastrointestinal Manifestations

Nonspecific gastrointestinal manifestations in SLE patients include nausea, vomiting and abdominal pain, and may reflect either general constitutional malaise or side effects of medication. Abdominal pain necessitates thorough evaluation since glucocorticoid therapy may mask a surgical abdomen. Sterile peritonitis may result from inflammation of serosal surfaces, but the possibility of bacterial peritonitis requires a diagnostic paracentesis. Bowel perforation, vasculitis with visceral infarction, and pancreatitis can cause an acute abdomen. Pancreatitis may result from corticosteroid or other drug (e.g., thiazide diuretics, azathioprine [Imuran]) treatment, hyperlipidemia, or active lupus per se. Liver enzyme abnormalities are common but usually reflect drug-related liver injury (e.g., fatty infiltration of the liver due to steroids or to nonsteroidal anti-inflammatory drugs).

Approach to Management

Since SLE is a chronic process with no known cure, the therapeutic strategy is to achieve adequate disease suppression within an acceptable range of drug-related side effects. Specific preventive measures—avoidance of direct sun exposure through use of proper clothing and sunscreens—although limited, are important. If the history suggests that certain environmental factors, such as situational stress or cold exposure (for patients with Raynaud's phenomenon), exacerbate disease or cause discomfort, it is prudent to minimize or avoid such environmental influences. The principles of good general medical care should also be followed.

The nature of specific symptoms, the evaluation of general disease activity, and the assessment of the severity of multiorgan system involvement all contribute to the formulation of the therapeutic plan. Infection, the leading cause of death in SLE patients, as well as other non-SLE processes, must be considered as a possible cause of each clinical presentation. General disease activity may be evidenced in objective findings such as the presence of fever, rash, oral or nasal ulcerations, alopecia, dermal vasculitis, pleuropericardial friction rubs, or synovial effusions and synovitis. Activity may also be apparent in laboratory tests with elevated antinuclear antibodies (ANA) and anti-dsDNA antibodies, low complement levels, one or more cytopenias, abnormal urinalysis, and an elevated erythrocyte sedimentation rate. Although individual patients differ, each may have characteristic patterns of findings that reliably reflect the activity of their disease.

After evaluation, two major issues should be considered prior to the formulation of an overall treatment plan. First, are there potentially life-threatening or seriously disabling manifestations that warrant aggressive therapy with its accompanying immediate and potential long-term side effects? Second, will therapy be directed at clinically manifest findings for which the therapeutic response can be clearly documented, or is the treatment directed at processes for which the physician must rely on intermediate and often inferential outcome parameters to assess the effects of therapy. For the former, medication can be titrated to the immediate clinical outcome; for the latter, general knowledge of the natural history of disease plays an important role in the specifics of the therapeutic plan.

Aspirin and other nonsteroidal anti-inflammatory drugs (NSAIDs) can often be used to control constitutional symptoms (fever, fatigue, and malaise), musculoskeletal findings (myalgia, arthralgia, and arthritis) and serositis (pleuritis, pericarditis, and sterile peritonitis). Although usually well tolerated, aspirin may be associated with elevated liver transaminase levels, and all NSAIDs may be associated with reversible renal impairment, especially in patients with renal disease. Some NSAIDs (including ibuprofen, sulindac, and tolmetin) may rarely cause idiopathic, reversible aseptic meningitis. Antimalarials, such as hydroxychloroquine, chloroquine and quinacrine, can be useful in some patients for whom constitutional and musculoskeletal symptoms are unresponsive to NSAIDs. Low-dose oral glucocorticoids are best reserved for refractory patients with significant impairment of activities of daily living.

Chronic cutaneous LE (discoid lesions) can usually be treated with topical fluorinated steroids. Occlusive dressings may enhance absorption, but extensive use of topical steroid preparations can cause atrophy and telangiectasia. Systemic use of antimalarial agents is often necessary for widespread cutaneous disease. Retinal toxicity, the most serious side effect of antimalarials, is rare, but can occur with both hydroxychloroquine and chloroquine. Pretreatment ophthalmologic examination and followup evaluations every 6 to 12 months are advisable. Responsive patients usually improve within 2 months. Quinacrine does not cause retinal toxicity, but it can lead to irreversible corneal opacities and yellowish skin discoloration in fair-skinned patients. Ophthalmologic monitoring is appropriate for quinacrine.

Subacute cutaneous lupus erythematosus (SCLE) is distinct from discoid disease, does not have a hypertrophic form, and does not usually lead to permanent scarring. Topical steroid compounds and systemic antimalarials, but not intralesional steroids, are appropriate for management of SCLE. Low-dose prednisone may be necessary on occasion. Because many patients with SCLE have systemic disease, the decision to use a brief course of oral prednisone may result primarily from consideration of the patient's composite clinical picture. In contrast to chronic discoid LE and SCLE, acute cutaneous LE occurs less in isolation and more in the setting of active systemic disease. With the exception of topical steroids and perhaps the use of dapsone for rare bullous disease, treatment is usually determined by other organ system involvement.

Active, severe major organ involvement in SLE is treated with high-dose systemic glucocorticoids (prednisone 1 to 1.5 mg per kg per day or equivalent). Initially, the glucocorticoids are given in two to three divided doses with subsequent consolidation to one single dose per day as disease activity is controlled. The total daily dose can be tapered as the overall clinical picture either allows or necessitates. An alternate-day schedule is desirable in order to minimize many of the steroid side effects, but it may not be feasible due to flareups of lupus activity on the alternate day. Some patients, including those with thrombocytopenia or with active glomerulonephritis and deteriorating renal function, are treated with three intravenous pulse doses of 1 g of methylprednisolone followed by maintenance oral gluococorticoids. Some immediate side effects of glucocorticoids may be avoided by "pulse" dosing, but it is not clear that longer term side effects such as avascular necrosis are also avoided.

The optimal therapeutic strategy is to use the smallest effective dose of glucocorticoids. With constitutional or non-major organ signs or symptoms (unresponsive to other measures), an improvement in those signs or symptoms with low-dose oral prednisone reflects the desired therapeutic outcome and allows prompt tapering of steroids. For example, a flareup of pericarditis with pericardial pain, incompletely responsive to NSAIDs, may be controlled with systemic steroids. Subsequently, the prednisone can be tapered to the lowest dose that, in conjunction with an NSAID, continues to control the pain. Among major hematologic manifestations, treatment of leukopenia is usually not indicated except in the rare instance of severe autoimmune neutropenia. In contrast, severe autoimmune hemolytic anemia or thrombocytopenia may require aggressive steroid treatment. Since the hematocrit and platelet count are readily measurable, the dose of steroids can be readily titrated to achieve the desired laboratory value. Patients with excessive steroid dependence are unable to taper steroids to an acceptable level for long-term therapy while maintaining a reasonable hematocrit or platelet count. These patients usually proceed to splenectomy, and perhaps other therapies in order to minimize steroid side effects. Other therapies may include cyclophosphamide, vincristine, intravenous gamma globulin, danazol, and plasmapheresis.

Therapy with corticosteroids, and other agents, is more controversial when the desired therapeutic outcome is not directly measurable or when the net outcome cannot be assessed until years later. In such cases the physician must rely on an understanding of the natural history of the end-organ manifestation. Obviously, this circumstance can be difficult in a disease as inherently variable as SLE. Kidney and nervous system disease are important examples.

The desired outcome in lupus nephritis is the preservation of renal function. However, the progression to hemodialysis is a long-term result that represents tissue damage accumulated over time. Suppression of ongoing tissue injury that precedes loss of renal function is, therefore, the immediate goal of therapy. Several general therapeutic approaches are available: first, to make a general prognostic assessment based on renal biopsy information and assign a long-term treatment plan using general knowledge of the natural history; second, to use laboratory tests that may reflect the underlying pathophysiologic process (anti-dsDNA antibodies, complement levels, circulating immune complexes) and adjust therapy to normalize these measures; and third, to use measures that may reflect ongoing end-organ damage (urinary sediment, decreasing renal function, increasing protein excretion) and adjust therapy to correct these abnormalities. In clinical practice, management decisions are usually based on an amalgam of these three approaches. The renal biopsy can give information about the nature (mesangial, membranous, proliferative), the extent (focal, diffuse), the inflammatory activity (inflammatory cells, segmental necrosis, epithelial crescents), and the chronicity or permanent damage (glomerular sclerosis, fibrous crescents, interstitial fibrosis) of a patient's kidney lesions. Generally speaking, patients with mesangial and limited disease have a better prognosis. Active lesions are more likely to respond to therapy, whereas chronic damage is irreversible. Patients with diffuse proliferative disease and substantial chronic scarring and fibrosis have a poor prognosis.

Patients with normal renal function, unremarkable urinary sediments, and minimal findings on renal biopsy do not require treatment for nephritis. For patients with serious but potentially treatable histologic lesions, prednisone, 60 to 80 mg per day, is usually given for 1 to 2 months. If renal function tests and immunologic parameters show improvement, the steroids are gently tapered with the goal of reaching a reasonable dose while maintaining the improvement in the laboratory tests. However, if the immunologic and renal function tests do not improve with high-dose steroids, prednisone is usually tapered while further therapy, such as a cytotoxic drug, may be added.

The largest experience with cytotoxic agents (cyclophosphamide, chlorambucil, and azathioprine) in lupus has focused on the renal manifestations. The optimal duration of therapy remains unclear but is probably at least 6 to 12 months and longer if disease remains active. These agents may suppress or prevent some disease flareups and have a somewhat lower rate of renal failure evident years after the beginning of treatment. However, the serious side effects of these drugs include bone marrow suppression, infection especially with herpes zoster, gonadal failure, and an increased risk of malignancy. Intravenous administration of "pulse" cyclophosphamide (beginning with 0.5 g per m^2 of cyclophosphamide) with forced diuresis may avoid the hemorrhagic cystitis, and appears to be more effective in preventing renal failure. For patients with life-threatening disease unresponsive to steroids, with an unacceptable level of steroid requirement or with an inability to tolerate intravenous cyclophosphamide, the use of oral azathioprine (2 to 3 mg per kg per day) or oral cyclophosphamide (1.0 to 2.0 mg per kg per day) is an acceptable alternative. Careful monitoring for side effects is always essential.

The activity of lupus nephritis is frequently episodic. Typically, oral prednisone or high-dose intravenous "pulses" of methylprednisolone (1 g daily for 3 days) is used for flareups of renal disease activity. Oral steroids are usually effective in normalizing immunologic tests, especially anti-dsDNA antibodies and complement, and in improving the urinalysis. Acute rapid deterioration of renal function may require intravenous steroids. Cytotoxic drugs are generally considered longer acting agents with a more delayed onset of action.

The management of central nervous system disease, or "CNS lupus," also requires the synthesis of intermediate, and often inferential, measures of efficacy to guide therapy. Essential to the therapeutic approach is the recognition that "CNS lupus" may refer to a variety of pathophysiologic events (seizures, psychosis, stroke, movement disorders) and may be mimicked by nonlupus processes (infection, steroid psychosis, metabolic abnormalities, hypertensive seizures). Seizures are treated with anticonvulsants, and psychosis is managed with appropriate psychotropic medications. If the patient is on high-dose corticosteroids, the drug itself may be causing psychological problems, and the physician must then consider tapering the dose to improve the emotional status. The underlying lupus activity is treated with glucocorticoids, and at times with the addition of cytotoxic drugs as outlined earlier. Unlike nephritis in which antibodies to dsDNA and hypocomplementemia often reflect disease activity, CNS lupus activity does not correlate well with laboratory tests. The role of MRI in assessing status and monitoring therapy is currently undefined and clinical evaluation remains the essential guide to therapy.

Experimental therapies for lupus include cyclosporine, plasmapheresis, and total lymphoid irradiation. However, in the overall management of lupus patients, these interventions do not have a significant role. Indeed, appropriate treatment of the lupus-related but disease-nonspecific clinical events is probably more important than experimental treatment of lupus-specific end-organ tissue injury. Infection is the leading cause of death among lupus patients and must always be considered. Hypertension is common in patients with renal disease and must be aggressively managed. Similarly, attention to coping skills and psychological adjustment to a relapsing chronic disease yields worthwhile benefits in terms of compliance, followup and quality of life.

Course and Prognosis

The overall prognosis of patients with SLE has improved substantially over the last 40 years in part because newer, more sensitive diagnostic tests have facilitated the recognition of milder, more benign forms of disease. However, improved general medical care for hypertension, infection, and renal failure, coupled with judicious use of steroids and immunosuppressive drugs, has also probably played an important role. Overall outcome depends on the pattern of organ system involvement. Patients with cutaneous lupus and mild musculoskeletal disease have an excellent prognosis, whereas patients with kidney and brain involvement have a shorter expected survival. The pattern of activity varies from patient to patient: some have a sustained progressive course, others an episodic relapsing course, while still others may enjoy prolonged remissions. Ten-year survival statistics depend on the composition of the patient population but in general it approximates 80 percent. The principal causes of death are infection and renal failure.

Bibliography

Balow, JE: Lupus nephritis. Ann Intern Med 106:79, 1987.

Canadian Hydroxychloroquine Study Group: Randomized study of the effect of withdrawing hydroxychloroquine sulfate in systemic lupus erythematosus. N Engl J Med 324:150, 1991.

Kimberly, RP: Lupus erythematosus—systemic and local forms. In: Kelley, WN (ed): Textbook of Internal Medicine. Phladelphia, JB Lippincott, 1989, p 996.

Kimberly, RP et al: High-dose intravenous methylprednisolone pulse therapy in systemic lupus erythematosus. Am J Med 70:817, 1981.

Klippel, JH: Systemic lupus erythematosus. Rheum Dis Clin North Am 14:1, 1988.

Lahita, RG: Systemic lupus erythematosus. New York, John Wiley & Sons, 1987.

Levey, AS, et al: Progression and remission of renal disease in the lupus nephritis collaborative study. Ann Intern Med 116: 114, 1992.

Ropes, MW: Systemic lupus erythematosus. Cambridge, Mass., Harvard University Press, 1976.

Tan, EM: Interactions between autoimmunity and molecular and cell biology: Bridges between clinical and basic sciences. J Clin Invest 84:1, 1989.

Tan, EM et al: The 1982 revised criteria for the classification of systemic lupus erythematosus. Arthritis Rheum 25:1271, 1982.

Chapter 10

Dermatomyositis and Polymyositis

LAWRENCE KAGEN, M.D.

Introduction

Polymyositis and dermatomyositis are chronic disorders of unknown cause characterized by inflammation of skeletal muscle. They occur in both children and adults, with a characteristic rash distinguishing dermatomyositis. A scheme for classification is shown in Table 10-1. This listing separates childhood dermatomyositis as well as myositis associated with neoplasm. In addition, inflammatory muscle disease occurs in the course of other connective tissue disorders such as progressive systemic sclerosis (PSS), systemic lupus erythematosus (SLE), rheumatoid arthritis, Sjögren's syndrome, and sarcoidosis, and these disorders are also segregated for diagnostic purposes. Recently a variant disease, inclusion body myositis, has been described which, because of certain diagnostic and clinical features, may also warrant specific segregation.

Most patients in category 5 (see Table 10-1), who have other connective tissue disorders, are women, and there is also a slight preponderance of women in categories 1 and 2. There is no female preponderance, however, in childhood dermatomyositis or in myositis with neoplasm. Polymyositis may occur at any age, but most cases are noted in the fifth to sixth decades of life. The incidence of polymyositis and dermatomyositis is not known with certainty, although estimates have indicated it may be in the range of five new cases per million population per year.[1-4]

Diagnosis rests on the demonstration of an acquired, chronic myopathy as indicated by clinical, laboratory, and electrophysiologic features, with biopsy evidence of inflammation of muscle. Characteristic dermatologic findings, if present, are of great significance.

Clinical Manifestations

Weakness

Weakness is the most prominent feature of patients with myositis, and is manifested symmetrically in the proximal musculature of the extremities, trunk, and neck. Difficulty in lifting or carrying packages, hanging up clothing, or combing or brushing the hair may indicate upper extremity involvement. Difficulty in walking, using stairs, or in arising from a seat may be the result of weakness of the lower extremities. Anterior neck flexor weakness produces inability to lift the head when supine. Difficulty arising from bed may reflect weakness of the musculature of the trunk. Muscle weakness may be quantified in several ways. Observing functional activities such as gait, transfer from seated and supine positions, and stair climbing, as well as recording changes in function by history, are of central importance. In addition, schemes of manual muscle

Table 10-1. Classification of Inflammatory Muscle Disorders

1. Polymyositis
2. Dermatomyositis
3. Dermatomyositis of childhood
4. Myositis with neoplasm
5. Myositis with other connective tissue disorders (e.g., progressive systemic sclerosis, systemic lupus erythematosus, rheumatoid arthritis, Sjögren's syndrome, sarcoid)
6. Inclusion body myositis

strength testing as well as of biomechanical measurement have been employed (Fig. 10-1). Table 10-2 presents a scheme for scoring of function. Distal musculature of the extremities is generally spared, except in severely affected patients. Facial weakness is extremely rare.

Approximately 10 to 15 percent have trouble swallowing. Dysphagia is usually associated with severe disease and may lead to aspiration of oral and pharyngeal contents into the airways. Dysphagia may arise from decreased strength of pharyngeal contractions, disordered esophageal peristalsis, tongue weakness, or improperly timed closure of the cricopharyngeus mechanism. Since surgical relief of cricopharyngeus obstruction is possible,[5] investigation of the mechanism of dysphagia by radiography or esophageal manometry is of importance in assessing therapeutic approaches.

Muscle Pathology

Necrosis, phagocytosis of necrotic myofibers, and perivascular and interstitial inflammation, along with evidence of myofiber regeneration, are the major findings in patients with inflammatory muscle disease. The inflammatory infiltrate, however, is the diagnostic hallmark, and it consists of small and large lymphocytes, macrophages, and occasionally plasma cells. Increase in collagen-containing connective tissue is also a feature, particularly with disease chronicity. Thickened bands of connective tissue, sometimes containing fat cells, may separate bundles of myofibers, or may isolate and replace necrotic myofibers. In patients with chronic disease, atrophy, fibrosis, and lipid accumulation are predominant elements. Although characteristic findings are present in most patients with polymyositis and dermatomyositis, a minority of biopsies (5 to 20 percent) may display normal findings or nonspecific changes. Therefore, muscle biopsy can present strong diagnostic evidence of the presence of inflammatory muscle disease, but a negative or nonspecific biopsy result does not of itself exclude this diagnosis.[3,6] Perifascicular atrophy, muscle infarction, and vasculopathic changes[19,20] are additional features in childhood dermatomyositis.

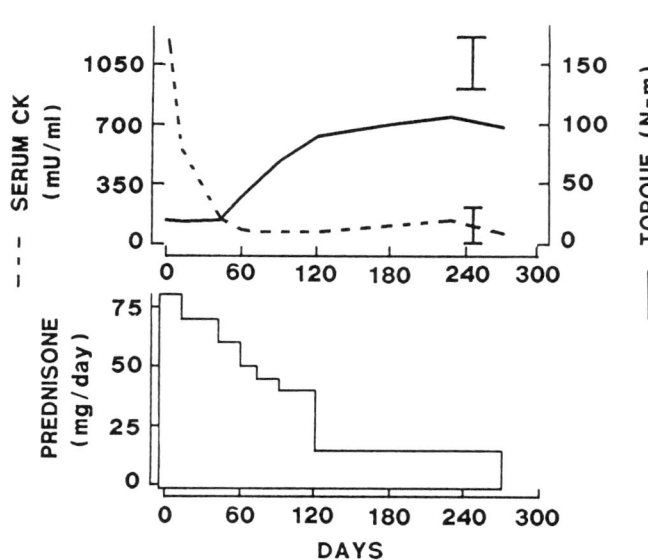

Table 10-2. Functional Assessment

Transferring from supine to sitting
Sitting unaided
Transferring from sitting to standing (low seat, standard chair)
Walking
Climbing stairs (ascend, descend)
Care of head and face (hair, toothbrushing)
Dressing (jacket or shirt, pants)
Lifting objects above shoulders

Rash

The rash of dermatomyositis in both children and adults is seen on the face, neck, chest, and extremities. On the face the skin appears deep violet-red,

Figure 10-1. Course of a patient with polymyositis demonstrating fall in serum creatine kinase (CK) followed by rise in strength during period of therapy. (*Upper panel*). Strength shown as isometric torque production of quadriceps femoris at 60° of knee flexion (*solid line*). Serum CK shown by dashed line. Brackets indicate normal range for strength and enzyme determinations. (*Lower panel*). Prednisone dose. Graphic display terminated after nine months; however, clinical course with tapering of therapy continued into the next year.

particularly in the periorbital areas. Scaling, ulceration, and telangiectasia may occur on the upper eyelids. Involvement of this type is referred to as heliotrope rash or lilac suffusion. Similar erythema may be noted on the forehead, neck, shoulders, and chest. On the skin of the extremities rash is most common over the extensor surfaces, especially the dorsa of the hands and fingers. Plaquelike patches of raised erythema appear over the wrists and knuckles. Patches of this sort can also be seen over the elbows, knees, and ankles. Rash also commonly involves the scalp and upper outer arms and thighs. In these areas, raised patches, or a macular, lividolike erythema is noted. In the nailbeds telangiectasia, enlarged capillary loops, and avascular areas can be seen in patients with either dermatomyositis or polymyositis. In some series, but not all, nailbed lesions have been associated with malignancies or with disease severity.[7,8] In children with dermatomyositis the severity of lesions may be correlated with the presence of widespread microangiopathy.[9]

Pulmonary Disease

Pulmonary disease (Table 10-3) may occur in patients with myositis in relation to several factors: respiratory muscle dysfunction with hypoventilation; chronic or acute aspiration associated with abnormalities of pharyngeal or esophageal musculature; infection secondary to hypoventilation, aspiration, or arising as a consequence of altered host susceptibility due to agents used in treatment; and rarely, drug hypersensitivity or toxicity, for example, to methotrexate or cyclophosphamide. In addition to these considerations, fibrosing alveolitis or interstitial pulmonary fibrosis may be a significant feature of disease in certain patients with polymyositis or dermatomyositis.

In approximately one half of these patients, pulmonary abnormalities may be observed prior to the appearance of myopathy. Cough and shortness of breath are the major symptoms, and physical examination reveals either normal breath sounds or fine, crepitant, basilar rales. The chest x-ray study may show diffuse, linear, interstitial thickening with an alveolar pattern of fibrosis. Occasionally enlargement of the right ventricle or prominent hilar markings may suggest increased pressure in pulmonary vessels. Pulmonary function tests demonstrate ventilatory restriction with reduction of total lung and vital capacities. Biopsies have demonstrated patchy areas of mononuclear cell infiltrates, alveolar cell hyperplasia, and alveolar septal fibrosis. Interstitial edema and arteriolar intimal and medial thickening have also been observed. The clinical course is variable. Some patients respond well to adrenal corticosteroid treatment, others have static abnormalities with little change over time, and some have progressive pulmonary involvement with changes of consolidation, "honeycombing," and respiratory insufficiency. Pulmonary vasculitis may be present in perhaps 20 percent of these patients and indicates a poor prognosis.[10,11] The Jo-1 antibody is present in 50 to 60 percent of patients with polymyositis and interstitial lung disease.[12,13]

Cardiac Findings

Electrocardiographic abnormalities, including dysrhythmias and heart block, may occur in patients with myositis (Table 10-4).[14,15] It is rare, however, for clinical features to be marked. Overall, perhaps 5 to 10 percent of patients have congestive heart failure, with complete heart block in a lesser number.[16] Postmortem evaluations have revealed myocarditis as well as myocardial fibrosis.[17,18]

Calcinosis

Soft tissue calcification may be a disabling complication in patients with myositis. It may be present deeply in the connective tissue around muscle, causing a woody induration, or it may be present superficially in masses under the skin. Calcinosis is most commonly noted during the course of childhood dermatomyositis, but may also be seen in adults, particularly those with overlap features of scleroderma. In this situation calcification may be present in superficial aggregates at the distal extremities or

Table 10-3. Pulmonary Manifestations

Hypoventilation
Aspiration (chronic or acute)
Infection
Drug related (methotrexate, cyclophosphamide)
Fibrosing alveolitis of myositis (associated antisynthetase syndrome)

Table 10-4. Cardiac Manifestations

1. Asymptomatic electrocardiographic abnormalities
2. Rarely, clinically evident cardiac dysfunction

near other areas of skin involvement. Medical therapies have been disappointing. Troublesome localized masses may be removed surgically.

Vascular Involvement

Vasculopathy is the striking feature of childhood dermatomyositis. There may be inflammation of vessels and, even in its absence, endothelial swelling, necrosis, and vessel obliteration may occur. The terminal attack components of the complement sequence may be found associated with the endothelium of affected vessels.[46] Capillaries, venules and small arteries of the skin, gastrointestinal tract, muscles, nerves, and fat are affected, as well as the capillary network of the nailbeds. Endothelial cells of affected vessels can be seen by electron-microscopy to contain cytoplasmic inclusions made up of aggregates of tubular structures. Thrombosis of affected small vessels may occur. The resulting ischemia of muscle can lead to infarction or perifascicular atrophy. In the bowel, ischemic vasculopathy may lead to perforation of the small intestine, a grave complication of childhood dermatomyositis. In the skin, ulcerating cutaneous vasculitis may occur, particularly with the presence of severe active disease.[19-21]

Laboratory Studies

Serum Enzymes and Myoglobin

Elevations of the activities of several sarcoplasmic enzymes occur during periods of disease activity and return toward normal during remission or periods of disease inactivity. Creatine kinase (CK), lactate dehydrogenase, aldolase, and aspartate aminotransferase are commonly monitored. In general, changes in CK levels are the most pronounced and clinically reliable. However, there are some situations in which this may not be the case. Rarely, in 1 to 5 percent of patients, the serum CK level may be normal and, even more infrequently, all serum enzyme levels tested may be normal throughout the course of illness.[16,22] Creatine kinase MB, the isoenzyme form usually thought of in connection with cardiac disease, may be elevated in the absence of demonstrable myocardial involvement[23-26] probably as the result of release from regenerating fibers in skeletal muscle. Hypermyoglobinemia also occurs in inflammatory muscle disease and its level may also be used to follow the course, as is done with the serum enzyme activities. Severe myoglobinuria is rare, but has been noted in association with renal failure.[27] Other factors, such as increased activity, alcohol intake, as well as hypothyroidism, commonly cause increases in muscle enzymes and myoglobin in the serum, so that the entire clinical picture must be considered in assessing these laboratory tests.

Pathogenesis

Since the cause of these entities is not known, ideas of pathogenesis remain imprecise and to a degree speculative. Current areas of interest are related to the possible involvement of immune mechanisms, the relationship of myositis to infectious agents, and its possible association with malignant neoplasms.

Immune Mechanisms, Humoral Factors, Antinuclear and Anticellular Reactions

Antibodies to nuclear components may be demonstrated in sera of patients with myositis with variable prevalence and titer. Most sera tested with sensitive assay methods have reactivity with nuclear components, and less frequently, cytoplasmic and nucleolar staining reactions may be observed in the fluorescent antinuclear antibody test. In addition staining of cytoplasmic filamentous structures, centromeric and small bright speckled patterns have been noted on occasion.[28] The relationship between serologic reactivity and clinical pattern of disease has been most explored with the anti-Jo-1 system in polymyositis, anti-Mi in dermatomyositis, and antinuclear-RNP in polymyositis–systemic lupus overlap syndromes. In general it seems apparent, however, that groups of patients with inflammatory muscle disease may exhibit antibodies of different specificities. In juvenile dermatomyositis a coarsely speckled antinuclear pattern may be seen.

The Mi antigen-antibody system has been further defined to include two specificities. Anti-Mi-1 does not seem directly related to myositis,[29] whereas anti-Mi-2 has been found almost exclusively in dermatomyositis, where its frequency may approach 20 percent.[30] The nature of the Mi-2 nuclear antigen is not at present known.

In polymyositis-scleroderma overlap syndrome, anti-PM-Scl may occur in nearly 10 to 20 percent of patients along with antibodies of other specificities. The PM-Scl antigen appears to be a nuclear component.[31,32]

Approximately 20 to 30 percent of patients with polymyositis, especially those with fibrosing alveolitis, have been found to have an antibody designated anti-Jo-1. The antigen in this case is histidyl-tRNA synthetase.[33] Patients with anti-Jo-1 have an increased frequency of pulmonary involvement,[6] occasional joint manifestations, Raynaud's phenomenon, and an association with HLA-DR3.[34] In one series of patients with polymyositis and fibrosing alveolitis, 68 percent had antibodies to Jo-1.[12] Other antibodies have been detected in the sera of patients with myositis against other RNA charging enzymes. Antithreonyl-tRNA synthetase (PL-7) and antialanyl-tRNA synthetase have been noted in 3 to 5 percent of patients, and other myositis sera have been recognized that precipitate tRNA, indicating that there may be other antibodies against tRNA-related antigens not as yet delineated.[35-37] Recently it has been suggested that patients with antisynthetase antibodies may comprise a clinical subset marked by pulmonary disease, Raynaud's phenomenon, arthralgia or arthritis, and a relapsing course.

In addition, patients with myositis associated with other connective tissue disorders may demonstrate other antibody specificities, such as anti-Ku in PSS and SLE, as well as antibodies to RNP, Scl-70, DNA, and La.

Inflammatory Cell Infiltrate

The inflammatory cell infiltrate in muscle of patients with polymyositis contains both lymphocytes and macrophages. Studies based on immunohistochemical markers suggest that cytotoxic CD8 lymphocytes may be a predominant element of the invading infiltrate in both polymyositis and inclusion body myositis. In dermatomyositis, however, the inflammatory infiltrate is richer in B lymphocytes at perivascular areas. In both dermatomyositis and polymyositis the relative proportion of T lymphocytes bearing CD8 and Ia markers increases from perivascular areas to the endomysium. Conversely the relative proportion of B lymphocytes and CD4-bearing lymphocytes decreases in this direction. From data derived from these studies, it has been suggested that in dermatomyositis, with higher percentages of B cells and relatively more CD4-bearing cells, humoral immune mechanisms may be of importance, whereas in polymyositis the predominance of cytotoxic CD8 cells in endomysial loci indicates a more central role for cell-mediated mechanisms.[38,39] Patterns of cellular inflammation involving perifascicular areas of muscle with atrophy correlate strongly with the presence of dermatomyositis.[40]

Mononuclear cells from patients with polymyositis and dermatomyositis liberate factors, after incubation with autologous muscle, that interfere with the calcium binding properties of the sarcoplasmic reticulum.[41] Taken together, therefore, the evidence would suggest that the inflammatory infiltrate may be the source of factors that impair the efficiency of muscle function, and perhaps produce tissue damage. The reason for the aggregation of these cells, however, at sites within muscle still is unknown. The role of autosensitized mononuclear cells as instigators of inflammation remains provocative and controversial. A recent study indicates that peripheral mononuclear cells from patients with dermatomyositis have damaging effects on cultured skin fibroblasts,[42] and inflammatory myopathy has been observed as a feature of the chronic graft-vs.-host disease in a patient after bone marrow transplantation from a sibling donor.[43]

Humoral Immunity and Antibodies to Muscle Components

Immunoglobulins as well as complement components have been found in muscle tissue of some patients with myositis. Not all investigators who have examined this question are in agreement with the findings or their possible meaning. Some have felt these proteins to be of pathogenic significance; others have found them to be nonspecifically deposited. Recently, however, antigens of the terminal membrane–attack complex of the complement system were noted associated with intramuscular arterioles and capillaries in dermatomyositis of children. These findings may be related to the vascular disease found in this disorder.[44-46]

Antibodies to myosin heavy and light chains, tropomyosin-troponin complex, troponin, myoglobin, filamin, and vinculin have been observed in sera of patients with both polymyositis and dermatomyositis.[47] The significance of these reactivities remains uncertain.

Experimental Allergic Myositis

Animals injected with emulsions of muscle in complete Freund's adjuvants have developed myositis. Experimental myositis of this type has been produced in strains of mice, guinea pigs, and rats. The active inciting material in muscle extracts is not known, although a recent study has indicated the myosin B fraction may be of importance.[48] Although experimental myositis may be patchy, focal and mild, these findings focus attention on the possible role of the immune system in producing or contributing to the clinical picture.

Infectious Agents

Several types of infectious agents and pathogenic organisms may cause inflammation and destruction of muscle. Viruses, bacteria, protozoa, and parasitic forms have all been observed to produce myopathy, although to the present there is no direct evidence indicating a primary role for infection in the etiology of chronic dermatomyositis and polymyositis. Nonetheless, the possibility that a myotropic agent in an appropriately susceptible host might play a role in instigating or exacerbating inflammatory myopathy is an intriguing notion.

Viruses

Several types of viruses cause muscle inflammation and damage, usually of a transient nature. Among the best characterized are coxsackie virus, echovirus, and influenza viruses. Viral myopathies have been described both in children and adults, in isolated cases, and in epidemiclike clusters.

Serologic studies have demonstrated elevations of antibody titers to coxsackie virus B in some adults and children with polymyositis and dermatomyositis.[49,50] In addition, it is possible to produce chronic inflammatory myositis in mice after infection with a particular strain of type 1 coxsackie virus B. In the animal disorder not all strains of type 1 coxsackie B are equally effective. Host genetic factors are of importance and live virus is required, as is competence of T-cell immune mechanisms.[52-55]

Other viruses have also been associated with myositis. Hepatitis B virus, herpes, Epstein-Barr, other picornaviruses—all have been reported in patients with muscle inflammation. Echovirus infection has been associated with inflammatory myopathy in a number of instances, including patients with X-linked hypogammaglobulinemia. In this condition recovery of virus as well as response to treatment with immunoglobulin preparations containing antibody to echovirus has been reported. Here, accurate diagnosis is of prime importance, since the conventional treatment of myositis with immunosuppressive medications may be detrimental.[56,57] Recently, myopathy has been observed in patients with acquired immune deficiency syndrome (AIDS), a viral infection.[58-60] It is not known for certain whether or to what degree secondary agents may play a role in this circumstance. In patients with AIDS, the use of AZT may contribute to mitochondrial abnormalities.

Experimental myositis has also been studied after infection of mice with Ross River virus and encephalomyocarditis virus.

All of the above indicates that infection with certain viruses may lead to inflammation and necrosis of muscle fibers and that host factors are important in the expression of disease. Further study to elucidate the relationship to chronic inflammatory myopathy is anticipated, as well as investigation into the role of antiviral agents in therapy.

Toxoplasma Gondii

This protozoan occurs commonly and may produce transient inflammation as well as persistent cysts in muscle. Case reports of severe chronic myositis after toxoplasma infection, as well as serologic evidence of recent infection with Toxoplasma gondii in certain patients with recent onset of polymyositis, have led to the possibility that this agent may be etiologically related to the manifestations of myositis, or that reactivation of toxoplasmosis may occur concurrent with inflammation in muscle.[61,62]

Bacterial Diseases

Although at present there is little reason to suspect bacteria or their products in the production of polymyositis or dermatomyositis, it is of interest that myositis has been described in Lyme disease with muscle invasion by *Borrelia burgdorferi*,[63] and that the Legionella organism has also been associated with a polymyositis like syndrome.[51] Bacterial pyomyositis, usually staphylococcal, is marked by abscesses in muscle occurring in otherwise healthy young people, generally in tropical climates, although cases in temperate zones have been described. Pyomyositis has been noted in association with HIV infection.[64] This information suggests that in certain hosts, perhaps with altered immune responses, particular bacteria may produce inflammatory myopathy. However, the relation of bacterial myositis to polymyositis is undetermined.

Genetics

Associations with HLA groups have been observed in some but not all series of patients studied. HLA-B8/DR3 has been noted in increased frequency in both dermatomyositis and polymyositis.[65,66] In addition, increased frequencies of HLA-B14 and HLA-B40 have also been observed. Using DNA genomic analyses of 20 children with dermatomyositis, 13 were found to have the extended haplotype B8, DR3, C4A*QO, C4B*1, C2*C, and B_f*S. In addition, a null allele for C4 was also present in five other children, three for C4A and two for C4B. In the entire group, therefore, 90 percent had the presence of a null allele for C4, suggesting either a direct relationship between the C4 gene and disease susceptibility, or a strong linkage disequilibrium between the C4 genes and those for susceptibility.[67] Of interest in this regard is the report of a patient with hereditary C2 deficiency and dermatomyositis.[68]

Association with Malignant Disease

Among the most provocative and controversial aspects of inflammatory muscle disease is its relationship to malignancy. The frequency of this association is not known precisely, although several series have indicated that it is approximately 15 to 20 percent in adults with dermatomyositis. A malignant disease association in children is rare, but it has been described. Most information on this concurrence is based on retrospective analysis of case reports and patient series, and it is possible that undue emphasis on this association has resulted therefrom. Moreover, the lack of prospectively obtained data casts doubt on the criteria used for diagnosis in groups of patients compared retrospectively. The selection of comparison groups has also not been the same in all retrospective studies. For these reasons there is disagreement on aspects of this issue. Nonetheless, a recent summary of current literature using standardized criteria for diagnosis of muscle disease suggested that roughly 20 percent of patients with dermatomyositis had associated malignancy. The frequency in polymyositis was less.[69] A retrospective survey of the older literature noted 258 cases of malignant disease concurrent with myositis. Most were seen in the fifth and sixth decades of life. The temporal relationship was reported in 167 patients: in 99, myopathy was noted first and the malignant process discovered later, usually within a year; in 17, both diseases were noted at the same time; and in 51, myopathy was recognized after the malignancy.[70] The most frequently seen tumors are cancers of the breast, lung, ovary, colon, and stomach. However, many types of neoplasms, carcinomas, sarcomas, as well as malignancies of the blood-forming and lymphatic organs have occurred. Adding to the impression of the significance of this relationship are case reports of patients with multiple neoplasms in whom exacerbation of dermatomyositislike signs were observed with tumor recurrence or appearance of a new tumor. The course of these two disorders is not always parallel, however. Independent remissions and exacerbations have been observed. One possible reason for the association of malignancy with myositis in a small subset of patients may relate to the antecedent use of cytotoxic or immunosuppressive agents. Seven such patients who had received azathioprine, cytoxan, and/or methotrexate have recently been reviewed.[69] At present, however, it is the general feeling that the potential benefits of therapy far outweigh the uncertain risk of malignancy in patients with myositis. In terms of a relationship between myositis and malignancy, because of the different kinds of malignancies observed, the varied times of appearance of one disease relative to the other, and the lack of a predictably direct relationship in the course of the two diseases, it is not likely that one is the direct cause of the other. It is possible that an alteration in the host, perhaps involving the immune system, may underlie susceptibility to these disorders. However, it should be borne in mind that the nature and extent of this relationship remains unknown.

Other Forms of Myositis

Inclusion Body Myositis

This is a chronic, slowly progressive, wasting disorder, usually of middle-aged or elderly men. There is no skin rash. There is often distal as well as asymmetric weakness without myalgia. Serum CK levels are generally only moderately elevated, and electromyography has revealed both myopathic (brief duration, polyphasic potentials) and neuropathic (fibrillation, long-lasting, large-amplitude potentials) features. Histologic evaluation demonstrates inflammatory infiltrates, chiefly with T-lymphocyte aggregates and myonecrosis, and inclusions in the sarcoplasm and nucleus. Rimmed vacuoles filled with basophilic granules are seen in frozen sections stained with hematoxylin and eosin. In paraffin-prepared sections the vacuoles may appear empty. The inclusions, when seen by electron-microscopy, are observed to contain masses of filamentous material, often in crystalline arrays. Their pathogenesis is not known, although a viral etiology has been proposed. Response to therapy, including corticosteroids and immunosuppressive agents, has been poor.[71-77]

Granulomatous Myopathy

Granulomatous infiltrates may be formed in muscle during the course of disorders such as sarcoidosis and Crohn's disease of the bowel. In addition, granulomatous myopathy may appear without signs of other disease. In this situation, granulomatous myositis is usually part of a clinical pattern of chronically progressive myopathy, occasionally complicated by dysphagia, which has been observed particularly in middle-aged women.

Eosinophilic Fasciitis, Myositis, and Eosinophilic Syndromes

Myositis may occur during the course of eosinophilic fasciitis. A recent postmortem study of this entity indicated inflammatory infiltrates in the epimysium in six of 15 cases; inflammation in the endomysium was present in ten of 15, and in the perimysium in all. Muscle fiber degeneration was present in 14 patients. Other studies have indicated a lesser frequency of involvement of muscle in these patients. Nonetheless, in most patients muscle tissue involvement appears indistinguishable miscroscopically from that of patients with polymyositis, except that in some cases eosinophilic infiltrates are found. Eosinophilic infiltration of muscle may also be a part of hypereosinophilic syndromes. In these cases involvement of other organs and of the central nervous system may occur. Cardiac and pulmonary involvement, with peripheral neuropathy, may complicate the clinical picture.[78-83]

The eosinophilia–myalgia syndrome secondary to the ingestion of chemically contaminated lots of tryptophan indicates a relationship of myositis and perimyositis to an ingested toxin.[110]

Treatment

Since the course of the disease may be protracted, a spirit of understanding between patient and physician is essential. Episodes of depression and frustration in relation to periods of exacerbation should be anticipated.

Physical Measures

Rest during periods of active inflammation and physical therapy to increase strength during periods of remission are indicated. Passive range of motion exercises can be used throughout to attempt to prevent development of contractures.

Pharmacologic Therapy

Since pharmacologic therapy falls short of cure, and is employed in an ongoing manner, it is important to assess disease activity and severity over time. This allows titration of medication in response to need. Exacerbation of disease may be heralded by arthralgia, return of rash, and increase of telangiectasia. Renewed weakness is a prime factor and should be evaluated in light of therapeutic changes and the clinical picture. Elevation of serum muscle enzymes, myoglobin and, to a lesser degree, of erythrocyte sedimentation rate may accompany or precede disease worsening. However, in chronically ill patients, these changes may be less dramatic than they were initially at the onset of illness. In addition, factors such as increased physical activity, trauma, intramuscular injections, or electromyographic studies may lead to increases in enzymes and myoglobin in the absence of progression of disease. All of this suggests the need for continued assessment, as well as careful interpretation of findings.

Corticosteroids

Corticosteroids are the mainstay of the pharmacologic approach to dermatomyositis and polymyositis in both adults and children. The usual practice is to begin oral therapy in the range of 40 to 80 mg per day of prednisone, or its equivalent, for approximately 4 to 6 weeks, or until maximum benefit is achieved. The dose is then gradually reduced, with careful monitoring of symptoms, physical findings, and laboratory test results. For children, doses of 1 to 2 mg per kg body weight per day are used initially. A recent review has suggested that the initial dose, its maintenance, and the rate of taper are most beneficial when CK levels are maintained in the normal range.[84,85,86] Although these general practices are based on clinical experience, there have not been controlled trials to indicate their superiority over other approaches. In this connection, alternate-day therapy as well as parenteral pulse therapy have been used with good results reported.[87,88] After initial therapy and taper, stable maintenance dosage, subsequent increases, or continued taper are decided by clinical response and ensuing course. Complications of corticosteroid use, including hypertension, cardiovascular decompensation, exacerbation of diabetes mellitus, osteoporosis, osteonecrosis susceptibility to infection, and changes in mood and physical appearance have been encountered. Occasionally there may be a question of whether protracted muscle weakness itself represents the effect of continued disease activity or of the atrophic effects seen in steroid myopathy. In this case, even after considering all available clinical evidence, a decision may be hard to reach, and the effect of change in steroid dose may be the best guide. In a recent series of 81 patients, over 60 percent achieved normal or near-normal strength after 3 to 4 months of steroid therapy. However, eight patients had vertebral compression fractures; seven had avascular necrosis of the head of the femur; seven had peptic ulcers; seven had cataracts; and four patients developed diabetes mellitus.[89]

Other Agents

In situations that are unresponsive to adequate corticosteroid therapy, life-threatening and progressive, or responsive to corticosteroids but with difficult or intolerable side effects, other agents have been added to therapy. To date, most experience has been gained with methotrexate and azathioprine, but 6-mercaptopurine, chlorambucil, cyclophosphamide, and cyclosporine have all been used with reported benefits. Overall, substantial corticosteroid sparing effects have been noted in approximately 40 to 50 percent or more of patients treated with these agents.

Methotrexate is usually given either orally in dose ranges of 7.5 to 30 mg once weekly, or intravenously in doses of 10 to 15 mg weekly, with gradual increments, if needed, to 30 to 50 mg. After 4 to 6 months, the dosage may be tapered consonant with the response and the clinical state. Hepatotoxicity with cell necrosis and tissue fibrosis, leukopenia, and other evidence of bone marrow suppression, gastrointestinal hemorrhage, stomatitis, skin effects, and increased susceptibility to infection, as well as pneumonitis and pulmonary fibrosis, are potential side effects. Although methotrexate is not a demonstrated carcinogen, possible teratogenicity must be considered.[90-92]

Azathioprine has also had demonstrated effectiveness. A controlled study indicated improvement in functional ability and need for a lower maintenance prednisone dose in patients receiving both azathioprine and prednisone.[93] The dose was 2 mg per kg per day with subsequent reductions over time. Treatment usually employs a gradually incrementing dosage to the range of 100 to 200 mg per day until maximum effect has been achieved. Bone marrow suppression, gastrointestinal intolerance, increased susceptibility to infection, and hepatotoxicity are potential side effects. In addition to teratogenicity, the development of neoplasia is a cause of concern. This association has not been completely evaluated in patients with myositis.

In addition, there have been reports of smaller numbers of patients successfully treated with combinations of immunosuppressive agents.[94,95] Plasmapheresis[96,97] as well as total body irradiation[98,99] have also been reported to be helpful in certain patients.

Recently, beneficial responses to intravenous infusions of gamma globulin have been observed in patients with inflammatory myopathy. If confirmed and expanded, these observations could have a great impact on the treatment of these disorders.[111,112]

Other Aspects

Rash. The course of the rash in dermatomyositis does not always parallel the course of the muscle disease. In some patients prominent rash may antedate demonstrable myositis for a long period. Sun protection and, in certain situations, hydroxychloroquine therapy may be helpful.[100] The rash generally improves with steroid treatment.

Calcinosis. Medical therapy for calcinosis has been disappointing. Surgical removal of troublesome deposits may be helpful.

Toxoplasmosis. Several patients with serologic evidence of toxoplasmosis have been treated (with sulfonamides, pyrimethamine, and folinic acid) without dramatic change in disease manifestations. However, such therapy should be considered under appropriate circumstances.

Prognosis

Over the years the prognosis of affected patients has appeared to improve. This may relate in part to earlier treatment or to treatment of milder cases. Nonetheless, both polymyositis and dermatomyositis remain serious, potentially fatal, disorders.

The chance for complete remission in children is good in over 50 percent of cases. Respiratory tract infection, cardiac failure, and gastrointestinal hemorrhage are unfavorable complications that may lead to fatality. Approximately 30 to 40 percent of children may have chronic disease with periods of exacerbation and remission. In this group calcinosis, soft tissue contractures, and muscle weakness all are sources of prolonged disability. The duration of disease activity generally may be from 2 to 4 years.[85,101-103] Late relapses have been noted.[104]

The prognosis in adults cannot be stated with precision, but may be statistically similar to that of children. However, this approximation does not include patients with malignancy, who have a poor outcome. Younger patients (under age 20) have a better chance of survival than those over age 55. Intercurrent infections, especially of the lower respiratory tract, dysphagia, chronic active disease, severe weakness, and cardiopulmonary involvement all have unfavorable influences on prognosis.[105,106] Mortality may be substantial in adults, and chronic illness marked by relapses, with long-term need for medication, is common. Perhaps 20 to 30 percent of patients demonstrate evidence of disease activity for over 10 years. A recent review of 25 patients indicated a disease-free remission rate of 42 percent after 4 to 5 years of treatment and 3 years of subsequent followup. There was a positive correlation between age at diagnosis, or onset, and the duration of illness, as assessed by period of treatment. Among ten patients who were well enough to discontinue treatment, those whose initial treatment began when they were over age 50 required 8 to 9 years before discontinuation of therapy.[107] In recent years, a trend to better survival has become apparent, with increased rates of medication-free remission of over 40 to 50 percent and a cumulative survival rate of 73 percent after 8 years.[6,108,109]

It should be kept in mind, however, that most of these figures are derived from retrospective reviews, and that current criteria for diagnosis and classification may still allow for considerable clinical heterogeneity, particularly among patients with polymyositis. All of this makes precise prediction of the clinical course in particular patients difficult.

References

1. Pearson, CM, and Bohan, A: The spectrum of polymyositis and dermatomyositis. Med Clin North Am 61:439, 1977.
2. Medsger, TA, Dawson, WN, and Masi, AT: The epidemiology of polymyositis. Am J Med 48:715, 1970.
3. DeVere, R, and Bradley, WG: Polymyositis: Its presentation, morbidity and mortality. Brain 98:637, 1975.
4. Pearson, CM: Polymyositis. Annu Rev Med 17:63, 1966.
5. Kagen, LJ, Hochman, RB, and Strong, EW: Cricopharyngeal obstruction in inflammatory myopathy (polymyositis/dermatomyositis). Arthritis Rheum 28:630, 1985.
6. Hochberg, MC, Feldman, D, and Stevens, MB: Adult onset polymyositis/dermatomyositis: An analysis of clinical and laboratory features and survival in 76 patients with a review of the literature. Semin Arthritis Rheum 15:168, 1986.
7. Feldman, D et al: Cutaneous vasculitis in adult polymyositis/dermatomyositis. J Rheumatol 10:85, 1983.
8. Ganczarczyk, ML, Lee, P, and Armstrong, SK: Nailfold microscopy in polymyositis and dermatomyositis. Arthritis Rheum 31:116, 1988.
9. Silver, RM, and Maricq, HR: Childhood dermatomyositis: Serial microvascular studies. Pediatrics 83:278, 1989.
10. Dickey, BF, and Myers, AR: Pulmonary disease in polymyositis/dermatomyositis. Semin Arthritis Rheum 14:60, 1984.
11. Lakhampal S et al: Pulmonary disease in polymyositis/dermatomyositis: A clinicopathological analysis of 65 autopsy cases. Ann Rheum Dis 46:23, 1987.
12. Bernstein, RM et al: Anti-Jo-1 antibody: A marker for myositis with interstitial lung disease. Br Med J 289:151, 1984.
13. Yoshida, S et al: The precipitating antibody to an acidic nuclear antigen, the Jo-1, in connective tissue diseases, a marker for a subset of polymyositis with interstitial pulmonary fibrosis. Arthritis Rheum 26:606, 1983.
14. Gottdiener, JS et al: Cardiac manifestations in polymyositis. Am J Cardiol 41:1141, 1978.
15. Stern, R et al: ECG abnormalities in polymyositis. Arch Intern Med 44:2185, 1984.
16. Bohan, A et al: A computer-assisted analysis of 153 patients with polymyositis and dermatomyositis. Medicine (Baltimore) 56:255, 1977.
17. Denbow, CE et al: Cardiac involvement in polymyositis. Arthritis Rheum 22:1088, 1979.
18. Haupt, HM, and Hutchins, GM: The heart and cardiac conducting system in polymyositis-dermatomyositis. Am J Cardiol 50:998, 1982.
19. Banker, BQ: Dermatomyositis of childhood. J Neuropathol Exp Neurol 34:46, 1975.
20. Crowe, WE et al: Clinical and pathogenetic implications of histopathology in childhood polydermatomyositis. Arthritis Rheum 25:126, 1982.
21. Bowyer, SL et al: Juvenile dermatomyositis: Histological findings and pathogenetic hypothesis for the associated skin changes. J Rheumatol 13:753, 1986.
22. Fudman, EJ, and Schnitzer, TJ: Dermatomyositis without creatine kinase elevation: A poor prognostic sign. Am J Med 80:329, 1986.
23. Brownlow, K, and Elevitch, FR: Serum creatine phosphokinase iso-enzyme (CPK_2) in myositis. JAMA 230:1141, 1974.
24. Goto, I: Creatine phosphokinase isoenzymes in neuromuscular disorders. Arch Neurol 31:116, 1974.
25. Larca, LJ, Coppola, JT, and Honig, S: Creatine kinase MB isoenzyme in dermatomyositis: A noncardiac source. Ann Intern Med 94:341, 1981.
26. Morton, BD, III, and Statland, BE: Serum enzyme alterations in polymyositis. Am J Clin Pathol 73:556, 1980.

27. Kagen, LJ: Myoglobinemia and myoglobinuria in patients with myositis. Arthritis Rheum 14:457, 1971.
28. Fritzler, MJ, Valencia, DW, and McCarty, GA: Speckled pattern antinuclear antibodies resembling anticentromere antibodies. Arthritis Rheum 27:92, 1984.
29. Targoff, IN, Raghu, G, and Reichlin, M: Antibodies to Mi-1 in SLE: Relationship to other precipitins and reactions with bovine immunoglobulin. Clin Exp Immunol 53:76, 1983.
30. Targoff, IN, and Reichlin, M: The association between M1-2 antibodies and dermatomyositis. Arthritis Rheum 28:796, 1985.
31. Targoff, IN, and Reichlin, M: Nucleolar localization of the PM-SCL antigen. Arthritis Rheum 28:226, 1985.
32. Treadwell, EL et al: Clinical relevance of PM-1 antibody and physiochemical characterization of PM-1 antigen. J Rheumatol 11:658, 1984.
33. Mathews, MB, and Bernstein, RM: Myositis autoantibody inhibits histidyl-tRNA synthetase: A model for autoimmunity. Nature 304:177, 1983.
34. Arnett, FC et al: The Jo-1 antibody system in myositis: Relationships to clinical features and HLA. J Rheumatol 8:925, 1981.
35. Mathews, MB et al: Anti-threonyl-tRNA synthetase, a second myositis-related autoantibody. J Exp Med 160:420, 1984.
36. Okada, N et al: Isolation of a novel antibody, which precipitates ribonucleoprotein complex containing threonine tRNA from a patient with polymyositis. Eur J Biochem 139:425, 1984.
37. Bunn, CC, Bernstein, RM, and Mathews, MB: Autoantibodies against alanyl-tRNA synthetase and tRNA Ala coexist and are associated with myositis. J Exp Med 163:1281, 1986.
38. Engel, AH, and Arahata, K: Mononuclear cells in myopathies. Hum Pathol 17:704, 1986.
39. Arahata, K, and Engel, AG: Monoclonal antibody analysis of mononuclear cells in myopathies. V. Ann Neurol 23:493, 1988.
40. Kalovidouris, AE et al: Relationships between clinical features and distribution of mononuclear cells in muscle of patients with polymyositis. J Rheumatol 15:1401, 1988.
41. Kalovidouris, A: Mononuclear cells from patients with polymyositis inhibit calcium binding by sarcoplasmic reticulum. J Lab Clin Med 107:23, 1986.
42. Saito, E et al: Damaging effect of peripheral mononuclear cells of dermatomyositis on cultured human skin fibroblasts. J Rheumatol 14:936, 1987.
43. Urbano-Marquez, A et al: Inflammatory myopathy associated with chronic graft-versus-host disease. Neurology 36:1091, 1986.
44. Whitaker, JN, and Engel, WK: Vascular deposits of immunoglobulin and complement in idiopathic inflammatory myopathy. N Engl J Med 286:333, 1972.
45. Fessel, WJ, and Raas, MC: Autoimmunity in the pathogenesis of muscle disease. Neurology 18:1137, 1968.
46. Kissel, JT, Mendell, JR, and Rammohan, KW: Microvascular deposition of complement membrane attack complex in dermatomyositis. N Engl J Med 314:329, 1986.
47. Koga, K et al: Western-blotting method for detecting antibodies against human muscle contractile proteins in myositis. J Immunol Methods 105:15, 1987.
48. Matsubara, S, and Takamori, M: Experimental allergic myositis: Strain 13 guinea pig immunised with rabbit myosin B fraction. Acta Neuropathol 74:158, 1987.
49. Christensen, JL et al: Prevalence of Coxsackie B virus antibodies in patients with juvenile dermatomyositis. Arthritis Rheum 29:1365, 1986.
50. Travers, RL et al: Coxsackie B neutralisation titres in polymyositis/dermatomyositis. Lancet i:1268, 1977.
51. CL Warner, PB Fayad and RR Heffner Jr. Legionella myositis. Neurol. 41:750, 1991.
52. Ray, CG, Minnich, LL, and Johnson, PC: Selective polymyositis induced by Coxsackie virus B_1 in mice. J Infect Dis 140:239, 1979.
53. Strongwater, SL et al: A murine model of polymyositis induced by Coxsackievirus B_1 (Tucson strain). Arthritis Rheum 27:433, 1984.
54. Ytterberg, SR: Coxsackie B_1 induced polymyositis: Acute infection with active virus is required for myositis. J Rheumatol 14:12, 1987.
55. Ytterberg, SR, Mahowald, ML, and Messner, RP: T cells are required for Coxsackievirus B_1 induced murine polymyositis. J Rheumatol 15:475, 1988.
56. Mease, PJ, Ochs, HD, and Wedgewood, RJ: Successful treatment of ECHO virus meningoencephalitis and myositis-fasciitis with intravenous immune globulin therapy in a patient with X-linked agammaglobulinemia. N Engl J Med 304:1278, 1981.
57. Crennan, JM et al: Echovirus polymyositis in patients with hypogammaglobulinemia. Am J Med 81:35, 1986.
58. Gonzales, MF et al: Subacute structural myopathy associated with human immunodeficiency virus infection. Arch Neurol 45:585, 1988.
59. Dalakas, MC et al: Polymyositis associated with AIDS retrovirus. JAMA 256:2381, 1986.
60. Stern, R, Gold, J, and DiCarlo, EF: Myopathy complicting the acquired immune deficiency syndrome. Muscle Nerve 10:318, 1987.
61. Phillips, PE, Kassan, SS, and Kagen, LJ: Increased toxoplasma antibodies in idiopathic inflammatory muscle disease. Arthritis Rheum 22:209, 1979.
62. Magid, SK, and Kagen, LJ: Serological evidence for acute toxoplasmosis in polymyositis-dermatomyositis: Increased frequency of specific antitoxoplasma IgM antibodies. Am J Med 75:312, 1983.
63. Atlas, E et al: Lyme myositis: Muscle invasion by Borrelia burgdorferi. Ann Intern Med 109:245, 1988.
64. Gaut, P, Wong, PK, and Meyer, RP: Pyomyositis in a patient with the acquired immunodeficiency syndrome. Arch Intern Med 148:1608, 1988.

65. Friedman, JM et al: Immunogenetic studies of juvenile dermatomyositis. Tissue Antigens 21:45, 1983.
66. Pachman, LM et al: HLA-B8 in juvenile dermatomyositis. Lancet ii:567, 1977.
67. Robb, SA et al: C4 complement allotypes in juvenile dermatomyositis. Hum Immunol 22:31, 1988.
68. Leddy, JP et al: Hereditary complement (C2) deficiency with dermatomyositis. Am J Med 58:83, 1975.
69. Callen, JP: Dermatomyositis. Dis Mon 33:242, 1987.
70. Barnes, BE: Dermatomyositis and malignancy. Ann Intern Med 84:68, 1976.
71. Carpenter, S et al: Inclusion body myositis: A distinct variety of idiopathic inflammatory myopathy. Neurology 28:8, 1978.
72. Chou, S-M: Inclusion body myositis: A chronic persistent mumps myositis? Hum Pathol 17:765, 1986.
73. Danon, MJ et al: Inclusion body myositis: A corticosteroid-resistant inflammatory myopathy. Arch Neurol 39:760, 1982.
74. Eisen, A, Berry, K, and Gibson, G: Inclusion body myositis (IBM): Myopathy or neuropathy? Neurology 33:1109, 1983.
75. Julien, J et al: Inclusion body myositis. J Neurol Sci 55:15, 1982.
76. Yunis, EJ, and Samaha, FJ: Inclusion body myositis. Lab Invest 25:240, 1971.
77. Lazaro, RP et al: Inclusion body myositis: Case reports and a reappraisal of an under-recognized type of myopathy. Mt Sinai J Med 53:137, 1986.
78. Huang, K-W, and Chen, X-H: Pathology of eosinophilic fasciitis and its relation to polymyositis. Can J Neurol Sci 14:632, 1987.
79. Layzer, RB, Shearn, MA, and Satya-Murti, S: Eosinophilic polymyositis. Ann Neurol 1:65, 1977.
80. Bjelle, A, Henriksson, K-G, and Hofer, P-A: Polymyositis in eosinophilic fasciitis. Eur Neurol 19:128, 1980.
81. Schumacher, HR: A scleroderma-like syndrome with fasciitis, myositis and eosinophilia. Ann Intern Med 84:49, 1976.
82. Serratrice, G et al: Relapsing eosinophilic perimyositis. J Rheumatol 7:199, 1980.
83. Sladek, GD et al: Relapsing eosinophilic myositis. J Rheumatol 10:467, 1983.
84. Dubowitz, V: Treatment of dermatomyositis in childhood. Arch Dis Child 51:494, 1971.
85. Rose, AL: Childhood polymyositis. Am J Dis Child 127:518, 1974.
86. Oddis, CV, and Medsger, TA: Relationship between creatine kinase level and corticosteroid therapy in polymyositis-dermatomyositis. J Rheumatol 15:807, 1988.
87. Uchino, M et al: High single-dose alternate-day corticosteroid regimens in treatment of polymyositis. J Neurol 232:175, 1985.
88. Yanigasawa, T et al: Methyl prednisolone pulse therapy in dermatomyositis. Dermatologica 167:47, 1983.
89. Tymms, KE, and Webb, J: Dermatopolymyositis and other connective tissue diseases: A review of 105 cases. J Rheumatol 12:1140, 1985.
90. Malaviya, AN, Many, A, and Schwartz, RS: Treatment of dermatomyositis with methotrexate. Lancet ii:485, 1968.
91. Metzger, AL et al: Polymyositis and dermatomyositis: Combined methotrexate and corticosteroid therapy. Ann Intern Med 81:182, 1974.
92. Jacobs, JC: Methotrexate and azathioprine treatment of childhood dermatomyositis. Pediatrics 59:212, 1977.
93. Bunch, TW: Prednisone and azathioprine for polymyositis: Long-term follow-up. Arthritis Rheum 24:45, 1981.
94. Tiliakos, NA: Low dose cytotoxic combination therapy in intractable dermatopolymyositis. Arthritis Rheum 30:S14, 1987.
95. Wallace, DJ, Metzger, AL, and White, KK: Combination immunosuppressive treatment of steroid-resistant dermatomyositis/polymyositis. Arthritis Rheum 28:590, 1985.
96. Bennington, JA, and Dau, PC: Patients with polymyositis and dermatomyositis who undergo plasmapheresis therapy: Pathologic findings. Arch Neurol 38:553, 1981.
97. Dau, PC: Plasmapheresis in idiopathic inflammatory myopathy. Arch Neurol 38:544, 1981.
98. Engel, WK, Lichter, AS, and Galdi, AP: Polymyositis: Remarkable response to total body irradiation. Lancet i:658, 1981.
99. Kelly, JJ et al: Response to total body irradiation in dermatomyositis. Muscle Nerve 11:120, 1988.
100. Woo, TY et al: Cutaneous lesions of dermatomyositis are improved by hydroxychloroquine. J Am Acad Dermatol 10:592, 1984.
101. Miller, JJ: Late progression in dermatomyositis in childhood. J Pediatr 83:543, 1973.
102. Hill, RH, and Wood, WS: Juvenile dermatomyositis. Can Med Assoc J 103:1152, 1970.
103. Spenser, CH et al: Course of treated juvenile dermatomyositis. J Pediatr 105:399, 1984.
104. Lovell, HB, and Lindsley, CB: Late recurrence of childhood dermatomyositis. J Rheumatol 13:821, 1986.
105. Carpenter, JR et al: Survival in polymyositis: Corticosteroids and risk factors. J Rheumatol 4:207, 1977.
106. Medsger, TA, Jr, Robinson, H, and Masi, AT: Factors affecting survivorship in polymyositis. Arthritis Rheum 14:249, 1971.
107. McKendry, RJ: Influence of age at onset on the duration of treatment in idiopathic adult polymyositis and dermatomyositis. Arch Intern Med 147:1989, 1987.
108. Hoffman, GS et al: Presentation, treatment, and prognosis of idiopathic inflammatory muscle disease in a rural hospital. Am J Med 75:433, 1983.
109. Baron, M, and Small, P: Polymyositis/dermatomyositis: Clinical features and outcome in 22 patients. J Rheumatol 12:283, 1985.

110. Hertzman, PA, Falk, H, Kilbourne, EM, Page, S, and Shulman, LE: The eosinophilia-myalgia syndrome. J Rheum 18:867, 1991.
111. Roifman, CM, Schaffer, FM, Wachsmuth, SE, Murphy, G, and Gelfand, EW: Reversal of chronic polymyositis following intravenous immune serum globulin therapy. Journal of American Medicine Association. 258:513, 1987.
112. Cherin, P, Herson, S, Wechsler, B, Piette, JC, Bletry, O, Coutellier, A, Ziza, JM, Godeau, P: Effect of intravenous gammaglobulin therapy in chronic refractory polymyositis and dermatomyositis. American Journal of Medicine. 91:162, 1991.

Chapter 11
The Spectrum of Scleroderma

E. CARWILE LEROY, M.D.

Introduction

Scleroderma can be both straightforward and complex; straightforward because one criterion of its classification (taut skin proximal to the metacarpophalangeal joints) defines involvement in more than 90 percent of generalized scleroderma patients, and complex because of a remarkable variation in the degree and rate of progression of both the taut, hidebound skin, from which the term scleroderma (hard skin) is derived, and the internal organ involvement as well.

Localized scleroderma is called morphea. Meticulous studies of morphea have defined up to eight subsets (isolated, guttate, other) distinguishing these patients from one another. For this discussion, suffice it to say that localized scleroderma is not associated with systemic involvement. Its diagnosis, classification, and management is left to dermatology colleagues. Suspicion is generated by an area of skin that the examiner is unable to pinch. Biopsy can be helpful but may not be necessary.

Linear scleroderma, also not associated with visceral involvement, usually occurs in a dermatome distribution, often begins early in life, and may hamper skeletal and muscular development sufficiently to lead to progressive limb atrophy of major functional and cosmetic importance. Unfortunately, management is largely supportive, wound healing in affected areas is impaired, and all limb structures, including bone, muscle, nerve, and blood vessels, are impressively atrophied.

Generalized morphea is more difficult to define because it bridges localized and systemic types of scleroderma. Patients, usually females in their active childbearing years, note increasing numbers of isolated patches of morphea that may coalesce. Fortunately, new lesions appear less frequently after childbearing ceases. An occasional patient with generalized morphea has visceral organ involvement. Comparisons of generalized morphea with diffuse fasciitis with eosinophilia have been made, which is comparing the idiopathic with the enigmatic.

Systemic sclerosis (SSc), the major generalized type of scleroderma, is being increasingly recognized in the population of all ages who have the episodic, triphasic (pallor and cyanosis associated with suffusion, pain, and erythema) vascular reaction termed Raynaud's phenomenon. In South Carolina, a carefully controlled population-based study found that 3 to 4 percent of persons over age 18, men or women, black or white, have Raynaud's phenomenon. The unexpectedly high frequency in men was explained by occupational exposure to vibration and manual labor. It is from the Raynaud's-positive population that virtually all SSc patients emerge. The identification of the patient destined to develop SSc from the Raynaud's population is the purview of the internist and rheumatologist. Since two recently perfected techniques are available as office procedures to assist in this identification, and since the process of identification itself contributes significantly in establishing the long-term outcome and in defining the two major subsets of SSc (see later discussion), this identification process is discussed in detail.

Clinical Manifestations

Early Detection: Raynaud's Phenomenon

As stated, the symptoms of Raynaud's phenomenon should be recurrent, the color changes should be biphasic or triphasic, and multiple digits should be symmetrically involved. To be definite, these changes should be observed by an experienced observer. Frequency and duration should be self-recorded. On physical examination, digital pits, consisting of keratotic excrescences that mark prior epidermal ulcerations, and digital webs under the nails, which have a similar ischemic implication, should be searched for and, when present, have a positive predictive implication for the development of SSc.

The single test that can best distinguish the Raynaud's patient who is destined to develop connective tissue disease, especially SSc, is a photographic recording of the rows of cutaneous capillary loops at the base of the fingernail skin, which only in this anatomic location are conveniently viewable along their long axis, in contrast to cutaneous capillary loops elsewhere that are seen only as the dome of the closed end of the capillary loop. The procedure is termed widefield nailfold capillary microscopy, the technical details have been meticulously defined, and the evaluation of the Raynaud's subject is incomplete without a permanent photographic record of nailfold capillaries. Abnormalities consist of dilated loops and/or areas of absent capillaries, called capillary destruction or dropout. In population-based studies, capillary-positive patients comprise less than 20 percent of Raynaud's patients; essentially all future SSc patients reside in the capillary-positive group. In clinic-selected groups, subject to varying referral bias, most Raynaud's patients may be capillary positive. It is remarkable how constant the abnormal nailfold capillary pattern is, since conversions from positive to negative and negative to positive are extremely rare. The time between onset of Raynaud's phenomenon and the development of full blown SSc can be quite variable, so that silent and watchful waiting seems more prudent than immediate labeling; nonetheless, the biologic continuum between capillary-positive Raynaud's patients and the limited version of SSc seems inescapable.

It should be recalled that the differential diagnosis of capillary-negative Raynaud's phenomenon is very broad and spans mechanical, primary vascular, intravascular, and rheumatic syndromes, for a discussion of which the reader is referred to more comprehensive texts.

A second major confirming technique for the identification of the Raynaud's patient who will ultimately develop connective tissue disease is to determine the autoimmune serology of the patient, specifically the titer of antinuclear antibodies (ANA). Originally introduced into the clinic for the diagnosis of systemic lupus erythematosus (SLE), early ANA determination used lower vertebrate tissue, such as mouse thymus or rat liver, which had the disadvantages consisting of cells which were nonhuman and nondividing. When it became apparent that some patients, particularly patients with diffuse connective tissue disease, have circulating antibodies to nuclear antigens that are reactive only during the nuclear reorganization that occurs during mitosis, new substrates were sought. The introduction of a human laryngeal carcinoma line (HEp-2), which divides rapidly in culture and thus demonstrates frequent cells undergoing mitosis, increased by several-fold the prevalence of ANA positivity in connective tissue patients, especially SSc.

On this basis, an ANA on an HEp-2 substrate is an important, if not essential, adjunct to the evaluation of the Raynaud's patient. With one exception, it remains to be documented definitively that the type of ANA positivity can predict the illness pattern, prognosis, or outcome of individual patients. The exception is the anticentromere antibody pattern (see next section).

Thus, the capillary-positive, HEp-2 ANA-positive Raynaud's patient is seen as on a path toward the ultimate development of SSc. Fortunately, most represent the limited end of the spectrum of SSc involvement and should be managed expectantly, without alarming the patient, for its eventual development.

Scleroderma Subsets

When a patient develops taut skin proximal to the knuckles, he or she has SSc. The next major question that faces the physician is determination of the type of SSc the patient has. Most important for the patient is to identify the minority of patients who have the diffuse variety, termed diffuse cutaneous systemic sclerosis (dSSc). The dSSc patient presents with a rather explosive onset of Raynaud's phenomenon associated with edema (nonpitting, occasionally slightly tender, without warmth or redness), usually of the hands and face but occasionally also of the legs and arms. This "early puffy" clinical pattern may or may not be associated with a positive ANA test that does not include the anticentromere antibody (ACA) pattern; ultimately (the gold standard criterion of dSSc), dSSc patients develop truncal skin tightening usually within 18 to 24 months. Steen and Medsger have shown that the presence of tendon friction rubs prior to the appearance of truncal taut skin can predict dSSc in about 75 percent of patients; that is,

75 percent of patients with tendon friction rubs but without truncal skin tautness developed truncal skin changes over the next few years (Medsger, 1989).

Why is it important to distinguish dSSc from other subsets of generalized scleroderma? Simply because the present or future development of organ involvement is substantially more likely in dSSc patients than in other SSc patients, and it is well documented that organ involvement dictates both the mortality and the morbidity of the disease. The patient with dSSc should probably be taught to take his or her own blood pressure weekly, should have several 24-hour urine collections per year for protein excretion and creatinine clearance, should have yearly pulmonary function tests with single-breath diffusion studies, and should undergo thorough cardiovascular evaluations including chest x-ray studies, electrocardiogram, echocardiogram, Holter monitoring, ventriculography, and stress thallium cardiac scans. Essentially 100 percent of SSc patients who die from their disease in the first 10 years of symptoms have the features of dSSc described above; conversely, over that same crucial first decade, most dSSc patients develop at least one significant organ involvement. This is not to say that other SSc patients do not develop significant organ involvement; they do. They do not as a rule, which has occasional exceptions, develop significant organ involvement that limits function in the first 10 years of symptoms, which includes the duration of symptoms of Raynaud's phenomenon only.

The majority of SSc patients have a pattern of illness quite different from dSSc. These predominately female patients, for whom the designation limited cutaneous systemic sclerosis (lSSc) or CREST (calcinosis, Raynaud's phenomenon, esophageal hypomotility, sclerodactyly, and/or telangiectasia) is used, usually begin to note cold- or stress-associated Raynaud's phenomenon in the second, third, or fourth decade of life, as occasionally did their mothers or their female siblings. Often viewed as a nuisance or "one of those things that runs in the family," they may not consult a physician for this complaint. Complaints of Raynaud's phenomenon and nothing more may predominate for years; regularly the entire first decade of symptoms is so characterized. Almost imperceptibly the clinical pattern changes to include digital pitting, digital ulcers, taut skin of the fingers and later of the hands, difficulty with swallowing (esophageal hypomotility), and difficulty with breathing (pulmonary hypertension and/or interstitial lung disease). Trigeminal neuralgia from fibrotic impingement of the facial nerve is a rare late feature of lSSc. Therefore, the organ involvement of lSSc patients is in the second, third, and fourth decades of symptoms.

It is helpful to identify lSSc patients as early in the onset of symptoms as possible. If the nailfold capillary examination shows capillary dilatation without capillary destruction and, in addition, if the ANA is positive and shows an anticentromere pattern, one can assume that this is lSSc and initiate a multisystem evaluation at the outset and at approximately 5- to 10-year intervals. It is convenient and efficient that the same two tools most useful in distinguishing the connective tissue disease patient from the Raynaud's population are also most valuable in separating dSSc from lSSc: careful skin examination coupled with nailfold capillary and HEp-2 ANA patterns.

Pathogenesis

Systemic sclerosis is one of the autoimmune disorders with distinctive serologic reactions as shown in Table 11-1. Its end result is an exuberant fibrotic reaction composed of the usual proportions of types I and III collagens, perhaps other collagens, fibronectin (either the usual or an altered molecule), and proteoglycans. This at first cellular and later largely matrix material fills both the subcutaneous space, where it obliterates capillaries, and the subendothelial or intimal space of small arteries and arterioles. The key questions, largely unanswered, are: what stimuli generate the scar tissue and why does the body not remove it?

Table 11-1. Autoantibodies Observed in Patients with Scleroderma

Anticentromere antibodies (ACA) (kinetochore proteins)*
Antinucleolar antibodies
   RNA polymerase 1 (pol 1)*
   Fibrillarin (U3 RNP protein complex)*
   Nucleolar 4-6S RNA
   7-2 RNA protein complex
   PM-Scl†
Antitopoisomerase I (topo I) (formerly Scl-70)*,‡
Anticollagen type IV*
Antilaminin*
Antiribonucleoprotein (RNP)†

*Rarely seen in other autoimmune diseases, hence, can be considered as specific disease markers.
†Commonly seen in overlap patients, as is anti-Ro.
‡Antisera containing antibodies to topo I uniformly show weak nucleolar staining due to nucleolar topo I.

The etiology of SSc is almost completely unknown. The search for a susceptible host continues and is presently centered on a set of major histocompatibility genes that exhibit linkage disequilibrium with selective class III genes that express null alleles for the A and B components of the fourth component of complement. This association is at present better demonstrated for lupus, which does not show exuberant scarring, than for SSc, which does. At present, an immunogenetic basis for SSc remains elusive.

Increasing interest in several environmental triggers of SSc was catalyzed by the 4000 new cases of sclerodermalike illness precipitated by the accidental ingestion of an adulterated rapeseed oil in the environs of Madrid in 1981. The list of known environmental triggers for SSc is shown in Table 11-2. One mechanism they have in common is the production of toxic oxygen-derived free radicals. Systematic historical and environmental searches for triggers of environmental scleroderma should be undertaken in both dSSc and lSSc patients.

Presently, pathophysiologic studies in SSc have taken several directions:

1. Fribroblast studies. All recent studies lead to the conclusion that coordinate transcriptional activation of several matrix genes occurs by a mechanism yet to be precisely defined. Transacting protein factors that initiate transcription by binding to each other possibly by leucine zipper interactions and by binding to promote enhancer upstream regions of the gene, possibly by zinc fingerlike structures, are being searched for. A single control point for the scleroderma lesion might be found by further definition of the regulation of transcription of the matrix genes involved.

   In addition to a matrix abnormality, SSc fibroblasts exhibit a cell growth abnormality characterized by an autocrine growth stimulus manifested by decreased receptor numbers to platelet-derived growth factor and increased expression of a proto-oncogene c-myc, a gene also showing increased expression in SSc mononuclear cells. If the transcriptional regulation of c-myc turns out to be related to the regulation of collagen or other matrix genes, by either a homeotic group gene control mechanism or by similar interactions with protein transcriptional activators, this transcriptional regulation control point would be a suitable target for therapeutic intervention in SSc. One of the cytokines known to inhibit mRNA for collagen, gamma-interferon, could be functioning by way of these pathways and is presently being studied in therapeutic trials of SSc. Much more detailed study is needed.

2. Endothelial cell studies. The endothelial cell from artery to capillary in SSc is modulated (activated perhaps, injured perhaps) to favor increased permeability, decreased nutritional blood flow, increased thrombogenicity, and decreased or altered fibrinolysis. Whether a soluble cytokine (interleukin-1, interleukin-6, tumor necrosis factor, lymphotoxin, transforming growth factor-beta) or a membrane bound activity requiring direct T-cell endothelial cell interaction modulates endothelial cell function is unclear. Whatever the future holds in the altered endothelial cell pathobiology of SSc, in order for therapies to be logically directed, much more will need to be known about the specific targets of the autoimmune modulation of the endothelium.

3. Immune studies. The helper-inducer interleukin-2 dependent subset of T cells (CD4) is hyperactive in SSc. Levels of this activity correlate positively with disease activity and progression. The precise stimulus for this autoimmune activity still awaits precise molecular definition. There are several excellent candidates, all of which are specific for SSc, including type IV collagen and laminin (both of which are components of the endothelium), the centromere/kinetochore region of the chromosome, and the nuclear housekeeping enzyme topoisomerase I. Specific definition of the presumed immunogenetic background favorable for the development of SSc, perhaps combined with an environmental triggering stimulus, are now achievable goals.

Clinical, cellular, and molecular research in SSc is ongoing. An intense, well-funded effort could hopefully bring the bench to the bedside in the 1990s.

Table 11-2. Environmental Triggers of Scleroderma

Silica dust
Vinyl chloride (and trichloroethylene)
Bleomycin, *cis*-platinum
Chronic graft-vs.-host disease (GVHD)
Toxic oil syndrome
Vibration exposure
Benzene (and phenylenediamines)
Epoxy resins
Carbidopa and hydroxytryptophan
Silicone mammoplasty

Diagnosis and Management

Vascular Impairment

All SSc patients have vascular impairment; even those who profess not to have symptoms of Raynaud's phenomenon can be shown to have abnormally increased vascular sensitivity to cold-induced vasospasm. Both arterial and capillary vascular beds are involved in, at first, functional and, later, structural derangements. Treatment choices depend on the severity of the vascular symptoms and signs. All patients should avoid extreme cold and undue stress. Dress should include extra layers over the trunk to induce peripheral vasodilatation. Meals should be light in volume and in richness to reduce the redirection of blood flow to the gut. Cigarettes are strictly forbidden; all stimulants except alcohol are discouraged. Exercise should be regular and relaxing. Biofeedback, meditation, and other techniques of behavioral conditioning may be helpful if the patient is self-motivated.

Medications are indicated in the patient with severe symptoms or with ischemic signs, including digital pits, webs, or ulcers or a history of digital tissue loss. The calcium channel blockers are the single most effective group of drugs, and nifedipine seems to be the drug of first choice, with diltiazem a close second choice. These agents have far fewer side effects than do drugs previously used for Raynaud's phenomenon alone, and are an important addition for the management of Raynaud's phenomenon in SSc when it is uncomplicated.

Persistent ulcers and impending tissue loss from digital gangrene should be managed emergently with admission to the hospital. The differential diagnosis includes thromboangiitis obliterans, polyarteritis nodosa, and the antiphospholipid antibody syndrome. Stellate ganglion blocks and the entire pharmacologic armamentarium of vasodilators (calcium channel blockers), antiplatelet agents (dipyridamole and aspirin), and erythrocyte distensibility enhancers (pentoxifylline [Trental]) should be used. Lasting effects of dorsal or digital sympathectomy are less predictable. Plasmapheresis has not been given an extensive trial as yet.

Pulmonary Involvement

Pulmonary involvement in SSc is both subtle and ominous. Subtle because symptoms and chest x-ray studies detect patients only in the later stages and ominous because interstitial lung disease is now the leading cause of death in SSc patients.

The various aspects of pulmonary scleroderma are interrelated, perhaps with the exception of pleural serositis. Acute pleurisy is rare, but chronic chest discomfort, sometimes with a deep inspiratory component, is common and small pleural effusions and pleural thickening not detected clinically are common on postmortem examination. Pleural involvement usually does not significantly impair function and its symptoms are usually manageable with non-steroidal anti-inflammatory agents; rarely are glucocorticoids (steroids) necessary.

Before continuing, perhaps two ancient myths should be deflated. The notions that taut chest skin leads to restrictive lung disease is illogical and without a basis in fact. Similarly, the notion that esophageal hypomotility and aspiration cause all SSc pulmonary fibrosis is also inconsistent with clinical or the histologic picture of either aspiration pneumonia or pulmonary fibrosis. In other clinical settings, patients may have the one without the other.

Pulmonary hypertension and interstitial lung disease are inextricably intertwined. The most acute presentation is the patient with early dSSc who becomes acutely dyspneic, with or without an orthopneic component, without antecedent respiratory symptoms. The lungs are usually clear on examination, the cardiac second sound (S2) in the pulmonic area is often accentuated with a relatively fixed split, and the chest x-ray study and electrocardiogram are often unremarkable. Echocardiogram with Doppler studies is the critical test to provide, at the same time, both qualitative and quantitative confirmation of pulmonary hypertension. We usually admit the patient because of the danger of sudden death, and treat with prednisone, 40 to 60 mg in divided daily doses, nifedipine 10 to 30 mg t.i.d., and dipyridamole 50 to 100 mg t.i.d. These acute patients usually have little to no ventilatory impairment and respond well to treatment, at least over the short term. Whether they are more prone to develop pulmonary fibrosis than the patient who has not had a clinically detected episode of acute pulmonary hypertension is uncertain. The likelihood of sudden death in the next two to five years is high.

The insidiously progressive feature of pulmonary scleroderma is interstitial lung disease, also called fibrosing alveolitis. The tools used to detect it are history (most patients are asymptomatic until late); physical examination (dry crackles, also called Velcro rales, are present late); gallium scan (insensitive but specific); computerized tomography of the lung (recommended by one investigative team); and bronchoalveolar lavage (BAL), clearly the present gold standard. Bronchoalveolar lavage is sufficiently sensitive and specific that is has redefined the natural history of pulmonary involvement in connective tissue diseases, much as the first widespread use of single-breath diffusion capacity did 4 decades ago, when studies showed that 75 to 80 percent of early SSc patients had diffusion capacity abnormalities at a time when they were asymptomatic and had normal chest x-ray results. It was never clearly shown that all patients with diffusion capacity abnormalities, essentially a measure of the balance between ventilation and perfusion, go on to develop pulmonary fibrosis.

The emerging story with BAL is most promising for supplying the first essential criterion for effective therapy, which is early detection. Active alveolitis is defined as increased concentrations of neutrophils, eosinophils, or lymphocytes as a percentage of total cells. An equally sensitive measure of alveolitis is to measure the state of activation of the alveolar macrophage, such as the production of fibronectin from short-term cultures of BAL cells. Whatever the most specific measure of alveolitis turns out to be, BAL is about twice as sensitive as history and physical examination, as forced vital capacity measurements, or as scans for the detection of pulmonary parenchymal inflammation. Thus, the data are rapidly accumulating to document the sensitivity of BAL in the detection of alveolitis; of perhaps equal clinical importance is the recent observation of Silver and colleagues that patients with alveolitis who underwent BAL 1 to 2 years ago continue to show signs of alveolitis on repeat BAL and these persistently alveolitis-positive SSc patients are the group who demonstrate deterioration in ventilatory function over a period of several years' observation. The existing information is sufficiently promising to propose that all dSSc patients undergo BAL to detect the alveolitis-positive subset who can then be treated with a variety of therapeutic interventions to demonstrate potential efficacy. At present no specific therapies can be enthusiastically recommended for pulmonary involvement probably largely because none have been started sufficiently early in the course of involvement. Two studies have shown a statistically but probably not a clinically significant improvement in pulmonary function after many months of D-penicillamine therapy. Had BAL been used in these patients the focus might well have been sharper and the results more definitive. It is encouraging to see different therapeutic modalities being applied to pulmonary scleroderma; unfortunately, no emphasis can yet be given to these therapies; they include prednisone and cyclophosphamide, cyclosporin A, and plasmapheresis. We will have to wait for the needed studies to be done; BAL should greatly improve the patient selection and the duration required to detect a response, since the presumption can now be made that agents that convert abnormal BAL findings to normal can and should prevent and may even reverse pulmonary fibrosis.

Gastrointestinal Features

With detailed investigation, virtually all SSc patients can be shown to have evidence of decreased intrinsic motility of the gastrointestinal tract. It is not uncommon that this involvement is completely asymptomatic. Therefore, it is acceptable, if the patient is without complaint, to defer detailed testing until symptoms of dysphagia, denoting esophageal involvement, are presented by the patient. It is recommended, as worthwhile preventive measures, to suggest that all SSc patients sleep with the front two bedposts elevated on 6-inch wooden blocks, easily purchased from the neighborhood home improvement emporium; that they remain upright for 4 hours after a heavy meal, and that they ingest 1 g of sucralfate (Carafate) in a slurry of water before retiring. Although it cannot be rigorously proved, it is reasonable that this regimen, strictly adhered to, will decrease the prevalence of reflux esophagitis and esophageal stricture.

Appropriate tests to evaluate esophageal function can start simply with a determination of esophageal transit time using quantitative esophageal scintigraphy. A normal time is a sufficient test to reassure the patient and to postpone further testing. If transit is slowed, a cine-esophagram is needed to ensure that lesions essentially unrelated but relatively common are not present, such as the upper, striated muscle dysfunction of dermatomyositis/polymyositis, the presence of a hiatal hernia or a diverticulum of some sort, or other infrequent causes of swallowing dysfunction. If the cine-esophagram is negative, and further definition is indicated, esophageal manometry is the standard for esophageal hypomotility and decreased lower esophageal sphincter tone. If signs of obstruction (vomiting soon after eating food which tastes much as it did when it left the mouth) are present, direct esophagoscopy is indicated immediately.

Drugs to improve esophageal function have been disappointing. Metoclopramide (Reglan) and cisapride affect smooth muscle function and may not be able to affect SSc smooth muscle, which is atrophic, electrically dysregulated, and ultimately fibrotic. In practice oral doses of these agents do not improve the propulsion of the SSc esophagus. Dopaminergic central nervous system hyperkinetic behavior responses limit patient acceptance of metoclopramide. A preliminary report suggests that cisapride, a drug being tested to increase intestinal motility in pseudo-obstruction, can increase the resting level of lower esophageal sphincter tone. Inhibitors of gastric acid secretion (H_2 blockers), including the newer agent omeprazole, are standard therapy in SSc patients with dysphagia.

Second to dysphagia with or without heartburn (in gastrointestinal symptoms in SSc) is constipation, a constipation/diarrhea cycle, or obstipation. Some patients are highly desirous of "normalizing" this pattern; some are tolerant of it. Fiber helps: stool softeners help; most important is to avoid constipating agents such as codeine or Lomotil, which can turn a nuisance complaint into an emergency setting of ileus, obstipation, and acute surgical intervention. Too many SSc patients have died of cardiopulmonary/renal failure precipitated by an acute, aggressive, surgical management approach to a chronic intestinal complaint.

Most serious, and fortunately least common, of the features of gastrointestinal SSc is the pattern of small bowel hypomotility, dilatation and distention, bacterial overgrowth, and malabsorption, a pattern formerly termed adynamic ileus and now brought together by the term *pseudo-obstruction syndrome*. Conservative management of this syndrome has always been less than satisfactory; alternating antibiotics, partially digested foodstuffs, and motility enhancers have been tried with only limited success. If the affected small bowel segment is short and the remainder long and normal, resection can be proposed. Careful study is needed to determine the successfully resectable patient; nonetheless, when successful the results can be rewarding. Today it is more acceptable to contemplate resection, after exhaustive efforts at conservative management, because patients who fail treatment by resection, as well as unresectable patients in general, have access to a modality that has made a major difference in the quality of these patients' lives, total parenteral nutrition (TPN). We know of patients who have completed a decade of active, dedicated living who take nothing by mouth and supply all nutritional needs by nocturnal intravenous alimentation through Hickman catheters at home. After an unpredictable year or two in which basic disease and logistic factors are sorted out, survival is stable at about 85 percent and quality of life is reported to be acceptable. This admitted halfway technology has been literally lifesaving for many SSc patients.

Cardiac Involvement

The heart may be primarily or secondarily affected by SSc. Pulmonary hypertension has been discussed earlier under pulmonary involvement and systemic hypertension is discussed later under renal impairment. SSc patients are affected by atherosclerosis as are their age- and sex-matched "healthy" peers; since SSc is distinctly, perhaps primarily, a microvascular disease, SSc patients do not respond well to coronary bypass; because of the intense microvascular involvement, SSc patients with atherosclerosis do not perfuse well after bypass and the incidence of intraoperative mortality is high. In fact, to turn the coin around, cardiac patients who complete the evaluation for chest pain with the diagnostic designation of small-vessel myocardial disease only (intramyocardial or microvascular myocardial involvement) should undergo nailfold capillary examination, an HEp-2 ANA determination, esophageal manometry, and pulmonary function tests with single-breath diffusion studies to see if they belong in the scleroderma spectrum of disease.

The most prevalent cardiac feature of SSc is pericardial effusion. Rarely, it is acute with positional pain and a pericardial friction rub; when these are present a short course of glucocorticoids may be indicated. Usually it is indolent and painless. The two most definite features of pericardial effusion in SSc are painless symmetric dependent edema that is too easy to attribute to direct cutaneous involvement (early puffy) and a propensity to develop renal failure over the next 6 months. Pulsus paradoxus is usually absent; the echocardiogram is again both qualitatively and quantitatively specific. Diuretic and cardiotonic therapy should be applied slowly; when the effusion is large and persistent, pericardial windows are indicated. Diuresis that induces volume depletion should not be undertaken in SSc patients whose creatinine clearance is less than 60 ml per minute. Calcium channel blockers and afterload reduction are often tried and usually safe, but their efficacy remains unproved. These cardiac features are common to all SSc patients.

Patients with dSSc have a greater than 90 percent prevalence of small-vessel myocardial involvement demonstrated by stress thallium scans with reperfusion studies. It hardly seems necessary to do the study on all dSSc patients unless cardiac symptoms and signs are present. Moreover, there is the increasing awareness that the thallium imaging technique is detecting lesions that have little clinical or prognostic implications, at least for short-term prognosis. More definite and immediately useful information can be obtained using ventriculography. Nonetheless, it is appropriate to treat dSSc patients with agents to reduce or eliminate thallium defects. The calcium channel blockers and, recently, afterload reduction using converting enzyme inhibitors (CEIs) both seem able to reduce thallium scan abnormalities acutely. It will be difficult to design the study that can answer the related questions: do thallium scan abnormalities predict clinical SSc myocardial involvement and can any agent prevent its development? Once left ventricular dysfunction without other cause occurs in the SSc patient, it is unclear whether any agent can change the progressive and unrelenting continuing reduction in cardiac output that is usually seen.

Renal Impairment

Once the scourge of SSc, accounting for the majority of disease-related deaths, the abrupt onset of hypertension, oliguria, azotemia, proteinuria, hyperreninemia, and intense renal cortical vasoconstriction leading if uninterrupted to renal cortical infarction and renal failure (scleroderma renal crisis) has become uncommon since the introduction of CEIs, which inhibit the conversion of angiotensin I to angiotensin II, including captopril, enalapril, and others. Since response to treatment is dependent on early therapeutic intervention, it is critical to identify these clinical features of scleroderma renal crisis as early as possible.

Most renal failure occurs in dSSc patients; thus, all dSSc patients should be watched closely for the development of hypertension (home blood pressure testing is recommended), proteinuria, and a reduction in renal function. Several 24-hour urine collections a year are indicated for protein exertion and for creatinine clearance. The blood for serum creatinine determination should also be sent for hemoglobin and hematocrit studies, and the smear inspected for fragmented erythrocytes, indicative of microangiopathic hemolytic anemia, a strong prognostic indicator of impending renal failure in SSc and probably the only truly prognostic indicator, since the other features are part and parcel of the syndrome itself. Our cutoff for concern in the normotensive, asymptomatic dSSc patient without microangiopathy, proteinuria, pericardial effusion, or left ventricular failure is a 20-ml reduction in creatinine clearance or a clearance of less than 60 ml per minute. In these patients, glucocorticoid therapy should be avoided, intravenous contrast material should not be used, elective surgery should be postponed, a careful reevaluation of hemodynamic status should be made, and treatment, usually with captopril, should be instituted. If serum creatinine is less than 3.5 mg per dl, this is usually adequate to improve renal function. With serum creatinine above 3.5 mg per dl, renal failure can ensue despite treatment. It requires many weeks, sometimes many months, for renal function to begin to return toward normal after CEI therapy is begun. This period of concerned waiting can be difficult. Nephrectomy is not indicated and dialysis, when needed, should be continued for 2 to 3 years before renal transplantation is proposed because some SSc patients are able to come off dialysis on their own.

Presently, the most difficult SSc patients to manage are those with combined myocardial, pulmonary, and renal involvement who have been on both calcium channel blockers and CEIs for some time. Careful management of volume status seems to help; protection from sudden changes in volume or cardiac output are essential.

Conclusion

The major question facing the physician who manages patients with SSc today is: does disease modifying therapy for SSc exist? The fact that valid points of view exist on both sides of this question affirms the need for better therapy, which affirms the need for more complete understanding of the steps involved in the immune responses, in the vascular abnormalities, and in the relentless fibrosis that characterize this disease, which in its most aggressive forms can present devastating prospects both psychologically and physiologically to those who have it.

Bibliography

Kahaleh, MB, and LeRoy, EC: The immune basis for human fibrotic diseases, especially scleroderma (systemic sclerosis). Clin Aspects Autoimmun 3:19, 1989.

LeRoy, EC: Systemic sclerosis (scleroderma). In: Wyngaarden, JB, and Smith, LH (eds): Cecil Textbook of Medicine, ed 18. Philadelphia, WB Saunders, 1988, pp 2018–2024.

LeRoy EC et al: Scleroderma (systemic sclerosis): Classification, subsets and pathogenesis. J Rheumatol 15:202, 1988.

LeRoy, EC et al: A strategy for determining the pathogenesis of scleroderma (systemic sclerosis): Is transforming growth factor beta the answer? Arthritis Rheum 32:817, 1989.

Medsger, TA, Jr: Systemic sclerosis (scleroderma), localized scleroderma, eosinophilic fasciitis, and calcinosis. In: McCarty, DJ (ed): Arthritis and Allied Conditions, ed 11. Philadelphia, Lea & Febiger, 1989, pp 1118–1165.

Silver, RM, and LeRoy, EC: Systemic sclerosis (scleroderma). In: Samter, M et al (eds): Immunological Diseases. Boston, Little, Brown, 1988, pp 1459–1499.

Chapter 12
Sjögren's Syndrome

STUART S. KASSAN, M.D., F.A.C.P.
HARALAMPOS M. MOUTSOPOULOS, M.D., F.A.C.P.

Introduction

Sjögren's syndrome is a slowly progressive, inflammatory autoimmune disease affecting primarily the exocrine glands. The glandular lesion was originally described by Mickulicz in 1882[1] and is characterized by lymphocytic replacement of the salivary epithelium and the presence of "epimyoepithelial islands."[2] The replacement of the functional epithelium by these lymphocytic infiltrations may lead to decreased or absent exocrine secretions resulting in mucosal dryness. Such is the case in fully developed Sjögren's syndrome, in which keratoconjunctivitis sicca, xerostomia, xerotrachea, atrophic gastritis, and vaginal dryness are often found.[3-5]

Sjögren's syndrome has a broad clinical spectrum. It may be observed alone, primary Sjögren's syndrome, or in association with any of the other autoimmune diseases, secondary Sjögren's syndrome.[4] Primary Sjögren's syndrome often begins as an organ-specific autoimmune disease termed either sicca complex or autoimmune exocrinopathy. In approximately one fourth of these patients,[4] the disease progresses to involve a major organ resulting in a systemic disorder of lungs, kidneys, muscles, and blood vessels.[3-5] In some patients it may evolve into a B-cell lymphocyte neoplasm.[6-8] Because of these findings, the study of this disease may identify the pathogenesis of autoimmune disease as well as the interrelationships between autoimmunity and the development of lymphoid malignancy.

The autoimmune hallmarks of the syndrome are twofold: a profound B-cell hyperreactivity with development of serum antibodies,[3] circulating immune complexes,[3,4] and cryoglobulins[3,4]; and the aforementioned glandular lymphocytic infiltrations.[3-5]

The cause of the disease remains unknown. The importance of genetic background in the development of the disorder is reinforced by the increased incidence of certain major histocompatibility complex (MHC) genes in patients with Sjögren's syndrome.[9-11]

Epidemiology

Sjögren's syndrome affects primarily females (9:1 female to male ratio), mainly in the fourth and fifth decades of life[12]; it can occur, however, at all ages. During the last year, five additional children with Sjögren's syndrome have been reported.[13] The predominance of males in the reported pediatric cases probably represents the small size of the reported cohort, since Sjögren's syndrome in adults is largely a disease of females. In half of the children the disease started before age 9; the youngest child with Sjögren's syndrome was 3 years old. In the remaining six children, Sjögren's syndrome was observed between ages 12 and 16.

The prevalence of Sjögren's syndrome in the general population is unknown. In rheumatology clinics, primary Sjögren's syndrome appears as often as systemic lupus erythematosus (SLE). Furthermore, approximately 30 percent of rheumatoid arthritis and scleroderma patients have at least histologic evidence of Sjögren's syndrome.[14] Since rheumatoid arthritis affects 2 to 3 percent of the world's population, Sjögren's syndrome is obviously a frequent medical problem.

Autopsy studies have revealed that approximately 2 to 3 percent of persons without connective tissue disease had unexplained focal lymphocytic infiltrates compatible with Sjögren's syndrome in the labial minor salivary glands.[15,16] On the other hand, a clinical study from Great Britain reported a 33.3 percent frequency of Sjögren's syndrome in a geriatric population. In this study, however, no histologic confirmation of the diagnosis was obtained.

Drosos and co-workers[17] examined 62 apparently healthy elderly volunteers for evidence of primary Sjögren's syndrome. The evaluation included Schirmer's test, slit-lamp examination after rose bengal staining of the cornea and conjunctiva, stimulated parotid flow rate, minor salivary gland biopsy, and testing of the patients' sera for antibodies to immunoglobulins, including rheumatoid factor, and to the cellular antigens ds-DNA and Ro (SS-A)/La (SS-B). Three persons met the diagnostic criteria for primary Sjögren's syndrome while five had histologic changes compatible with Sjögren's syndrome but did not meet the author's criteria for the diagnosis. It should be emphasized that all subjects were asymptomatic and none had antibodies to Ro (SS-A)/La (SS-B) cellular antigens. National studies of unselected large numbers of persons of all ages are needed to address the question of prevalence.

Pathogenesis

The study of the pathogenesis of Sjögren's syndrome must take into account numerous factors that may impact on the development of the disease. These may include immunologic aberrations with B-lymphocyte hyperreactivity and the development of oligoclonal or monoclonal proteins, genetic influences, and possibly viral-mediated dysregulation of the immune system.[18]

B-Cell Hyperreactivity

Humoral Studies

Hypergammaglobulinemia has been recognized as a serologic hallmark of Sjögren's syndrome since 1958.[19] The elevated immunoglobulin levels in patients with Sjögren's syndrome contain antibodies directed against non-organ-specific antigens such as immunoglobulins (rheumatoid factor); cellular antigens such as Ro (SS-A), La (SS-B), and rheumatoid arthritis precipitine RAP (RANA [rheumatoid arthritis nuclear antigen], SS-C) and organ-specific antigens such as salivary gland, thyroid gland, and gastric mucosa.[4] The incidence of autoantibodies differs between patients with primary Sjögren's and those with secondary Sjögren's syndrome. The polyclonal B-cell hyperreactivity does not seem to be random. The presence of autoantibodies in patients with primary Sjögren's syndrome correlates well with earlier disease onset, longer disease duration, major salivary gland enlargement, the intensity of lymphocytic infiltration of minor labial salivary glands, and the presence of extraglandular manifestations, such as splenomegaly, lymphadenopathy, and vasculitis.[20-22]

Genetic analyses have yielded results that stress the importance of the MHC gene composition for specific antibody production.[23] Specifically, gene interaction at the HLA-DQ locus appears to direct, in part, the anti-Ro (SS-A) and anti-LA (SS-B) antibody production in patients with primary Sjögren's syndrome but not in those with secondary Sjögren's syndrome.[24] No conclusive evidence, however, for a true pathogenetic relationship between these autoantibodies and tissue destruction has been demonstrated. The presence of cryoglobulinemia, however, found in 30 percent of primary Sjögren's patients, correlates with the presence of antibodies and extra-glandular manifestations.[25] No such correlation is found with the presence of circulating immune complexes, which exists in 80 percent of primary Sjögren's patients.

The presence of serum and urine oligoclonal or monoclonal light chains of immunoglobulins has been found in primary Sjögren's patients with systemic manifestations but without an overt lymphoid malignancy.[26,27] This has been detected using a high-resolution electrophoretic technique combined with immunofixation. These findings suggest that primary Sjögren's patients, with systemic manifestations of disease, express both polyclonal B-cell hyperreactivity and oligoclonal or monoclonal B-cell reactivity before an overt lymphoid malignancy is apparent.[18]

Cellular Studies

The activated B cells in patients with Sjögren's syndrome seem to "home" to organs such as exocrine glands.[18,28] Specifically, unlike SLE patients, peripheral blood as well as bone marrow B-lymphocytes from Sjögren's patients and controls do not spontaneously secrete increased amounts of immunoglobulins.[28] In contrast, B cells infiltrating the minor labial salivary glands synthesize increased amounts of immunoglobulins with rheumatoid factor activity.[29] Thus, the exocrine gland tissues in

Sjögren's syndrome may be a major site of B-lymphocyte activation. The B-cell population with the CD_5 surface molecule is the proliferating cell in B-lymphocytic leukemia.[18,30] In patients with Sjögren's syndrome, increased levels of CD5-positive B cells are found in the major salivary glands and in the peripheral blood.[31] Higher levels of these B cells were found among Sjögren's patients with monoclonal proteins compared to those without such proteins.

Thus, in Sjögren's syndrome, one could postulate a progression of evolutionary stages of B-cell activation, the most reproducible aberration of immunoregulation seen in Sjögren's syndrome.[18] Stage I begins as a polyclonal activation. Stage II evolves to produce a polyclonal-oligoclonal-monoclonal activation, and stage III ends this evolutionary process in a malignant monoclonal proliferation.

Altered T-Cell Function

In 1980 lymphocyte studies in patients with Sjögren's syndrome demonstrated no abnormality of absolute numbers of T cells, T-cell subsets, or T suppressor cell function as compared with controls.[32] An immunoglobulin-mediated decrease in number of T suppressor cells was found in patients with primary Sjögren's syndrome who manifested systemic disease. Bakshi and associates[33] have shown an increase in B cells with a decrease in T cells (both T helper and T suppressor cells), whereas others have failed to document these changes in patients with Sjögren's syndrome.[34] This wide variation in results may point to a relative heterogeneity in Sjögren's patients in general.

Studies of the composition of immunocompetent cells found in salivary glands have demonstrated (with monoclonal antibodies) a predominantly T helper/inducer cell phenotype.[34,35] The T suppressor to T helper cell ratio is approximately 1:5 and B cells represent approximately 20 percent of total lymphocytes.[35] Studies investigating the role of defective T-cell immunoregulation on the B-cell hyperreactivity in the salivary glands of Sjögren's patients demonstrated that the infiltrating salivary-gland T cells do not exhibit aberrant function[36] but rather, altered B-cell function (activation) may be found, as noted above.

Overall, the effects of such an intrinsic B-cell abnormality with B-cell hyperreactivity may result in the known increased predisposition for Sjögren's patients (both primary and secondary) to develop non-Hodgkin's lymphomas, B-cell lymphomas, and Waldenström's macroglobulinemia.[18]

Clinical Manifestations

Diagnostic criteria for Sjögren's syndrome have been suggested in numerous reports.[3,37] All diagnostic criteria, however, are empirical, not based on statistical analysis of the data, and represent the opinion of the investigator. Thus, we are left with the definition of Sjögren's syndrome proposed by Bloch and colleagues[3]: "Ss consists of a triad; keratoconjunctivitis sicca, xerostomia, and rheumatoid arthritis or other connective tissue syndrome. Salivary or lacrimal gland enlargement may or may not be present." This definition, however, leaves criteria for diagnosing keratoconjunctivitis and xerostomia unspecified, as discussed later.

More recently, Fox and co-workers[38] have defined four criteria for the diagnosis of "definite" Sjögren's syndrome: (1). Keratoconjunctivitis sicca, defined by a positive Schirmer's test (complete wetting of a strip of filter paper of less than 9 mm in 5 minutes) and the presence of positive rose bengal corneal staining on slit-lamp examination. (2). Xerostomia with basal and stimulated salivary flow rates. (3). Labial salivary gland biopsy demonstrating lymphocytic infiltrates in which at least two lymphocytic foci per 4 mm^2 area are found. (4). Rheumatoid factor positivity (greater than 1:160 titer), antinuclear antibody positivity (greater than 1:160 titer), and/or SS-A or SS-B antibody positivity. The presence of only three of these criteria would constitute "possible" Sjögren's syndrome. Applying Fox's criteria,[38] one should be cautious since this set of criteria diagnoses as definite Sjögren's syndrome only a subgroup of patients with florid disease.

In general, two forms of Sjögren's syndrome have been identified: primary and secondary Sjögren's syndrome.[9,39] Primary Sjögren's syndrome occurs without another associated connective tissue disease. In secondary Sjögren's syndrome the disease manifests in association with rheumatoid arthritis or any of the other connective diseases. Various clinical, serologic, and genetic differences between primary and secondary Sjögren's syndrome patients have been identified as discussed later in the text.

Glandular Involvement

Oral Involvement

Xerostomia (dry mouth) is one of the hallmarks of Sjögren's syndrome, both primary and secondary. The oral manifestations may be subtle or overt complaints centering around mouth soreness, difficulty swallowing, change in taste, trouble with speech, and acceleration of developing dental caries. In some cases intraoral involvement is manifested by Candida overgrowth of the oral mucosa.[40]

Extraorally, parotid and/or submandibular gland enlargement with or without inflammation is a frequent finding in Sjögren's patients. Most patients manifest bilateral involvement of the salivary glands, but they may present initially with unilateral pain, swelling, and/or erythema. In some patients, secondary infection may also occur.

Clinical methods for documenting salivary gland involvement include: (1) measurement of salivary flow rates (stimulated or unstimulated)[40,41]; (2) sialography using radiocontrast[40,42]; (3) sequential salivary scintigraphy using ^{99m}Tc sodium pertechnetate[38,40,43]; (4) sialochemical measurements[44]; and (5) minor salivary gland biopsy.[40,45] The minor salivary gland biopsy seems to be the "gold standard" for demonstrating evidence of focal sialadenitis and probably represents the most disease-specific abnormality in Sjögren's patients.[40,45] The histologic finding of more than one lymphocytic focus per 4 mm^2 area has been used as the "threshold for significance"[45] in patients with Sjögren's syndrome. In some studies abnormal lip biopsies are found in a relatively high percentage of patients with SLE[46] or patients who have progressive systemic sclerosis and Sjögren's syndrome without clinical findings of xerostomia. Thus, early in the disease process, a true correlation may not exist between the clinical signs or symptoms of Sjögren's syndrome and biopsy findings.

Eye Involvement

Henrik Sjögren, the Swedish ophthalmologist, noted in 1933[47] that keratoconjunctivitis sicca was indeed associated with arthritis and arthralgias and in some cases, dry mouth. The dry eye in Sjögren's syndrome may be asymptomatic for years before symptoms begin to appear.[48] When symptoms do begin, patients may note a feeling of grittiness or a sandy sensation in the eyes when they arise in the morning. They often experience "ropey" or thickened conjunctival secretions.

Tears are made up of three layers: the mucus layer, the aqueous layer and the lipid layer. Keratoconjunctivitis sicca is a disorder of mainly the aqueous layer of the tears.[48,49] The aqueous layer of tears is the thickest of the three layers and is secreted by the lacrimal glands. Other contributing factors in the pathogenesis of keratoconjunctivitis sicca may include abnormalities of eyelid function[50] (i.e., age- or trauma-related) and corneal surface irregularities,[51] both of which may also exacerbate the keratoconjunctivitis that occurs in these patients.

The methods for the diagnosis and study of keratoconjunctivitis sicca have included (1) Schirmer's test,[52] (2) rose bengal corneal and conjunctival staining,[53] (3) tear break-up time,[54] (4) study of the chemistry of tears,[55] and (5) microscopic study of the corneal endothelium and epithelium.[51] The Schirmer's test and the rose bengal corneal staining test are the most commonly employed to diagnose the presence of keratoconjunctivitis sicca. Schirmer's test, with or without local anesthetic, measures the amount (measured in millimeters) of wetting of a strip of filter paper in 5 minutes when it is slipped beneath the lower eyelid.[52] The use of local anesthetic in this test measures basal tear secretions without local irritation caused by the filter paper.[56] The rose bengal stain of the cornea identifies, using slit-lamp examination, damaged or devitalized areas of the cornea, and filaments (epithelial-covered strands of mucus) attached to the cornea (termed filamentary keratitis).[53]

Corneal involvement in Sjögren's syndrome may be severe. Sterile corneal infiltrates may develop and corneal ulceration may occur; associated perforation may result.[49] Superficial corneal infection, blepharitis, and conjunctivitis may also occur due to a deficiency of lysozyme and other antibacterial components of tears in Sjögren's patients.[49,50]

Differential Diagnosis of Eye Involvement in Sjögren's Syndrome. Dry eyes and mouth as well as parotid or major salivary gland enlargement may occur in sarcoidosis.[52,57] In fact, these may be the initial manifestations of the disease. Usually, however patients with sarcoidosis and sicca complex do not have autoantibodies and the labial minor salivary gland biopsy is diagnostic, revealing noncaseating granulomas instead of focal lymphocytic infiltrates.[58] Other medical conditions that may mimic the eye signs in Sjögren's syndrome are amyloidosis,[59] lipoproteinemias, chronic graft-vs.-host-disease[60] and human immunodeficiency virus (HIV) infections.[61]

Extraglandular Involvement

About one-fourth of SS patients present with extraglandular involvement. These patients complain more often of fatigue, low grade fever, arthralgias, and myalgias. Raynaud's phenomenon occurs in approximately 35 percent of pSS patients and usually precedes sicca manifestations by many years.[61a]

Respiratory System Involvement

Pulmonary involvement in Sjögren's syndrome (primary or secondary) is frequent but often not clinically significant. Manifestations may include xerotrachea,[62] recurrent pulmonary infections,[63] obstructive impairment of the large airways, small airway disease,[64] and interstitial lung disease.[64]

Xerotrachea results from a decrease in mucous gland secretions in the tracheobronchial tree. Clinical manifestations consist of severe cough stimulated by the dry mucous membrane that results. The abnormality has been documented by bronchoscopy[62,65] and biopsy findings show inflammatory change.[65]

Recurrent respiratory tract infections may be caused by the bronchial dryness that results from decreased exocrine secretions from the mucous glands of the trachea and bronchi but may not be due to the underlying disease process itself.[66] Mucuciliary clearance rates may be normal in Sjögren's patients and frequent pneumonias are not found in a significant percentage of patients with Sjögren's syndrome.[67]

Large airway obstructive disease in Sjögren's syndrome is not frequent,[66] occurring in 20 percent or less of primary Sjögren's and 46 percent of secondary Sjögren's patients.[66] Some studies have found a somewhat higher incidence of obstructive disease (nearly 50 percent of patients with primary Sjögren's syndrome). This divergence of findings is not well explained.

Small airway disease has been reported in both primary and secondary Sjögren's syndrome.[64,65,67] Histologic findings of mononuclear cell infiltration have also been documented in two such cases. Papathanasiou and investigators,[66] however, found no difference in small airway involvement between primary and secondary Sjögren's syndrome and age- and sex-matched controls.

The most common pulmonary manifestation in Sjögren's is diffuse interstitial lung disease.[62,64,68] Two patterns of involvement have been described[68]: interstitial fibrosis, and lymphoid interstitial disease. Overlap between these two forms of disease is common. Involvement may be patchy, with normal lung diffusing capacities early in the disease process.[62,64] The presence of lymphoid nodules in the lung may represent the presence of pseudolymphoma or lymphoma with histopathologic findings that may not clarify the distinction.[62,69] Such problems in pathologic diagnosis make accurate prognoses and treatment decisions difficult.

Gastrointestinal Involvement

Sjögren's syndrome patients may manifest alterations of the gastrointestinal and hepatic systems.[70] Esophageal involvement may produce dysphagia contributed to by xerostomia[63] and/or other symptoms of esophageal dysmotility.[71] One recent study demonstrated altered esophageal motility in one third of primary Sjögren's patients; these findings did not correlate with activity of disease or the presence or absence of anti-Ro (SS-A) or anti-La (SS-B) antibodies.

Gastric involvement may be manifested by symptoms of dyspepsia and nausea.[72] Histologic evaluation of the gastric mucosa has demonstrated atrophic gastritis and T helper lymphocytic infiltration.[72] Other findings, for example, elevated serum gastrin levels,[72] decreased acidity of gastric secretions, and decreased serum vitamin B_{12} levels,[72] have been demonstrated in patients with Sjögren's syndrome. In general, no significant histologic or biochemical differences between primary and secondary Sjögren's syndrome have been demonstrated.[72]

The small bowel also may be affected in patients with Sjögren's syndrome. Nutritional deficiencies have been reported in Sjögren's syndrome[73] as has the coexistence of celiac disease.[74] The incidence of the latter association is unknown.

Abnormal pancreatic function in Sjögren's syndrome has been noted to produce few symptoms.[75] Rarely, acute pancreatitis and asymptomatic hyperamylasemia have been reported.[76]

Liver involvement in Sjögren's patients has encompassed a wide spectrum including hepatomegaly (in up to 58 percent[70]) and abnormal liver function tests (in up to one third of patients).[70,77,78] In one study by Golding and associates[79] in 1970, 40 percent to 70 percent of patients with chronic active hepatitis, primary biliary cirrhosis and cryptogenic cirrhosis had clinical evidence of xerostomia and xerophthalmia. The relative high coexistence of primary biliary cirrhosis with signs and symptoms of Sjögren's syndrome[80] supports the autoimmune nature of both of these disease processes in which a common postulated mechanism is damage to the ductular epithelium[70,81] resulting in a "dry gland syndrome."[81]

Renal Disease

Renal involvement in Sjögren's syndrome may be latent or overt.[82] The most common form of renal disease is interstitial nephritis in which the interstitial lymphocytic infiltration is often associated with tubular atrophy and fibrosis. The manifestations of interstitial nephritis in Sjögren's syndrome include hyposthenuria, renal tubular acidosis (Type 1), distal and less commonly, Fanconi's syndrome. Renal tubular acidosis, often latent, may be present in 20 to 30 percent of Sjögren's patients.[82,83] Tubular dysfunction may also present with hyposthenuria. Infrequently, nephrocalcinosis may be seen. Nephrogenic diabetes insipidus has been found in 16 percent of Sjögren's patients in one study.[3] The cause for this has been postulated to be the result of renal tubular acidosis (hypokalemic tubular injury) and/or the inflammatory process associated with interstitial lymphocytic infiltration often found in patients with Sjögren's syndrome. In addition to the renal tubular acidosis, interstitial nephritis in Sjögren's syndrome may result in tubular necrosis, hyalinization of glomeruli, and renal insufficiency.

Immune complex glomerulonephritis has been described in Sjögren's syndrome in limited reports.[84] Some cases have been associated with circulating immune complexes, mixed cryglobulinemia, macrobulinemia, and clinical symptoms of extraglandular involvement with signs of peripheral vasculitis.[84] Pathologic changes on renal biopsy have included changes of membranous, membranoproliferative, and proliferative glomerulonephritis.[84-86]

Vasculitis

Systemic vasculitis in Sjögren's syndrome may be manifested by small, medium and, rarely, large vessel involvement.[87] Major organ involvement has been demonstrated in Sjögren's patients and may affect the peripheral and central nervous system, lung, kidney, gastrointestinal tract, pancreas, liver, spleen, and salivary glands.[87] A wide spectrum of clinical vasculitis has been reported.[87] Because the vasculitis in Sjögren's syndrome involves mainly the small vessels, the more common clinical presentation is one of slow progression.[87] In those patients with medium and/or large vessel vasculitic involvement,[87,88] a more fulminant and clinically significant progression of disease is seen.

Alexander and associates[89,90] have described two distinct histopathologic types of inflammatory vascular disease in primary Sjögren's syndrome: neutrophilic inflammatory vascular disease, and mononuclear inflammatory vascular disease. Both types of vasculitic involvement may result in end-organ damage. Neutrophilic inflammatory vascular disease has been associated with seropositivity for anti-Ro (SS-A) and anti-La (SS-B) antibodies, and rheumatoid factor. The mononuclear inflammatory vascular disease, however, is associated with seronegativity for these antibodies. These differences imply varying immunopathogenetic mechanisms for the two clinically similar manifestations of the disease; possibly the mononuclear seronegative form of the disease may be a precursor for the seropositive neutrophilic "phase" of the vasculitic process in Sjögren's syndrome.[87]

Tsokos and co-workers,[91] however, described four patterns of vessel involvement in patients with Sjögren's syndrome. These include leukoclastic and lymphocytic vasculitis, acute necrotizing angiitis, and endarteritis obliterans involving small and medium-size arteries.

Cutaneous vasculitic disease in Sjögren's syndrome has been recognized in up to 30 percent of patients.[3,21] The manifestations of cutaneous vasculitis include palpable purpura, petechial lesions, urticaria and, less commonly, erythema multiforme, subcutaneous nodules, and necrotizing panniculitis.[87]

Peripheral nerve involvement as a result of vasculitis of the vasa nervorum has been reported[21,92,93]; nerve biopsies have demonstrated vascular inflammation. The most frequent vasculitic infiltrate in Sjögren's patients seems to be a mononuclear infiltrate as opposed to the neutrophilic inflammatory infiltrate seen in leukocytoclastic vasculitis.[87] Manifestations of peripheral nerve involvement include polyneuropathy (sensory), mononeuritis multiplex, peripheral entrapment syndromes, and cranial nerve involvement, most commonly trigeminal neuropathy.[87,92,94]

Central nervous system involvement has been demonstrated by investigators at Johns Hopkins and may have various manifestations, including focal deficits, diffuse involvement (e.g., encephalopathy, aseptic meningitis, dementia, and psychiatric manifestations[93,94]), and spinal cord involvement (e.g., transverse myelitis and myelopathy).[93-95] In some Sjögren's patients, clinical changes reminiscent of and indistinguishable from multiple sclerosis have been found.[93]

Another study of 105 patients with Sjögren's syndrome (50 with primary Sjögren's, 55 with secondary Sjögren's syndrome) and showed that 18 had neurologic abnormalities.[96] The majority of the neurologic manifestations were mild, confined to the patient group with Sjögren's syndrome and another connective tissue disorder (secondary Sjögren's syndrome), and characteristic of the underlying connective tissue disorder. Only three patients with primary

Sjögren's syndrome presented central nervous system (CNS) abnormalities (transient ischemic attacks, vertigo, and repeated episodes of transient loss of consciousness). Brain computed tomography (CT) scans in these patients were without abnormalities. In all patients the symptoms disappeared without residual disability. Thus, this group of investigators questioned the seriousness and progressiveness of CNS lesions reported in patients with primary Sjögren's syndrome by the Johns Hopkins group and suggested that the differences can be attributed to racial differences in the groups tested or to the biased collection of patients by the Baltimore investigators due to their recognized interest in the CNS disease of primary Sjögren's syndrome.

Overt clinical myositis in Sjögren's syndrome is a fairly uncommon manifestation of the disease.[87] In some cases, however, a low-grade myopathy may be found; muscle biopsy changes of lymphocytic infiltration with little or no muscle necrosis has been described.[97] Inflammatory vascular changes on muscle biopsy in Sjögren's patients is, however, well-documented in the presence or absence of histologic myositis.[3,92,98] Immunofluorescent studies on muscle biopsy specimens from Sjögren's patients have demonstrated epimyseal and connective tissue staining for immunoglobulin and vascular deposit in some, of IgG, IgM or C3.[87,88] Electron microscopy has demonstrated changes of the microvasculature that include intracytoplasmic inclusions and subendothelial deposits of electron-dense material.

Sjögren's Syndrome—Occurring with Other Autoimmune Diseases

Sjögren's Syndrome with Rheumatoid Arthritis

Secondary Sjögren's syndrome (that entity which exists with other connective tissue diseases) has been reported to coexist with rheumatoid arthritis (RA), SLE, progressive systemic sclerosis (PSS), mixed connective tissue disease (MCTD), polymyositis (PM), polyarteritis nodosa (PAN), and primary biliary cirrhosis.[3,13,99,100] Where primary Sjögren's syndrome starts on the clinical spectrum and where secondary Sjögren's syndrome begins is sometimes difficult to ascertain, especially in the settings of Sjögren's syndrome with RA and Sjögren's syndrome with SLE.[100] This problem arises especially in patients whose disease begins as secondary Sjögren's syndrome and who later develop manifestations of the other connective tissue diseases.

Maini[100] illustrates such a relationship with the arthropathy of Sjögren's syndrome and RA or other connective tissue disease in which three forms of joint involvement can be found: (1) arthropathy of primary Sjögren's syndrome (associated with arthralgias, myalgias, and mild synovitis); (2) RA with Sjögren's syndrome (associated with erosive polyarthritis with or without the extra-articular features of classic RA); and (3) arthropathy of other autoimmune diseases associated with secondary Sjögren's syndrome (associated with the arthropathy found in SLE, PSS, primary biliary cirrhosis etc.) and the classical features of the respective primary disease.

In RA associated with secondary Sjögren's syndrome, certain differences have been elucidated to distinguish this entity from primary Sjögren's syndrome. In most patients with RA associated with secondary Sjögren's syndrome, articular symptoms precede signs and symptoms of Sjögren's syndrome and usually progress to a more severe erosive arthritis.

In RA extra-articular manifestations of disease are also different from those found in primary Sjögren's syndrome and include rheumatoid nodules, digital infarcts, pericarditis, mononeuritis multiplex, Felty's syndrome, and the late development of amyloidosis.[39,100]

Sicca manifestations are offered spontaneously by only 5 percent of unselected consecutive RA patients. If one applies, however, a specific questionnaire, approximately 20 percent of RA patients answer affirmatively to having the symptoms of dry eyes and dry mouth. The feeling of dry eyes is elicited much more frequently than xerostomia, and parotid of other major salivary gland enlargement is uncommon.[118] In contrast, 20 percent of unselected scleroderma patients spontaneously offer sicca complaints, equally from the eyes and mouth, and parotid gland enlargement occurs in these patients with an incidence similar to that seen in PSS patients.[17] It should be noted that sicca complaints and manifestations in scleroderma patients may be due to fibrosis of the exocrine glands. This occurs in approximately 25 percent of the patients and is attributed to the scleroderma process itself.

Ss with SLE/MCTD

The overlap and/or coexistence of Ss with SLE points up certain similarities and differences between pSs, sSs with SLE/MCTD, and SLE alone. The true incidence of Ss features in SLE patients is about 25 percent.[140] However, the frequency of developmental SLE after the initial diagnosis of Ss is between 1 percent and 9 percent.[4,63,140]

The similarities between pSs and SLE alone include polyarthritis (nonerosive), rash, vasculitis, glomerulonephritis, and central nervous system involvement.[4] In contrast, features of lymphadenopathy, hepatosplenomegaly, interstitial renal disease, pulmonary involvement, and cutaneous and peripheral nerve vasculitis are seen with greater frequency and severity in pSs than in SLE.[3,4,27,129,140] In some cases the clinical findings of Ss may be subclinical and/or mildly symptomatic.[55] Reports of MCTD with Ss are few.[141,142]

Serologically a high incidence of patients with pSs develop antibodies to the extractable nuclear antigens Ro and La.[4] These antibodies are also present in SLE; anti-La is more commonly positive in primary Sjögren's syndrome and Sjögren's syndrome with SLE as compared with SLE alone.

Genetic studies have established phenotypic differences between primary and secondary Sjögren's syndrome, but certain similarities are found between primary Sjögren's syndrome and SLE. Both of these latter groups have increased frequencies of HLA-B$_8$, HLA-DRw3, and the B-lymphocyte alloantigen Ia-715.[104,105] This seems to enhance the theory that primary Sjögren's syndrome and SLE may share a common pathophysiology.

Sjögren's Syndrome with Progressive Systemic Sclerosis

Patients with PSS have been noted, by histologic criteria, to have a 17 to 35 percent incidence of Sjögren's syndrome. Other clinical features of Sjögren's syndrome have been found in even greater percentages of PSS patients.

Clinical differences have also been noted between PSS alone and PSS occurring with secondary Sjögren's syndrome. In the latter, purpura, lymphadenopathy, hepatomegaly, splenomegaly, and interstitial renal disease are features not shared with the former (PSS without Sjögren's syndrome.)[106] Vasculitis also is infrequent in PSS alone, yet in PSS occurring with Sjögren's syndrome, those patients with positive anti-Ro antibodies have a higher risk of developing vasculitis. Many of these patients have features of the CREST syndrome (calcinosis, Raynaud's phenomenon, esophageal dysfunction, sclerodactyly, and telanglectsia) with manifestations of vasculitic involvement that include mononeuritis multiplex, visceral ischemia, and cutaneous ulcers.[107] Hepatic disease (specifically primary biliary cirrhosis) occurs more frequently in PSS associated with secondary Sjögren's syndrome than in Sjögren's syndrome alone.[106] Also, a higher proportion of secondary Sjögren's patients have the CREST syndrome.[107]

The relationship between PSS and Sjögren's syndrome and the immune system is illustrated by the reports of graft-vs.-host disease[108] following allogeneic bone marrow transplantation in which the development of PSS and a Sjögren's-like syndrome developed. Both disorders have also been reported following breast augmentation with silicone preparations; possible human adjuvant disease was proposed as the cause for this process.[106,109]

Malignancy in Sjögren's Syndrome

The spectrum of benign to malignant disease in Sjögren's syndrome has been addressed in numerous reports and reviews.[4-7,110] In the study of Kassan and colleagues,[6] in a population of 136 female Sjögren's patients, both primary and secondary, 15 cases of cancer (excluding skin cancers) were observed in an average followup period of 8.1 years per patient. There were seven cases of non-Hodgkin's lymphoma and eight cases of other malignancies. The overall relative risk for the development of lymphoma (observed/expected) was 43.8. The relative risk for other malignancies was not statistically significant. Those at greatest risk were those with parotid swelling, lymphadenopathy, and splenomegaly.

An actual history of this "immunoregulatory disease" is a slowly evolving one in which the autoimmune features of the disease may precede the development of malignancy by up to 20 years.[111] This evolution has been described as theoretically passing through three stages: (1) the autoimmune exocrinopathy stage, (2) the pseudolymphoma stage, and (3) the lymphoma stage.

The first or autoimmune exocrinopathy stage manifests features of Sjögren's syndrome, in which extraglandular involvement is not found and lymphocytic infiltrates are histologically benign. Hypergammaglobulinemia and seropositivity for anti-Ro and anti-La antibodies may be found. The pseudolymphoma stage exhibits features of extraglandular involvement in which lymphadenopathy, splenomegaly, pulmonary infiltrates, and renal infiltrates may be found. The histologic picture is one of atypical lymphoid infiltrates. In addition to hypergammaglobulinemia and seropositivity for anti-Ro and anti-La antibodies, monoclonal gammopathies may also be found.[110-112] The lymphoma stage may be of two types: (1) undifferentiated B-cell lymphoma,[15] or (2) pleomorphic lymphomas with or without a monoclonal macrogammaglobulinemia.[111] In the former, hypergammaglobulinemia may be noted, as well as seropositivity to various antibodies.

The sites of lymphomatous involvement may include salivary glands (rarely) or other organs including kidney, gastrointestinal tract, and lung.[111]

Immunohistologic studies have described in situ salivary gland B-cell immunocytomas or immunoblastic lymphomas producing, locally, monoclonal IgM kappa immunoglobulin.[113]

Monoclonal immunoglobulins may be produced very early in the salivary glands of Sjögren's patients.[110,111] Using a high-resolution agarose gel electrophoresis technique,[114,115] 67% of 21 American patients with primary Sjögren's syndrome were found to have monoclonal protein with lambda light chains.[26] In that study, 100 percent of those Sjögren's patients with glandular involvement alone had evidence of monoclonal proteins.

The foregoing data and other studies have demonstrated that in Sjögren's syndrome, B-cell activation may begin locally at the salivary gland level with later progression to extraglandular sites where malignant evolution may occur. The high incidence of monoclonal protein production in Sjögren's patients also suggests that both a monoclonal and polyclonal B-cell activation may be present very early in these patients.[111]

Laboratory Tests

A mild normochromic, normocytic anemia is present in one fourth of Sjögren's patients and leukopenia occurs in 30 percent. Thrombocytopenia, although infrequent in primary Sjögren's patients, can precede by years the sicca manifestations. An elevated erythrocyte sedimentation rate is a very common manifestation (80 percent of patients). In contrast, C-reactive protein levels are not elevated in primary Sjögren's patients.[116]

Because Sjögren's syndrome is a disease characterized by B-cell activation, autoantibody production is not unanticipated. Antinuclear antibody positivity is found in close to three fourths of Sjögren's patients,[3,94,117,118] in which immunofluorescent patterns may be homogeneous, speckled, and/or nucleolar. Numerous antitissue antibodies have also been identified and include antibodies to mitochondria,[94] histone, vimentin, erythrocyte, thyroglobulin,[117,119] and salivary gland.[118,120]

Two antibodies to extractable nuclear antigens have been found in a high proportion of Sjögren's patients, namely, anti-Ro (SS-A), and anti-La (SS-B).[117,121,122] These antibodies are not specific for Sjögren's syndrome and may be found in numerous other autoimmune diseases, specifically SLE, RA, primary biliary cirrhosis, idiopathic thrombocytopenic purpura, chronic active hepatitis, and polymyositis.

Theoretically, autoantibodies may be intimately involved in the immunopathogenesis of disease.[117] Close relationships between anti-Ro (SS-A) antibodies and various disease manifestations in Sjögren's syndrome have been reported.[20,21] Alexander and investigators[21] found that Sjögren's patients with anti-Ro positivity had an increased incidence of vasculitis, salivary gland enlargement, lymphadenopathy, and purpura. These patients were also found to have a greater incidence of leukopenia, anemia, and positive tests for rheumatoid factor, hypergammaglobulinemia, cryoglobulinemia, and hypocomplementemia.

Overall, the anti-Ro (SS-A) and anti-La (SS-B) antibodies are most specific for Sjögren's syndrome and SLE[21] and are found in 40 to 45 percent of Sjögren's and 25 to 30 percent of SLE patients.[21,123] The anti-La (SS-B) antibody is found in 40 to 50 percent of Sjögren's and 10 percent of SLE patients.[20,123] Control populations of patients without evidence for connective tissue disease had an incidence of only 0.1 percent for the anti-Ro (SS-A) antibody.[123] No such large control populations for the anti-La (SS-B) antibody have been studied.

Immunogenetic studies have shown that anti-Ro (SS-A) positivity has an increased frequency of correlation with HLA-DR2, HLA-DR3 and HLA-Dw62.[123,125] In contrast, the anti-La (SS-B) antibody has an increased association with the HLA-DR3 and not the HLA-DR2 phenotype.[124,125] Thus, on the basis of these studies, one might speculate that the clinical similarities between anti-Ro–positive SLE and anti-Ro–positive Sjögren's patients may occur as a result of shared immunogenetic factors.

Other immunogenetic studies have demonstrated an increased frequency of HLA antigens, HLA-B8, HLA-DR3 and HLA-Dw52 in patients with primary Sjögren's syndrome as compared with control populations.[9,11,126,127] In addition, there are different antigen frequencies when comparing primary and secondary Sjögren's syndrome.[4,119] There is an increased frequency of HLA-DR4 in secondary Sjögren's syndrome with RA.[9] HLA-DRw52 was found in greater frequency for both primary and secondary Sjögren's syndrome.[125] Thus, these HLA typing studies and family studies[11] of Sjögren's patients demonstrate that major histocompatibility complex antigens are genetic markers for these diseases[126] and probably play a contributing and not primary role in the disease process.[126] Theoretically, various combinations of HLA-DR antigens provide the genetic setting for the immune response that may result in the development of Sjögren's syndrome. Other triggering mechanisms may contribute to the development of Sjögren's syndrome in other autoimmune diseases, notably viral infections.

Treatment

Sjögren's syndrome often proves to be a most difficult disease to treat. Close attention to the various manifestations of the disease are the mainstays of treatment. Careful followup at periodic intervals, including observation by a rheumatologist, an ophthalmologist, and a dentist, are important in attempting to "troubleshoot" for potential problems before or when they occur. Clinical and laboratory evaluations performed serially may aid in the early detection of glandular and extraglandular complications as well as the possible development of malignancy.

The treatment of the glandular manifestations of Sjögren's syndrome includes trying to alter the environment to avoid drying conditions. In addition, avoidance or withdrawal, if feasible, of medications that exacerbate mucous membrane dryness (e.g., anticholinergic agents, antihistamines, antidepressants, antispasmodics, and antiparkinsonian agents) is advisable. Local lubrication for the eyes is accomplished by the use of artificial tears or lubricating ointments. Sometimes these agents cause local irritation due to various preservatives. In these instances other therapies may be used, including the use of a slow-release tear (Lacrisert, Merck Sharp and Dohme, Rahway, N.J.), inserted into the conjunctival sac, or punctal occlusion, which is used mainly in the most severe cases. Other agents such as pilocarpine and bromhexine have also been reported as helpful in some patients as stimulants of automatic function, but they have not been used widely. Other experimental approaches have included dilute sodium hyaluronate as a 10 percent solution for topical use.[125] Fox and collaborators[127] have also used an artificial tear preparation in a procedure that utilizes the patient's own serum in such a solution.

Treatment of the oral manifestations of Sjögren's syndrome has met with less success than the ocular treatments. As with the treatment of xerophthalmia, elimination of exacerbating factors is imperative. This includes cessation of smoking, drugs with drying effects, and conditions that predispose to mouth breathing. Sugarless candies and gums as well as other potential secretagogues may be helpful in stimulating salivary flow. In some cases, however, these agents may precipitate an acute obstructive parotitis in more advanced cases of parotid involvement. Artificial salivary substitutes have been used when mucin-containing agents may be more effective[128] because they provide greater lubricating, cleansing, and antibacterial activity. Local dental stannous fluoride applications may also retard the progressive development of dental caries. Parasympathomimetic agents have been used locally or systemically with limited success in stimulating salivary flow. Bromhexine, a mucolytic agent, has been tried[129] and will soon undergo clinical trials in the United States under "orphan drug" status. A battery powered electronic salivary gland stimulator is also available and causes a local stimulation of salivary secretions. Vaginal manifestation of Sjögren's syndrome include dryness and local irritation. Local measures, such as moisturizing creams and lubricating jelly have been used. In post-menopausal women estrogen deficiency may worsen the preexistent condition, and local and/or systemic estrogen replacement may also be helpful.

One effort at systemic therapy involved hydroxychloroquine; ten Sjögren's syndrome patients with primary Sjögren's syndrome were treated with 200 mg daily of hydroxychloroquine for 1 year.[130] The treatment effectiveness in these patients was judged by following another ten Sjögren's patients without treatment. It was observed that hypergammaglobulinemia was partially corrected and IgG antibodies to La (SS-B) antigen were decreased. Furthermore, in hydroxychloroquine-treated patients, the erythrocyte sedimentation rate decreased and the hemoglobin levels increased. Little change, however, was noted in lacrimal and salivary gland function.[130] Preliminary data should be reevaluated in a double blind fashion in a larger number of patients.

In previous studies cyclosporin A and decadurabolin were tried in a double-blind fashion to determine their efficacy and safety in patients with primary Sjögren's syndrome.[131,132] The cyclosporine A treated group reported that they had an improvement in their xerostomia, while dry eyes and parotid gland enlargement remained unchanged. Furthermore, flow rates of tears and saliva did not improve in the drug vs. the placebo group. Thus, in the face of the drug's potent side effects and the minimal therapeutic effect shown in this study, cyclosporin A cannot be recommended for the treatment of Sjögren's syndrome.[132]

Some evidence suggests that estrogens promote autoimmune processes whereas androgens can supress them. Wandrolone decanoate (Deca-Durabolin) is a long-acting anabolic steroid that has been found to improve lupus like disease in experimental animal models and particularly to decrease lymphocytic infiltrates in the salivary glands of these animals.[133] This observation prompted Drosos and colleagues[132] to study the effects of intramuscular Deca-Durabolin (100 mg for 2 weeks) versus placebo in PSS patients. It was found that patients administered Deca-Durbolin showed a moderate subjective improvement in xerostomia and a significant decrease in the erythrocyte sedimentation rate. However, the objective parameters of dry eyes and mouth remained unchanged.

Treatment of extraglandular disease may be indicated for major organ involvement. Interstitial lung disease with pneumonitis and lymphocytic infiltration may require lung biopsy and subsequent steroid and/or immunosuppressant therapy. Renal disease, as previously discussed, may take the form of interstitial nephritis, immune complex glomerulonephritis, or cryoglobulinemia-induced glomerular disease. Treatment of these disorders may involve the use of corticosteroids as well as cytotoxic drug therapy dictated by the severity of disease.

The level of treatment of the vasculitic sequelae of Sjögren's syndrome is based on the severity of disease and the presence of visceral involvement, which is similar to the approach to the treatment of vasculitis associated with any of the other autoimmune diseases.

The treatment of pseudolymphoma is often complicated by the difficulty encountered in distinguishing benign from malignant disease histologically. In some cases, truly benign lesions of pseudolymphoma may be sufficiently invasive as to require aggressive intervention with systemic corticosteroids and, rarely, with cytotoxic agents. The treatment of true lymphomas in these patients does not differ from established regimens.

References

1. Mickulicz, J: Uber eine ergenartige symmettrische Erkrankung ber Tranen-umb Mundespeicheldrusen beitz z Chir Fetser f. Stuttgart, Theodor Billroth, 1882, p 610.
2. Morgan, WS, and Castleman, B: A clinicopathologic study of "Mickulicz disease." Am J Pathol 29: 471, 1953.
3. Bloch, KJ et al: Sjögren's syndrome: A clinical, pathological and serological study of 62 cases. Medicine 44: 187, 1965.
4. Moutsopoulos, HM et al. Sjögren's syndrome (sicca syndrome): Current issues. Ann Intern Med 92: 212, 1980.
5. Strand, V, and Talal, N: Advances in the diagnosis and concept of Sjögren's syndrome (autoimmune exocrinopathy). Bull Rheum Dis 30: 1046, 1980.
6. Kasan, SS et al: Increased risk of lymphoma in sicca syndrome. Ann Intern Med 89: 888, 1978.
7. Talal, N, and Bunim, JJ: Development of malignant lymphoma in the course of Sjögren's syndrome. Am J Med 36: 529, 1964.
8. Zulman, J, Jaffe, R, and Talal, N: Evidence that the malignant lymphoma of Sjögren's syndrome is a monoclonal B-cell neoplasm. N Engl J Med 299: 1215, 1978.
9. Moutsopoulos, HM et al: Genetic differences between primary and secondary sicca syndrome. N Engl J Med 301: 761, 1979.
10. Papasteriades, C et al: HLA-alloantigen associations in Greek patients with Sjögren's syndrome. J Autoimmun 1: 85, 1988.
11. Mann, DL, and Moutsopoulos, HM: HLA-DR alloantigens in different subsets of patients with Sjögren's syndrome and in family members. Ann Rheum Dis 42: 533, 1983.
12. Pavlidis, NA, Karsh, J, and Moutsopoulos, HM: The clinical picture of primary Ss: A retrospective study. J Rheumatol 9: 685, 1982.
13. Kraus, A, and Alarcon-Segovia, D: Primary juvenile Sjögren's syndrome. J Rheumatol 15: 803, 1988.
14. Drosos, AA et al: Sjögren's syndrome in progressive systemic sclerosis. J Rheumatol 15: 965, 1988.
15. Scott, J: Qualitative and quantitative observations on the histology of human labial salivary glands obtained post mortem. J Biol Buccale 8: 187, 1980.
16. Takeda, Y, and Komori, A: Focal lymphocytic infiltration in the human labial salivary glands: A post mortem study. J Oral Pathol 15: 83, 1986.
17. Drosos, AA et al: Prevalence of primary Sjögren's syndrome in an elderly population. Br J Rheumatol 27: 123, 1988.
18. Moutsopoulos, HM, and Manoussakis, MN: Immunopathogenesis of Sjögren's syndrome: "Facts and Fancy." Autoimmunity 5: 17–24, 1989.
19. Bloch, KJ et al: Sjögren's syndrome. I. Serologic reactions in patients with Sjögren's syndrome without rheumatoid arthritis. Arthritis Rheum 3: 287, 1960.
20. Alexander, EL et al: Ro (SSA) and La (SSB) antibodies in the clinical spectrum of Sjögren's syndrome. J Rheumatol 9: 239, 1982.
21. Alexander, EL et al: Sjögren's syndrome: Association of anti-Ro (SSA) antibodies with vasculitis, hematologic abnormalities and serologic hyperreactivity. Ann Intern Med 98: 155, 1983.
22. Manoussakis, MN et al: Serological profiles in subgroups of patients with Sjögren's syndrome. Scand J Rheumatol 61 (Suppl): 89, 1986.
23. Harley, JB: Autoantibodies in Sjögren's syndrome. In Talal, N, Moutsopoulos, HM, and Kassan, SS (eds): Sjögren's Syndrome: Clinical and Immunologic Aspects. Berlin, Springer-Verlag, 1987, p 218.
24. Harley, JB et al: Gene interaction at HLA-DQ enhances autoantibody production in primary Sjögren's syndrome. Science 232: 1145, 1986.

25. Tzioufas, AG et al: Cryoglobulins in autoimmune rheumatic diseases: evidence for circulating monoclonal cryoglobulins in patients with primary Sjögren's syndrome. Arthritis Rheum 29: 1098, 1986.
26. Moutsopoulos, HM et al: High incidence of free monoclonal lambda light chains in the sera of patients with Sjögren's syndrome. J Immunol 130: 2663, 1983.
27. Moutsopoulos, HM et al: Demonstration and identification of monoclonal proteins in the urine of patients with Sjögren's syndrome. Ann Rheum Dis 44: 109, 1985.
28. Fauci, AS and Moutsopoulos, HM: Polyclonally triggered B-cells in the peripheral blood of normal individuals and patients with SLE and primary Sjögren's syndrome. Arthritis Rheum 24: 577, 1981.
29. Anderson, LG et al: Salivary gland immunoglobulin and rheumatoid factor synthesis in Sjögren's syndrome. Natural history and response to treatment. Am J Med 53: 456, 1972.
30. Plater-Zyberk, C et al: A rheumatoid arthritis B-cell subset expresses a phenotype similar to that in chronic lymphocytic leukemia. Arthritis Rheum 28: 971, 1985.
31. Dauphinee, M, Tovar, Z, and Talal, N: B-cells expressing CD_5 are increased in Sjögren's syndrome. Arthritis Rheum 31: 642, 1988.
32. Moutsopoulos, HM, and Fauci, AS: Immunoregulation in Sjögren's syndrome. Influence of serum factors on T-cell subpopulation. J Clin Invest 65: 519, 1980.
33. Bakhshi, A et al: Lymphocyte subsets in Sjögren's syndrome: A quantitative analysis using monoclonal antibodies in the fluorescence-activated cell sorter. J Clin Lab Immunol 10: 63, 1983.
34. Fox, RI et al: Salivary gland lymphocytes in primary Sjögren's syndrome lack lymphocyte subsets defined by Leu-7 and Leu-11 antigens. J Immunol 135: 207, 1985.
35. Moutsopoulos, HM et al: HLA-DR expression by labial salivary gland tissues in Sjögren's syndrome. Scand J Rheum 61 (Suppl): 67, 1986.
36. Dalavanga, YA, Drosos, AA, and Moutsopoulos, HM: Labial salivary gland immunopathology in Sjögren's syndrome. Scand J Rheum 61 (Suppl): 67, 1986.
37. Daniels, TE, and Talal, N: Diagnosis and differential diagnosis in Sjögren's syndrome. In Tatal, N, Moutsopoulos, HM, and Kassan, SS (eds): Sjögren's Syndrome: Clinical and Immunologic Aspects. Berlin, Springer-Verlag 1987, p 193.
38. Fox, RI et al. Sjögren's syndrome: Proposed criteria for classification. Arthritis Rheum 29: 577, 1986.
39. Moutsopoulos, HM et al: Differences in the clinical manifestations of sicca syndrome in the presence and absence of rheumatoid arthritis. Am J Med 66: 73, 1979.
40. Daniels, TE: Oral manifestations of Sjögren's syndrome. In Talal, N, Moutsopoulos, HM, and Kassan, SS (eds): Sjögren's Syndrome. Clinical and Immunologic Aspects. Berlin, Springer-Verlag, 1987, p 15.
41. Chisholm, DM, and Mason, DK: Salivary gland function in Sjögren's syndrome. A review. Br Dent J 135: 393, 1973.
42. Chisholm, DM et al: Hydrostatic sialography as an index of salivary gland in Sjögren's syndrome. Acta Radiol 11: 577, 1971.
43. Stephen, KW et al. Diagnostic value of quantitative scintiscaning of the salivary glands in Sjögren's syndrome and rheumatoid arthritis. Clin Sci 41: 555, 1971.
44. Baum, BJ, and Fox, PC: Chemistry of saliva. In Tatal N, Moutsopoulos, HM, and Kassan, SS (eds): Sjögren's Syndrome. Clinical and Immunologic Aspects. Berlin, Springer-Verlag 1987, pp 34.
45. Daniels, TE, Labial salivary gland biopsy in Sjögren's syndrome. Assessment as a diagnostic criterion in 362 suspected cases. Arthritis Rheum 27: 147, 1984.
46. Alarcon-Segovia, D et al: Sjögren's syndrome in systemic lupus erythematosus–clinical and subclinical manifestations. Ann Intern Med 81: 577, 1974.
47. Sjögren, H: Auf Kennentnis der Kertoconjunctivitis sicca keratitis filiformis bei Hypofunction der Tramendrusen. Acta Ophthalmol 11 (suppl): 1, 1933.
48. Shearn, MA: Sjögren's Syndrome. Philadelphia, WB Saunders, 1971, p 33.
49. Kincaid, MC: The eye in Sjögren's syndrome. In Tatal, N, Moutsopoulos, HM, and Kassan, SS (eds): Sjögren's Syndrome: Clinical and Immunologic Aspects. Berlin, Springer-Verlag 1987, p 25.
50. Lemp, MA: Diagnosis and treatment of tear deficiencies. In Daune, TD, and Jaeger, EA (eds): Clinical Ophthalmology. Philadelphia, Harper & Row, 1985, Vol 4, Chap 14, p 1.
51. Lemp, MA, and Gold, JD: An in vivo study of the corneal surface in keratoconjunctivitis sicca. Trans Ophthalmol Soc UK 104: 436, 1985.
52. Lamberts, DW: Keratoconjunctivitis sicca. In Smolin, G, and Thoft, RA (eds): The Cornea. Boston, Little Brown, 1983, p 293.
53. Van Bijstervald, OP: Diagnostic tests in the sicca syndrome. Arch Ophthalmol 82: 10, 355, 1969.
54. Holly, FJ, and Lempe, MA. Tear physiology in dry eyes. Surv Ophthalmol 22: 69, 1977.
55. Seal, DV: The effect of aging in disease on tear constituents. Trans Ophthalmol Soc UK 104: 355, 1985.
56. Muenzler, WS: The dry eye: A working outline of etiology, symptoms, diagnosis and treatment. Geriatr Ophthalmol 2: 19, 1985.
57. Greenberg, G et al: Enlargement of parotid gland due to sarcoidosis. Br J Med 2: 861, 1964.
58. Giotaki, H et al: Labial minor salivary gland biopsy: A highly discriminatory diagnostic method between sarcoidosis and Sjögren's syndrome. Respiration 50: 102, 1986.
59. Simon, BG, and Moutsopoulos, HM. Primary amyloidosis resembling sicca syndrome. Arthritis Rheum 22: 932, 1979.

60. Gratwhol, AA et al. Sjögren-type syndrome after allogenic bone marrow transplantation. Ann Intern Med 87: 703, 1977.
61. Ulirsch, RC, and Jaffe, ES: Sjögren's syndrome-like illness associated with the AIDS-related complex. Hum Pathol 18: 1063, 1987.
61a. Skopouli, FN et al: Raynaud's phenomenon in primary Sjögren's syndrome. J Rheumatol 17: 618, 1990.
62. Constantopoulos, SH, and Moutsopoulos, HM: The respiratory system in Sjögren's syndrome. In Tatal, N, Moutsopoulos, HM, and Kassan, SS (eds): Sjögren's Syndrome: Clinical and Immunologic Aspects. Berlin, Springer-Verlag, 1987, p 83.
63. Shearn, MA: Sjögren's syndrome. Med Clin North Am 61: 271, 1977.
64. Constantopoulos, SH, Papdimitriou, CS, and Moutsopoulos, HM: Respiratory manifestations in primary Sjögren's syndrome. Chest 88: 226, 1985.
65. Dariffi, F et al: Pulmonary involvement in Sjögren's syndrome. Respiration 46: 82, 1984.
66. Papathanasiou, MP et al: Reappraisal of respiratory abnormalities in primary and secondary Sjögren's syndrome: A controlled study. Chest 90: 370, 1986.
67. Vitali, C et al: Lung involvement in Sjögren's syndrome: A comparison between patients with primary and secondary Sjögren's syndrome. Ann Rheum Dis 44: 455, 1985.
68. Hunninghake, GW, and Fauci, AS: State of the art: Pulmonary involvement in the collagen vascular diseases. Am Rev Respir Dis 119: 471, 1979.
69. Marchevsky, A et al: Localized lymphoid nodules of lung: A reappraisal of the lymphoma versus pseudolymphoma dilemma. Cancer 51: 2070, 1983.
70. Trevino, H, Tsianos, EB, and Schenker, S: Gastrointestinal and hepatobiliary features in Sjögren's syndrome. In Tatal, N, Moutsopoulos, HM, and Kassan, SS (eds): Sjögren's Syndrome: Clinical and Immunologic Aspects. Berlin, Springer-Verlag, 1987, p 89.
71. Ramirez-Mata, M, Pena-Ancira, FF, and Alarcon-Segovia, D: Abnormal esophageal motility in primary Sjögren's syndrome. J Rheumatol 3: 63, 1976.
72. Maury, CPJ, Tornroth, T, and Teppo, AM: Atrophic gastritis in Sjögren's syndrome: Morphologic, biochemical and immunologic findings. Arthritis Rheum 28: 388, 1985.
73. Rafle, RB: Sjögren's disease associated with a nutritional deficiency syndrome. Br Med J 1: 1140, 1950.
74. MacLaurin, BP, Matthews, N. and Kilpatrick, JA: Coeliac disease associated with autoimmune thyroiditis, Sjögren's syndrome and a lymphocytic serum factor. Aust N Z J Med 4: 405, 1972.
75. Dreiling, DA, and Soto, JML: The pancreatic involvement in disseminated "collagen" disorders: Studies of pancreatic secretion in patients with scleroderma and Sjögren's "disease." Am J Gastroenterol 66: 546, 1976.
76. Tsianos, EB et al: Serum isoamylases in patients with autoimmune rheumatic diseases. Clin Exp Rheumatol 2: 235, 1984.
77. Webb, J et al: Liver disease in rheumatoid arthritis and Sjögren's syndrome: Prospective study using biochemical and serological markers of hepatic disfunction. Ann Rheum Dis 34: 70, 1975.
78. Voigel, C, Wittenborg, A, and Reichart, P: The involvement of the liver in Sjögren's syndrome. J Oral Surg 50: 26, 1980.
79. Golding, PL et al: "sicca complex" in liver disease. Br Med J 4: 340, 1970.
80. Bodenheimer, HC, and Shaffner, F: Primary biliary cirrhosis and the immune system. Am J Gastroenterol 72: 285, 1979.
81. Epstein, O, Thomas, HC, and Sherloc, S: Primary biliary cirrhosis in a dry gland syndrome with features of chronic graft-versus-host disease. Lancet i: 1166, 1980.
82. Kassan, SS, and Talal, N: Renal disease with Sjögren's syndrome. In Tatal, N, Moutsopoulos, HM, and Kassan, SS (eds): Sjögren's Syndrome: Clinical and Immunologic Aspects. Berlin, Springer-Verlag, 1987, p 96.
83. Talal, N, Zisman, E, and Schur, P: Renal tubular acidosis, glomerulonephritis and immunologic factors in Sjögren's syndrome. Arthritis Rheum 11: 774, 1968.
84. Moutsopoulos, HM et al: Immune complex glomerulonephritis in sicca syndrome. Am J Med 64: 955, 1978.
85. Hardin, JA: Case records of the Massachusetts General Hospital. N Engl J Med 292: 1285, 1975.
86. Meltzer, M et al: Cryoglobulinemia: A clinical and laboratory study. II. Cryoglobulins with rheumatoid factor activity. Am J Med 40: 837, 1966.
87. Alexander, EL: Inflammatory vascular disease in Sjögren's syndrome. In Tatal, N, Moutsopoulos, HM, and Kassan, SS (eds): Sjögren's Syndrome: Clinical and Immunologic Aspects. Berlin, Springer-Verlag, 1987, p 102.
88. Alexander, EL et al: Necrotizing arteritis in spinal subarachoid hemorrhage in Sjögren's syndrome. Ann Neurol 11: 632, 1982.
89. Alexander, EL, and Provost, TT: Cutaneous manifestations of primary Sjögren's syndrome: A reflection of vasculitis in association with anti-Ro (SSA) antibodies. J Invest Dermatol 80: 386, 1983.
90. Molina, R, Provost, TT, and Alexander, EL: Two histopathologic prototypes of inflammatory vascular disease in Sjögren's syndrome: Differential association with seroactivity to rheumatoid factor and antibodies to Ro (SSA) and with hypocomplementemia. Arthritis Rheum 28: 1251, 1985.
91. Tsokos, M, Lazarou, S, and Moutsopoulos, HM: Vasculitis in primary Sjögren's syndrome: Histologic classification and clinical presentation. Am J Clin Pathol 86: 26, 1986.
92. Kaltreider, HB, and Talal, N: The neuropathy of Sjögren's syndrome: Trigeminal nerve involvement. Ann Intern Med 70: 751, 1969.
93. Alexander, EL et al: Neurologic complications of primary Sjögren's syndrome. Medicine 61: 247, 1982.

94. Alexander, EL: Neuromuscular complications of primary Sjögren's syndrome. In Tatal, N, Moutsopoulos, HM, and Kassan, SS (eds): Sjögren's Syndrome: Clinical and Immunologic Aspects. Berlin, Springer-Verlag, 1987, p 61.
95. Alexander, EL et al: Primary Sjögren's syndrome with central nervous system dysfunction mimicking multiple sclerosis. Ann Intern Med 104: 323, 1986.
96. Binder, A, Snaith, ML, and Isenberg, D: Sjögren's syndrome: A study of its neurological complications. Br J Rheumatol 27: 275, 1988.
97. Whaley, K et al: Sjögren's syndrome. II. Clinical associations and immunological phenomena. Q J Med 42: 513, 1973.
98. Shearn, MA: Sjögren's Syndrome. Philadelphia, WB Saunders, 1971, p 117.
99. Bloch, J, and Bunim, JJ: Sjögren's syndrome and its relation to connective tissue disease. J Chron Dis 16: 915, 1963.
100. Maini, RN: The relationship of Sjögren's syndrome to rheumatoid arthritis. In Tatal, N. Moutsopoulos, HM, and Kassan, SS (eds): Sjögren's Syndrome: Clinical and Immunologic Aspects. Berlin, Springer-Verlag, 1987, p 165.
101. Kassan, SS, and Talal, N: Sjögren's syndrome with systemic lupus erythematosus/mixed connective tissue disease. In Tatal, N, Moutsopoulos, HM, and Kassan, SS (eds): Sjögren's Syndrome: Clinical and Immunologic Aspects. Berlin, Springer-Verlag, 1987, p 177.
102. Alarcon-Segovia, D: Symptomatic Sjögren's syndrome in mixed connective tissue disease. J Rheumatol 3: 191, 1976.
103. Sharp, GC: Mixed connective tissue disease. Bull Rheum Dis 25: 828, 1975.
104. Reinertson, JL et al: B-lymphocyte alloantigens associated with systemic lupus erythematosus. N Engl J Med 299: 515, 1978.
105. Moutsopoulos, HM et al: B-lymphocyte antigens in sicca syndrome. Science 199: 1441, 1978.
106. Medsger, TA, Jr: Sjögren's syndrome and systemic sclerosis (scleroderma). In Tatal, N, Moutsopoulos, HM, and Kassan, SS (eds): Sjögren's Syndrome: Clinical and Immunologic Aspects. Berlin, Springer-Verlag, 1987, p 182.
107. Oddis, CV et al: Vasculitis in systemic sclerosis: A subset of patients with the CREST variant, Sjögren's syndrome and neurologic complications. Arthritis Rheum 29: S43, (abstract), 1986.
108. Lawley, TJ et al: Scleroderma, Sjögren-like syndrome and chronic graft-versus-host disease. Ann Intern Med 87: 707, 1977.
109. Okano, Y, Nishikai, M and Sato, M: Scleroderma, primary biliary cirrhosis, in Sjögren's syndrome after cosmetic breast augmentation with silicone injection: A case report of possible human adjuvant disease. Ann Rheum Dis 43: 520, 1984.
110. Anderson, LG, and Talal, N: The spectrum of benign to malignant lymphoproliferation in Sjögren's syndrome. Clin Exp Imnol 9: 199, 1972.
111. Tzioufas, AG, Moutsopoulos, H, and Talal, N: Lymphoid malignancy in monoclonal proteins. In Tatal, N, Moutsopoulos, HM, and Kassan, SS (eds): Sjögren's Syndrome: Clinical and Immunologic Aspects. Berlin, Springer-Verlag, 1987, p 129.
112. Talal, N, Sokoloff, L, and Barth, WF: Extrasalivary lymphoid abnormalities in Sjögren's syndrome (reticulum-cell-sarcoma, "pseudolymphoma," macroglobulinemia). Am J Med 43: 50, 1967.
113. Schmid, U, Helbron, D, and Lennart, K: Development of malignant lymphoma in myeopithelial sialadenitis (Sjögren's syndrome). Pathol Anat 395: 11, 1982.
114. Papadopoulos, NM, and Kintzios, JA: Differentiation of pathological conditions by visual evaluation of serum protein electrophoresis patterns. Proc Soc Exp Biol Med 123: 927, 1967.
115. Papadopoulos, NM, Elin, RJ, and Wilson, DM: Incidence of gamma globulin banding in the healthy population by high-resolution electrophoresis. Clin Chem 28: 707, 1982.
116. Moutopoulos, HM et al: Serum C-reactive protein in primary Sjögren's syndrome. Clin Exp Rheumatol 1: 57, 1983.
117. Harley, JB: Autoantibodies in Sjögren's syndrome. In Tatal, N, Moutsopoulos, HM, and Kassan, SS (eds): Sjögren's Syndrome: Clinical and Immunologic Aspects. Berlin, Springer-Verlag, 1987, p 218.
118. Bloch, K et al: Unusual occurrence of multiple tissue component antibodies in Sjögren's syndrome. Trans Assoc Am Physicians 73: 166, 1960.
119. Virji, Ma: Circulating prostatic acid phosphatase-immunoglobulin complexes in Sjögren's syndrome. Clin Chim Acta 151: 223, 1985.
120. Feltkamp, TEW, and Van Rossum, AL: Antibodies to salivary duct cells, and other autoantibodies in patients with Sjögren's syndrome and other idiopathic autoimmune diseases. Clin Exp Immunol 3: 1, 1983.
121. Akizuki, M et al: Purification of an acidic nuclear protein antigen and demonstration of its antibodies in subsets of patients with sicca syndrome. J Immunol 119: 932, 1977.
122. Alspaugh, M, and Maddison, PJ: Resolution of the identity of certain antigen-antibody systems in systemic lupus erythematosus and Sjögren's syndrome: An interlaboratory collaboration. Arthritis Rheum 22: 796, 1979.
123. Provost, TT, Alexander, EL, and Reichlin, M: The relationship between anti-Ro (SSA) precipitin positive Sjögren's syndrome and antibody positive lupus erythematosus. In Tatal, N, Moutsopoulos, HM, and Kassan, SS (eds): Sjögren's Syndrome: Clinical and Immunologic Aspects. Berlin, Springer-Verlag, 1987, p 244.
124. Alvarellos, A et al: Relationship of HLA-DR and MT antigens to antibody expression in systemic lupus erythematosus. Arthritis Rheum 26: 1533, 1983.
125. Wilson, R et al: Sjögren's syndrome: Influence of multiple HLA-D region alloantigens on clinical and serological expression. Arthritis Rheum 27: 1245, 1984.

126. Mann, DL: Immunogenetics of Sjögren's syndrome. In Tatal, N, Moutsopoulos, HM, and Kassan, SS (eds): Sjögren's Syndrome: Clinical and Immunologic aspects. Berlin, Springer-Verlag, 1987, p 235.
127. Fox, RI et al: Beneficial effect of artificial tears made with autologous serum in patients with keratoconjunctivitis sicca. Arthritis Rheum 27: 459, 1984.
128. Talal, N, and Moutsopoulos, HM: Treatment of Sjögren's syndrome. In Tatal, N. Moutsopoulos, HM, and Kassan, SS (eds): Sjögren's Syndrome: Clinical and Immunologic Aspects. Berlin, Springer-Verlag, 1987, p 292.
129. Nahir, AM et al: Effect of prolonged bromhexine therapy on Sjögren's syndrome. Isr J Med Sci 17: 403, 1981.
130. Fox, RI et al: Treatment of primary Sjögren's syndrome with hydroxychloroquine. Am J Med 85: 62, 1988.
131. Drosos, AA et al: Cyclosporin-A (CyA) in primary Sjögren's syndrome: A double blind study. Ann Rheum Dis 45: 732, 1986.
132. Drosos, AA et al: Nandrolone decanoate (Deca-Durabolin) in primary Sjögren's syndrome: A double blind pilot study. Clin Exp Rheumatol 6:53, 1988.
133. Schot, LPC, Verheul, HM, and Schnurs, AHWM: Effect of nandrolone decanoate on Sjögren's syndrome-like disorders in NZB/NZW mice. Clin Exp Immunol 57: 571, 1984.

Chapter 13
Immunosuppressive Therapy in the Treatment of Joint and Connective Tissue Disorders

DAVID P. RECKER, M.D.
JOHN H. KLIPPEL, M.D.

Introduction

Studies of immunosuppressive drugs in the rheumatic diseases span nearly 4 decades starting with early studies of nitrogen mustard in rheumatoid arthritis[1] and immune complex glomerulonephritis[2] and methotrexate in rheumatoid and psoriatic arthritis.[3] The rationale for the use of immunosuppressives in the rheumatic diseases assumes a pivotal role of the immune system in pathology. Suppression of immune function would be expected to mitigate pathologic states mediated by immune abnormalities, leading to eventual clinical improvement. The scope of clinical experience with immunosuppressives has expanded to cover most of the rheumatic diseases. Documentation of efficacy by randomized controlled trials, however, has been adequately assessed only for several of the major diseases. Moreover, it has become readily apparent that complications associated with immune suppression as well as toxicities unique to individual agents are far from trivial. The basic role of the immune system as a host defense mechanism against infection becomes compromised with an increased susceptibility to both common and, in particular, opportunistic infections. Infections with immunosuppressive agents in the rheumatic diseases are compounded by a heightened predisposition to infection inherent in the basic disease process. Finally, there has been major concern regarding the potential for an increased risk for tumor development either from direct drug-induced mutagenesis or the loss of surveillance function for malignancies. Certainly for several of the immunosuppressive agents used hematologic and lymphoreticular malignancies appear to be increased.

Indications for Immunosuppressives

There are very restricted approved indications for immunosuppressive drugs in the rheumatic diseases. Therefore, in general, use of these agents are considered investigational and require informed consent and, ideally, an organized research protocol. Proper concern for potential toxicities has generally limited the use of immunosuppressive drugs to patients with (1) severe, advanced forms of disease who have failed conventional treatments, and (2) patients at high risk for morbid or fatal outcomes. Recognized examples of the latter would include rheumatoid vasculitis, systemic lupus with progressive nephritis or central nervous system disease, polymyositis with cardiopulmonary complications, or forms of systemic vasculitis such as Wegener's granulomatosis.

Historically, there has been little interest in the use of immunosuppressive drugs in patients with early or mild forms of rheumatic disease. The high likelihood of spontaneous improvements or benefit with conventional, less toxic forms of therapy has been used as an argument against aggressive approaches to early disease management. However, under the assumption that the immune system plays an important primary role in the mediation of inflammation in the rheumatic diseases, it is reasonable to postulate that suppression of immune function might be most effective and maximally beneficial at an early stage of disease. Currently, early aggressive drug interventions in the rheumatic diseases is a subject of considerable interest. In the future, it is possible that immunosuppressive drug therapy may become an important aspect of early primary drug management.

Immunosuppressive Drugs

Drugs that directly interact with or interfere with the function of deoxyribonucleic acids (DNA), ribonucleic acids (RNA), or processes involved in cellular division or protein synthesis are of potential use as immunosuppressive agents. The majority of drugs with these properties have been developed for the purpose of treatment of malignant disorders. The effects on the immune system are by and large nonspecific, but some chemotherapies have greater effects on immune function than others. Among the many drugs available, experience in rheumatology has included drugs from several different categories: nitrogen mustard alkylating agents, analogs of natural purines, antagonists of folic acid, and inhibitors of select lymphokine transcription.

Nitrogen Mustard Alkylating Agents

Alkylating agents are compounds with highly reactive alkyl radicals that form covalent bonds with electron-rich sites of nucleic acids, cellular proteins, and membranes. Alkylating agents function throughout all phases of the cell cycle, including the resting (Go) phase. The major site of alkylation of DNA is at the highly neutrophilic 7-nitrogen position of the purine base guanine leading to the formation of a quaternary ammonium. This produces miscoding errors through the substitution of incorrect base pairs. Nitrogen mustard alkylating drugs have two or more alkylating groups and are referred to as bifunctional agents. As a result of this property, internal cross-linkages within the DNA as well as between phosphate groups of the DNA backbone are formed to produce major alterations of the double helical structure. These effects may be lethal to the cell or simply inhibit cell replication or DNA transcription. Alkylation and covalent cross-linkage of ribonucleic acids, intracellular enzymes, and both internal and external cellular membranes further disrupt cell function. The multiple mechanisms through which alkylating agents act make this class of drugs the most highly efficient of all immunosuppressive agents. The most commonly used alkylating agents in the rheumatic diseases are both derivatives of the bifunctional nitrogen mustard alkylating drug mechlorethamine.

Cyclophosphamide

Substitution of a cyclic phosphamide for the N-methyl group of mechlorethamine produces the stable, inert alkylating agent cyclophosphamide (Table 13-1). The drug is well absorbed from the gastrointestinal tract with peak serum levels during the first hour following the dose. The kinetics of oral and intravenous drug administration are similar with a serum half-life of about 6 hours. Cyclophosphamide is metabolized in the liver by microsomal mixed function oxidase (P-450) enzymes. Metabolism may be affected by drugs that inhibit or stimulate oxidative enzymes. The principle intermediate alkylating metabolite, aldophosphamide, is nonenzymatically cleaved to carboxyphosphamide and the potent alkylating compound phosphoramide mustard. These metabolites, in addition to alkylation, have the capacity to phosphorylate molecular structures of the cell. Metabolites and small amounts of unchanged drug are excreted by the kidneys; dosage adjustments are necessary in patients with renal impairment.

In addition to the nonspecific effects produced by the cytotoxicity of cyclophosphamide on cells of the immune system, more selective functional properties have been described. Long-term, low-dose oral cyclophosphamide has been associated with reduced immunoglobulin levels, impairments of in vitro mitogen-stimulated B-cell function, and impaired induction of T suppressor cell activity. Patients with systemic lupus erythematosus treated with high-dose intravenous cyclophosphamide have been found to have reductions of absolute B cells and both CD4+ and CD8+ T cells.[4]

Perhaps most convincing evidence that immunosuppressive drugs can alter the clinical course of rheumatic diseases derives from studies of cyclophosphamide in rheumatoid arthritis,[5-11] systemic lupus erythematosus,[12-14] polymyositis,[15] and Wegener's granulomatosis.[16] In rheumatoid arthritis, multiple randomized controlled trials conducted throughout the 1970s demonstrated low-dose, oral

Table 13-1. Cyclophosphamide, a Nitrogen Mustard Alkylating Agent

Pharmacology	
Route/Dose:	Oral (1–4 mg/kg daily)
	Intravenous (0.5–1.0 g/m^2) diluted in saline and infused over 30 to 60 minutes every 1 to 3 months.
Drug Interactions:	Altered metabolism by drugs that inhibit (e.g., allopurinol, chloroquine, phenothiazine) or stimulate (e.g., corticosteroids, barbiturates, sex hormones) hepatic oxidative enzymes.
Contraindications	Pregnancy, infection, malignancy, renal insufficiency.
Randomized Trials	
Rheumatoid Arthritis: Vs.	Placebo: Cooperating Clinics (1970),[5] Lidsky (1973),[6] Levy (1975),[9] Smyth (1975),[10] Townes (1976)[11]
	Gold: Gumpel (1975),[7] Currey (1974)[8]
	Azathioprine: Currey (1974)[8]
Systemic Lupus:	Donadio (1981),[13] Austin (1986)[14]
Major Toxicities	Bone marrow suppression, infection, bladder hemorrhage, fibrosis and carcinoma, testicular and ovarian fibrosis, malignancies.

cyclophosphamide to be superior to placebo, gold, and azathioprine (Table 13-1). Moreover, evidence suggests that it is one of the few drugs able to prevent joint erosions.[5]

Cyclophosphamide has been carefully studied in long-term trials in lupus nephritis. Donadio and colleagues[12] evaluated a 6-month course of low-dose oral cyclophosphamide in lupus patients with diffuse proliferative nephritis. Analysis at 4 years reported a lower incidence and average rate of clinical recurrence of active nephritis yet failed to detect any significant effect on the loss of renal function, including complete progression to end-stage renal failure. Subsequent analysis after 6 years average followup again failed to reveal differences in the frequencies of end-stage renal failure in patients treated with prednisone (32 percent) and those treated with cyclophosphamide (35 percent).[13] A similar study conducted at the National Institutes of Health after a median followup of 75 months reported less progression of chronic scarring in the kidney[16] and a reduced risk of end-stage renal failure[14] in patients treated with immunosuppressive drugs. Of the various regimens evaluated, intermittent, high-dose, intravenous cyclophosphamide was found to be most effective in the prevention of renal failure. Bolus intravenous cyclophosphamide has also been reported to be beneficial in the management of both neuropsychiatric and hematologic complications of lupus.

The role of bolus cyclophosphamide in the management of other rheumatic diseases has been less well studied. It would appear to be effective in the management of systemic rheumatoid vasculitis, but, interestingly, it has little or no influence on synovitis.[17] Studies in polymyositis have reported conflicting results.[15,18]

The toxicities of cyclophosphamide are substantial, and have greatly limited use of the drug. The cytotoxic effects are most commonly expressed on the bone marrow with the development of leukopenia or anemia. Blood counts with chronic oral drug administration need to be monitored regularly. Cumulative drug effect on the bone marrow produces slowly progressive leukopenia or anemia over the course of months or years. Bolus intravenous cyclophosphamide produces a dose-dependent leukopenia with the nadir occurring in the period 8 to 12 days following drug administration. During this time, serial white blood cell counts should be obtained with adjustment of the subsequent dose accordingly. As a general rule, the absolute white blood cell count should not be depressed below 2000 cells per mm^3, nor the absolute neutrophil count below 1000 cells per mm^3.

Cyclophosphamide damages gonadal tissue to produce ovarian failure, oligospermia, or azoospermia. Sections of the ovary reveal destruction of follicles and fibrosis of the interstitium. Serum levels of follicle stimulating and luteinizing hormones are increased and estradiol levels fall leading to signs and symptoms of menopause. In males, the primary damage is to the germinal epithelial lining layer of the seminiferous tubules. This is associated with marked elevations of serum follicle stimulating hormone, a measurement useful in monitoring effects on the testes. Recovery of spermatogenesis or ovarian function after cyclophosphamide is unpredictable, although it has occurred months or even years after the drug has been discontinued. It is likely that drug dose, duration of therapy, patient age, and vulnerability of different phases of the ovarian cycle in the instance of intermittent therapy are important factors in the development of and recovery from cyclophosphamide-induced gonadal toxicity. The teratogenic effects of cyclophosphamide mandate that the drug not be used during pregnancy. During active drug therapy, effective measures of birth control are essential.

Cyclophosphamide is associated with several forms of bladder toxicities including hemorrhagic cystitis, fibrosis, and transitional and squamous cell carcinoma.[19] The metabolite acrolein appears to be the major irritant responsible for acute cystitis. Liberal fluid intake of at least several liters daily to assure brisk diuresis is a simple and important preventive measure. In addition, it is likely that the concomitant use of mesna (2-mercaptoethanesulfonate) will become an important adjunct for the prevention of cyclophosphamide-induced bladder complications. Both cumulative drug dose and duration of continuous drug administration are important risk factors for bladder fibrosis and malignancy. The finding of hematuria, particularly of new onset after prolonged drug administration, warrants evaluation by urine cytology and cystoscopy for possible malignant change. There is a tenfold to 100-fold increased risk for the development of bladder cancer following oral cyclophosphamide.[20]

Quantitative data to document the magnitude of risk for other malignancies with cyclophosphamide is incomplete. Increases in late malignancies following oral cyclophosphamide therapy of rheumatoid arthritis have identified an approximate fivefold increase in non-Hodgkin's lymphoma and leukemia.[21] Other studies have estimated the relative risks compared to normal controls for all types of malignancies at 2.2 and 3.7.[22] A comparison to age-, sex-, and disease-matched rheumatoid controls not treated with cyclophosphamide found a similar increased relative risk of 4.1; four hematologic or lymphoreticular malignancies were noted (expected 0.27). The increase in the rate of malignancies in the period 7 to 9 years postinitiation of cyclophosphamide would be compatible with a dose-dependent, time-lag model of tumor induction. A single case of acute, nonlymphocytic leukemia following bolus cyclophosphamide has been reported.[23]

Rarely, cyclophosphamide has been associated with other toxicities, particularly with high-dose therapy, including hepatic toxicity, interstitial pneumonitis, and cardiotoxicity.

Chlorambucil

Chlorambucil is an aromatic bifunctional alkylating agent produced by the replacement of the N-methyl group of mechlorethamine with phenylbutyric acid. The drug is given orally, typically at a dose of 0.1 to 0.2 mg per kg daily. Serum drug half-life is approximately 90 minutes; both methylation and beta-oxidation are involved in drug metabolism.

Chlorambucil has been less well studied than cyclophosphamide, but the efficacy of the two drugs would appear to be comparable. Selection between the two drugs is based more on regional preferences and toxicity profiles than efficacy differences. Chlorambucil has been reported to be effective in rheumatoid arthritis[24] and systemic lupus erythematosus.[25] A randomized, double-blind study of chlorambucil in scleroderma failed to detect any benefit.[26]

Many of the potential toxicities of chlorambucil are similar to those observed with cyclophosphamide, including hematologic complications, infections, and ovarian and testicular failure. Bladder toxicities are not a feature of the drug. On the other hand, it would appear that chlorambucil is associated with a much higher risk for the development of malignancies, particularly leukemias. The association is strongest for acute myeloblastic leukemia, although lymphoblastic, monocytic, myelomonocytic, and megakaryocytic leukemias have been reported.

Purine Analogs

The cellular mechanisms of action of analogs of purines involve alterations of nucleotide synthesis and interconversions as well as structure and function of both DNA and RNA. Purine analogs are metabolized to monophosphate ribonucleotides that are poor substrates for the enzymes responsible for the formation of both diphosphates and triphosphates. The resultant accumulation of the monophosphates produces a feedback inhibition on the conversion of phosphoribosyl pyrophosphate to ribosylamine 5-phosphate, a rate-limiting substrate for the further biosynthesis of purine nucleotides. In addition, formation of adenine and guanine nucleotides are affected by the inhibition of inosinic acid conversion by monophosphates. Finally, the triphosphate analogs that are formed become incorporated into DNA, ultimately leading to RNA miscoding and subsequent faulty transcription.

Purine analogs affect both immune and inflammatory pathways. Lymphocytopenia with a reduction in both T and B cells develops. Although the induction of primary delayed hypersensitivity responses is impaired by the drug, there is no effect on established hypersensitivity responses. Immunoglobulin synthesis is suppressed, including antibody responses to secondary immunizations. The anti-inflammatory effects are likely secondary to suppression of monocyte function, including inhibition of monocyte production.

Azathioprine

The major purine analog used clinically is azathioprine, a mercaptopurine prodrug (Table 13-2). Azathioprine is a nitroimidazole derivative of the thiol analog of hypoxanthine, 6-mercaptopurine. Unlike mercaptopurine, azathioprine is well absorbed from the gastrointestinal tract with peak serum levels occurring 1 to 2 hours after administration. The drug is converted in vivo by sulfhydryl compounds such as glutathione, resulting in a slow release of mercaptopurine within tissues. Conversion of mercaptopurine to the nucleotide level by oxidation and methylation pathways results in disruption of cellular metabolism through interference with polynucleotide synthesis and metabolism as well as alterations of DNA and RNA function. The metabolites of azathioprine are excreted by the kidneys and reductions of the usual drug doses are required in patients with impaired renal function.

The enzymatic oxidation of mercaptopurine to 6-thiouric acid can be blocked by the xanthine oxidase inhibitor allopurinol. This results in enhancement of the myelosuppressive and immunosuppressive actions of the drug. Therefore the usual dose of azathioprine must be reduced by about one third if given simultaneously with allopurinol.

Azathioprine is perhaps the most widely used immunosuppressive drug in the management of rheumatic diseases. Randomized studies in rheumatoid arthritis have demonstrated azathioprine to be superior to placebo and to have comparable efficacy to gold, chloroquine, and D-penicillamine (Table 13-2).[7,27-34] However, an analysis of the combined data from these studies concluded that azathioprine was a valuable agent in management.[39] Commonly cited indications for azathioprine in lupus are for the treatment of nonrenal disease manifestations and as a corticosteroid-sparing agent. Neither of these uses has been satisfactorily studied. Combinations of azathioprine with heparin[37] and antilymphocyte globulin[40] have been evaluated in investigational studies in lupus.

Azathioprine combined with high-dose prednisone has been studied in the treatment of polymyositis.[41] Improvements in muscle histopathology and muscle strength at 3 months were comparable in groups treated with azathioprine-prednisone and prednisone alone. A reassessment at 3 years, however, revealed significantly less functional disability and a lower prednisone requirement in patients treated with azathioprine.

Table 13-2. Azathioprine, a Purine Analog

Pharmacology	
Route/Dose:	Oral (1–4 mg/kg daily)
Drug Interactions:	Inhibition of xanthine oxidase blocks oxidative pathway and shunts mercaptopurine metabolism to methylation pathway.
Contraindications	Infection, malignancy, pregnancy (?)
Randomized Trials	
Rheumatoid Arthritis: Vs.	Placebo: Barnes (1969),[27] Levy (1972),[28] Hunter (1975),[30] Goebel (1976)[31]
	Gold: Currey (1974),[8] Dwosh (1977)[33]
	Cyclophosphamide: Currey (1974),[8] Levy (1975)[29]
	Chloroquine: Dwosh (1977)[33]
	D-Penicillamine: Berry (1976),[32] Paulus (1984)[34]
Psoriatic Arthritis:	Levy (1972)[28]
Systemic Lupus Erythematosus:	Szejnbok (1971),[35] Donadio (1972),[36] Cade (1973),[37] Hahn (1975),[38] Austin (1986)[14]
Polymyositis:	Bunch (1981)[41]
Major Toxicities	Gastrointestinal, myelosuppression, infection, hepatitis, pancreatitis, malignancy.

Azathioprine has a suppressive effect on both myeloid and erythroid elements of the bone marrow. Macrocytosis with megaloblastic erythroid changes of the marrow may occur unrelated to deficiencies of folic acid or vitamin B_{12}. Blood counts must be monitored regularly to detect hematologic abnormalities early and dose adjustments made accordingly. The development of leukopenia or anemia may be abrupt and profound. Bone marrow toxicity from azathioprine is generally reversible with discontinuation of the drug or reduction of the dose.

Azathioprine can produce hepatitis, presumably on a hypersensitivity basis. This is often accompanied by fever, diffuse abdominal pain, and a maculopapular skin eruption. Liver enzymes, particularly the pyruvic and glutamic oxaloacetic transaminases, are markedly elevated; levels of alkaline phosphatase are typically normal. Changes on liver biopsy include hepatocellular necrosis and mild biliary stasis. Although liver changes are usually reversible on stopping the drug, cases of hepatic fibrosis following azathioprine therapy have been reported.

Azathioprine would appear to confer an increased risk for the development of malignancies. In a study of nontransplant patients treated with azathioprine, although the overall frequency of malignancy was comparable to controls, the number of patients observed to develop non-Hodgkin's lymphoma was substantially above that expected.[42] In addition, a fourfold increase in cervical atypia following azathioprine has been reported.[43]

Folic Acid Antagonists

Analogs of folic acid interfere with the biosynthesis of purine nucleotides, thymidylate, and ultimately DNA and RNA, by acting as competitive inhibitors of the enzyme dihydrofolate reductase (DHFR). Folic acid is an essential vitamin of the B complex. It is actively transported into cells, converted to dihydrofolate, and reduced to tetrahydrofolic acid by DHFR. Tetrahydrofolate serves as a coenzyme onto which single carbon fragments are added for transfer as part of multiple cellular biosynthetic reactions. Analogs of folic acid, all of which are 4-amino folate derivatives, have an affinity for dihydrofolate reductase that is orders of magnitude greater than that of the natural substrate. The binding of this critical enzyme by the analog inhibits the formation of the natural tetrahydrofolate and all subsequent synthetic reactions involving single carbon transfers.

Methotrexate

Although there are several clinically important folate antagonists, methotrexate (amethopterin) is by far the most widely used. It differs from folic acid only by the addition of a methyl group at the N^{10} position and the substitution of an amino group for the hydroxyl group at the C^4 position on the pteridine ring. Low doses of methotrexate are well absorbed from the gastrointestinal tract, with peak serum drug concentrations at 2 hours and a serum half-life of 5 to 6 hours. Both methotrexate and its poly-g-glutamyl derivative are active inhibitors of DHFR. The latter form also inhibits thymidylate synthetase and, thus, purine biosynthesis. Only a small fraction of methotrexate is metabolized in the liver, principally to the inactive product 7-hydroxymethotrexate. One-half of the drug circulates bound to plasma proteins. The drug is excreted predominantly by the kidneys where it undergoes glomerular filtration, reabsorption, and secretion within the proximal tubules.

Low-dose methotrexate has significant anti-inflammatory properties likely resulting from impairments of neutrophil chemotaxis, reduced monocyte migration, and down-regulation of the production of leukotriene B_4. The influences of low-dose methotrexate on immune function are less clear; antiproliferative effects on immune cells and suppression of antibody synthesis have been described.

Methotrexate has been used in the treatment of most of the rheumatic disorders including rheumatoid and psoriatic arthritis,[44-52] polymyositis,[53] Reiter's syndrome,[54] and systemic lupus erythematosus (Table 13-3).[55] Dose schedules involving oral or parenteral drug therapy have been recommended. It is entirely unclear whether there are important differences in clinical efficacy or drug toxicities among the various regimens. Drugs that displace methotrexate from serum proteins or interfere with renal excretion should be avoided. Many of the severe toxicities reported with methotrexate have developed as a consequence of failure to recognize the influence of other drugs on methotrexate levels. The teratogenicity of methotrexate mandates that pregnancy be excluded prior to the initiation of therapy and that effective means of birth control be practiced throughout therapy.

Methotrexate has been best studied in rheumatoid arthritis in which randomized controlled trials have clearly documented low-dose methotrexate to be far superior to placebo and have comparable efficacy to other second-line agents such as parenteral gold, oral gold, and azathioprine (Table 13-3). There is no

Table 13-3. Methotrexate, a Folic Acid Anatagonist

Pharmacology	
Route/Dose:	Oral, intramuscular, or intravenous routes; dose schedules in common use include: Intermittent, divided dose, oral schedule over 36 hours each week, typically 2.5–5 mg at 12-hour intervals. Single weekly oral, intramuscular, or intravenous dose of 10–15 mg orally or 25–50 mg parenterally.
Drug Interactions:	Displaced from serum proteins by salicylates and other nonsteroidal anti-inflammatory drugs, phenytoin, sulfonamides, tetracycline, and other drugs. Organic acids, probenecid, and thiazide diuretics interfere with renal excretion.
Contraindications	
Absolute:	Pregnancy, acute/chronic liver disease, alcoholism, infection.
Relative:	Renal dysfunction, pulmonary fibrosis, anemia, leukopenia, thrombocytopenia.
Randomized Trials	
Rheumatoid Arthritis: Vs.	Placebo: Thompson (1984),[44] Andersen (1985),[45] Weinblatt (1985),[46] Williams (1985)[47] Gold: Suarez-Almazor (1988),[48] Morassut (1989),[49] Weinblatt (1989)[50] Azathioprine: Hamdy (1987)[51]
Psoriatic Arthritis:	Willkens (1984)[52]
Major Toxicities	Gastrointestinal, mucosal ulceration, hepatotoxicity, hypersensitivity pneumonitis, myelosuppression.

convincing evidence, however, that methotrexate retards erosions. Moreover, disease relapses even after prolonged courses of drug therapy are typical.

Adverse effects from methotrexate are significant and limit long-term therapy. In patients with rheumatoid arthritis, during the first 2 years of drug treatment approximately one third of patients are forced to discontinue therapy secondary to the development of drug complications.[56] The most frequent toxicities occur as a result of drug effects on rapidly proliferating tissues. Gastrointestinal symptoms, including nausea and vomiting, abdominal pain, anorexia, diarrhea, and stomatitis are common, particularly during the 24- to 48-hour period after drug administration. Reductions of drug dosage or folic acid supplementation often leads to improvement of symptoms.

Elevations of serum transaminase levels may be detected in approximately one third of patients treated with low-dose oral methotrexate. In general, enzyme elevations return to baseline within 5 to 7 days. Chronic or excessively high elevations of enzymes are indications for withholding the drug and reintroducing it at a lower dose once the enzymes have returned to normal. The extensive experience with low-dose methotrexate in psoriasis, however, has clearly documented a risk of serious hepatic injury ranging from fibrosis to cirrhosis. Abnormalities of serum liver enzymes are not reliable markers of these complications and liver biopsy is recommended after 1.5-g cumulative doses of methotrexate to detect occult liver injury. The role of pretreatment liver biopsy in patients treated with methotrexate is not clear. The Health and Public Policy Committee of the American College of Physicians has recommended pretreatment biopsy only for patients with known or suspected preexisting liver disease.[57] On the other hand, the American College of Gastroenterology Committee on FDA-related Matters suggests that pretreatment biopsy be performed on all rheumatoid patients treated with methotrexate.[58] In rheumatoid arthritis, evidence of minor hepatic fibrosis following methotrexate has been documented in several studies, with a suggestion of increasing frequency with increased cumulative doses of the drug. Factors thought to be associated with an increased risk of methotrexate hepatotoxicity include preexisting liver disease, alcoholism, and increased patient age.

An acute inflammatory pneumonitis consistent with a hypersensitivity reaction to methotrexate and unrelated to cumulative drug dose has been described.[59] A prodrome of fever and malaise typically precedes the nonproductive cough, dyspnea, and diffuse alveolar and interstitial infiltration apparent on chest radiograph. The entire process resolves spontaneously on discontinuing the drug, although corticosteroids are thought to be beneficial in patients with very acute and rapidly progressive pulmonary involvement. There is no evidence of chronic pulmonary injury associated with long-term methotrexate administration.

Hematologic toxicity from methotrexate is uncommon; scattered case reports of leukopenia, thrombocytopenia, and pancytopenia have been described. Sustained elevations of mean corpuscular volume has been thought to be a predictor of hematologic toxicity.

The extensive, long-term clinical experience with low-dose methotrexate in psoriasis has not revealed convincing evidence for an increased risk of malignancy. In a large retrospective study, 14 patients treated with methotrexate were identified who had developed a malignancy.[60] This was not significantly greater than the number expected in normal controls (expected 6.8, relative risk 2.1). However, among the observed malignancies were an acute granulocytic leukemia and a lymphoma, relatively unusual types of malignant processes that have been associated with other immunosuppressive drugs.

Cyclosporine

The cyclosporines are metabolic products of the fungi Trichoderma polysporum and Cylindrocarpon lucidium. Nine cyclosporines have been isolated, A through I, but only A, C, and G possess immunologic activities. Cyclosporine is unique among immunosuppressives in that its immunosuppressive properties are secondary to selective suppression of T-cell activity; it has virtually no primary effect on polymorphonuclear leukocytes, macrophages, or other phagocytic cells. The effects on immune function are primarily mediated by preventing the activation phase of T cells by inhibition of production and secretion of interleukin-2 (IL-2), interleukin-1 (IL-1), and other lymphokines, at the transcriptional level. Processes dependent on IL-2 secretion including the induction of cytotoxic T lymphocytes, activation of T suppressor cells, and release of gamma-interferon and B-cell activating factors are most influenced.[61] Clinical immunologic diseases such as graft rejection, graft-vs.-host disease, and various autoimmune syndromes dependent on these immune functions have the potential to be modified by cyclosporine. Because of its lipophilic nature, cyclosporine must be solubilized in olive oil for oral administration and castor oil for intravenous use.

Clinical studies of cyclosporin A have reported improvements in multiple rheumatic diseases, including rheumatoid arthritis,[62-65] psoriatic arthritis,[66] Sjögren's syndrome,[67] scleroderma,[68] and polymyositis (Table 13-4).[69] The drug has been most extensively evaluated in rheumatoid arthritis, in which randomized controlled trials of 4 to 6 months' duration have clearly documented drug efficacy. Recent studies have focused on low doses of the drug (5 mg per kg daily or less) in an effort to minimize side effects (see discussion further in text). The clinical effects in rheumatoid arthritis induced by cyclosporin A are rapidly reversed on discontinuation of the drug. Thus, chronic drug administration to maintain clinical benefit is required. Currently, there is limited information on the efficacy or safety of chronic low-dose cyclosporin A administration in rheumatoid arthritis.

There are multiple potential toxicities associated with cyclosporin A (Table 13-4). Clearly, the major concern has involved nephrotoxicity, observed in virtually every clinical study published to date. Impairments of renal function appear to be dose dependent and reversible on discontinuation of the drug. The use of the drug in doses greater than 10 mg per kg daily has been associated with glomerular sclerosis and interstitial fibrosis.[70] The changes result from pathology at the arteriolar level with ischemia, likely mediated by an alteration in the relative intrarenal prostacyclin–thromboxane A balance. Other

Table 13-4. Cyclosporin A, an Inhibitor of Lymphokine Transcription

Pharmacology	
Route/Dose:	Oral, optimal dose not established; likely 5 mg/kg daily, or less. Current recommendation that dose be adjusted to achieve trough serum level (RIA) of 50–200 mg/ml.
Drug Interactions:	Increase levels: High-dose prednisone, cimetidine, ketoconazole. Decrease levels: Diphenylhydantoin, rifampin, trimethoprim.
Contraindications	Renal insufficiency, pregnancy, infection, malignancy.
Randomized Trials	
Rheumatoid Arthritis:	Forre (1987),[62] Yocum (1988),[63] Dougados (1988),[64] Tugwell (1990)[65]
Sjögren's Syndrome:	Drosos (1986)[67]
Major Toxicities	Nephrotoxicity, hypertension, hepatotoxicity, tremors, paresthesias, convulsions, gingival hyperplasia, hirsutism, lymphoproliferative disorders, hyperuricemia.

nephrotoxic drugs, including aminoglycosides, amphotericin B, melphalan, trimethoprim, nonsteroidal anti-inflammatory drugs, and radiopharmaceuticals, have been shown to potentiate the vasoconstrictive effects of cyclosporine. There has been no direct correlation between cyclosporin-induced hypertension and nephrotoxicity; however, hypertension may be an important additive complication that contributes to the nephropathology.

Cyclosporine has been associated with other toxicities. Up to 20 percent of patients treated with cyclosporine have had hepatotoxicity, and hypertrichosis has developed in up to 50 percent. An increased incidence of choledocholithiasis has been observed with chronic drug administration. Gingival hyperplasia may be minimized with careful attention to dental hygiene. Neurotoxicity including tremor, headache, flushing, sleep disturbance, and seizures has been seen in 20 percent of renal and liver transplant patients. Hyperuricemia from decreased renal urate clearance is often observed and may be associated with gouty arthropathy.

The potential role of cyclosporin in tumor induction has been complicated by the frequent use of multiple other immunosuppressive agents. Most of the reported malignancies associated with the drug have been lymphomas or lymphoproliferative disorders. The finding of pure B-cell neoplasia and the incorporation of Epstein-Barr viral genome into tumor cell DNA[71] suggests the unopposed clonal expansion of virus-infected B lymphocytes.

Combination Chemotherapy

There is currently limited information on the effects of combinations of immunosuppressive agents in the rheumatic diseases, an approach used with great success in oncology. Among the various rationales proposed for combination chemotherapy, the elimination of an underlying malignant lymphoproliferative process and synergistic combinations to reduce drug doses and thus dose-dependent toxicities are the most attractive. In favor of the former are a number of clinical case studies documenting the remarkable improvement in rheumatic diseases in patients treated with oncology regimens for malignant disorders. It is far less certain, however, that effective synergistic drug combinations have been identified. To date, small experiences with combination chemotherapy have been reported in rheumatoid arthritis,[72] systemic lupus erythematosus,[14] and inflammatory myopathies.[73] In rheumatoid arthritis, impressive clinical improvements, including a high rate of complete disease remissions and healing of joint erosions, have been described with combinations of cyclophosphamide, azathioprine, and hydroxychloroquine.[72] However, serious toxicities were observed with the combination, including the development of four malignancies.

References

1. Jimenez-Diaz, C et al: Treatment of rheumatoid arthritis with nitrogen mustard: Preliminary report. JAMA 147:1418, 1951.
2. Baldwin, DS et al: Effect of nitrogen mustard on clinical course of glomerulonephritis. Arch Intern Med 92:162, 1953.
3. Gubner, R, August, S, and Ginsberg, V: Therapeutic suppression of tissue reactivity. II. Effects of aminopterin in rheumatoid arthritis and psoriasis. Am J Med Sci 221:176, 1951.
4. McCune, WJ et al: Clinical and immunologic effects of monthly administration of intravenous cyclophosphamide in severe systemic lupus erythematosus. N Engl J Med 318:1423, 1988.
5. Cooperating Clinics Committee of the American Rheumatism Association: A controlled trial of cyclophosphamide in rheumatoid arthritis. N Engl J Med 283:883, 1970.
6. Lidsky, MD, Sharp, JT, and Billings, S: Double-blind study of cyclophosphamide in rheumatoid arthritis. Arthritis Rheum 16:148, 1973.
7. Gumpel, JM et al: A double-blind comparative trial of cyclophosphamide and gold in rheumatoid arthritis. Ann Rheum Dis 33:574, 1974.
8. Currey, HLF et al: Comparison of azathioprine, cyclophosphamide and gold in treatment of rheumatoid arthritis. Br Med J 3:763, 1974.
9. Levy, J, Paulus, HE, and Barnett, R: Comparison of azathioprine and cyclophosphamide in the treatment of rheumatoid arthritis. Arthritis Rheum 18:412, 1975.
10. Smyth, CJ et al: Cyclophosphamide therapy for rheumatoid arthritis. Arch Intern Med 135:789, 1975.
11. Townes, AS, Sowa, JM, and Shulman, LE: Controlled trial of cyclophosphamide in rheumatoid arthritis. Arthritis Rheum 19:563, 1976.
12. Donadio, JV, Jr et al: Treatment of diffuse proliferative nephritis with prednisone and combined prednisone and cyclophosphamide. N Engl J Med 299:1151, 1978.
13. Donadio, JV, Jr, Holley, KE, and Ilstrup, DM: Adrenocorticoid and cytotoxic drug treatment of lupus nephropathy. In Zurukzoglu, W et al (eds): Advances in Basic and Clinical Nephrology. Basel, S Karger, 1981, pp 643–648.
14. Austin, HA et al: Therapy of lupus nephritis: Controlled trial of prednisone and cytotoxic drugs. N Engl J Med 314:614, 1986.

15. Bombardieri, S et al: Cyclophosphamide in severe polymyositis. Lancet i:1138, 1989.
16. Fauci, AS et al: Wegener's granulomatosis: Prospective clinical and therapeutic experience with 85 patients for 21 years. Ann Intern Med 98:76, 1983.
17. Scott, DGI, and Bacon, PA: Intravenous cyclophosphamide plus methylprednisolone in treatment of systemic rheumatoid vasculitis. Am J Med 76:377, 1984.
18. Cronin, ME et al: The failure of intravenous cyclophosphamide therapy in refractory idiopathic inflammatory myopathy. J Rheumatol 16:1225, 1989.
19. Pedersen-Bjergaard, J et al: Carcinoma of the urinary bladder after treatment with cyclophosphamide for non-Hodgkin's lymphoma. N Engl J Med 318:1028, 1988.
20. Plotz, PH et al: Bladder complications in patients receiving cyclophosphamide for systemic lupus erythematosus or rheumatoid arthritis. Ann Intern Med 91:221, 1979.
21. Baker, GL et al: Malignancy following treatment of rheumatoid arthritis with cyclophosphamide: Long-term case-control follow-up study. Am J Med 83:1, 1987.
22. Baltus, JAM et al: The occurrence of malignancies in patients with rheumatoid arthritis treated with cyclophosphamide: A controlled retrospective follow-up. Ann Rheum Dis 42:368, 1983.
23. Gibbons, RB, and Westerman, E: Acute nonlymphocytic leukemia following short-term, intermittent, intravenous cyclophosphamide treatment of lupus nephritis. Arthritis Rheum 31:1552, 1988.
24. Cannon, GW et al: Chlorambucil therapy in rheumatoid arthritis: Clinical experience in 28 patients and literature review. Semin Arthritis Rheum 15:106, 1985.
25. Snaith, MI et al: Treatment of patients with systemic lupus erythematosus including nephritis with chlorambucil. Br Med J 2:197, 1973.
26. Furst, DE et al: Immunosuppression with chlorambucil, versus placebo, for scleroderma: Results of a three-year, parallel, randomized, double-blind study. Arthritis Rheum 32:584, 1989.
27. Barnes, CG et al: Azathioprine: A controlled, double-blind trial in rheumatoid arthritis. Ann Rheum Dis 28:327, 1969.
28. Levy, J et al: A double-blind controlled evaluation of azathioprine treatment in rheumatoid and psoriatic arthritis. Arthritis Rheum 15:116, 1972.
29. Levy, J, Paulus, HE, and Bangert, R: Comparison of azathioprine and cyclophosphamide in the treatment of rheumatoid arthritis. Arthritis Rheum 18:412, 1975.
30. Hunter, T et al: Azathioprine in rheumatoid arthritis. Arthritis Rheum 18:15, 1975.
31. Goebel, KM et al: Disparity between clinical and immune responses in a controlled trial of azathioprine in rheumatoid arthritis. Eur J Clin Pharmacol 9:405, 1976.
32. Berry, H et al: Azathioprine and penicillamine in treatment of rheumatoid arthritis: A controlled trial. Br Med J 1:1052, 1976.
33. Dwosh, IL et al: Azathioprine in early rheumatoid arthritis: Comparison with gold and chloroquine. Arthritis Rheum 20:685, 1977.
34. Paulus, HE et al: Azathioprine versus D-penicillamine in rheumatoid arthritis patients who have been treated unsuccessfully with gold. Arthritis Rheum 27:721, 1984.
35. Sztejnbok, M et al: Azathioprine in the treatment of systemic lupus erythematosus: A controlled trial. Arthritis Rheum 14:639, 1971.
36. Donadio, JV, Jr et al: Treatment of lupus nephritis with prednisone and combined prednisone and azathioprine. Ann Intern Med 77:829, 1972.
37. Cade, R et al: Comparison of azathioprine, prednisone, and heparin alone or combined in treating lupus nephritis. Nephron 10:37, 1973.
38. Hahn, BH, Kantor, OS, and Osterland, CK: Azathioprine plus prednisone compared to prednisone alone in the treatment of systemic lupus erythematosus: Report of a prospective controlled trial in 24 patients. Ann Intern Med 83:597, 1975.
39. Felson, DT, and Anderson, J: Evidence for the superiority of immunosuppressive drugs and prednisone alone in lupus nephritis: Results of a pooled analysis. N Engl J Med 311:1528, 1984.
40. Hollingsworth, P et al: Intensive immunosuppression versus prednisolone in the treatment of connective tissue diseases. Ann Rheum Dis 41:557, 1982.
41. Bunch, TW: Prednisone and azathioprine for polymyositis: Long-term follow-up. Arthritis Rheum 24:45, 1981.
42. Kinlen, LJ et al: Cancer in patients treated with immunosuppressive drugs. Br Med J 282:474, 1981.
43. Nyberg, G, Eriksson, O, and Westberg, NG: Increased incidence of cervical atypia in women with systemic lupus erythematosus treated with chemotherapy. Arthritis Rheum 24:648, 1981.
44. Thompson, RN et al: A controlled two-centre trial of parenteral methotrexate therapy for refractory rheumatoid arthritis. J Rheumatol 11:760, 1984.
45. Andersen, PA et al: Weekly pulse methotrexate in rheumatoid arthritis. Ann Intern Med 103:489, 1985.
46. Weinblatt, ME et al: Efficacy of low-dose methotrexate in rheumatoid arthritis. N Engl J Med 312:818, 1985.
47. Williams, HJ et al: Comparison of low-dose oral pulse methotrexate and placebo in the treatment of rheumatoid arthritis: A controlled clinical trial. Arthritis Rheum 28:721, 1985.
48. Suarez-Almazor, ME et al: A randomized controlled trial of parenteral methotrexate compared with sodium aurothiomalate. J Rheumatol 15:753, 1988.
49. Morassut, P et al: Gold sodium thiomalate compared to low dose methotrexate in the treatment of RA—a randomized double blind 26-week trial. J Rheumatol 16:302, 1989.

50. Weinblatt, ME et al: Oral methotrexate versus gold therapy (auranofin) in active rheumatoid arthritis: A 36-week multicentre trial. Arthritis Rheum 32:S43, 1989.
51. Hamdy, H et al: Low-dose methotrexate compared with azathioprine in the treatment of rheumatoid arthritis: A twenty-four week controlled clinical trial. Arthritis Rheum 30:361, 1987.
52. Willkens, RF et al: Randomized, double-blind, placebo controlled trial of low-dose pulse methotrexate in psoriatic arthritis. Arthritis Rheum 27:376, 1984.
53. Metzger, AL et al: Polymyositis and dermatomyositis: Combined methotrexate and corticosteroid therapy. Ann Intern Med 81:182, 1974.
54. Lally, EV, and HO, G: A review of methotrexate therapy in Reiter's syndrome. Semin Arthritis Rheum 15:139, 1985.
55. Rothenberg, RJ et al: The use of methotrexate in steroid-resistant systemic lupus erythematosus. Arthritis Rheum 31:612, 1988.
56. Alarcon, GS, Tracy, IC, and Blackwood, WD: Methotrexate in rheumatoid arthritis: Toxic effects as the major factor limiting long-term treatment. Arthritis Rheum 32:671, 1989.
57. Health Policy Committee of the American College of Physicians: Methotrexate in rheumatoid arthritis. Ann Intern Med 107:418, 1987.
58. American College of Gastroenterology: Methotrexate-induced chronic liver injury: Guidelines for detection and prevention. Am J Gastroenterol 88:1337, 1988.
59. Cannon, GW et al: Acute lung disease associated with low-dose pulse methotrexate therapy in patients with rheumatoid arthritis. Arthritis Rheum 26:1269, 1983.
60. Bailin, PL et al: Is methotrexate therapy for psoriasis carcinogenic? A modified retrospective-prospective analysis. JAMA 232:359, 1975.
61. Kahan, BD: Cyclosporine. N Engl J Med 321:1725, 1989.
62. Forre, O et al: An open controlled randomized comparison of cyclosporine and azathioprine in the treatment of rheumatoid arthritis. Arthritis Rheum 30:88, 1987.
63. Yocum, DE et al: Cyclosporin A in severe, treatment-refractory rheumatoid arthritis: A randomized study. Ann Intern Med 109:863, 1988.
64. Dougados, M, Awada, H, and Amor, B: Cyclosporin in rheumatoid arthritis: A double blind, placebo controlled study in 52 patients. Ann Rheum Dis 47:127, 1988.
65. Tugwell, P et al: Low-dose cyclosporin in patients with rheumatoid arthritis. Lancet 335:1051, 1990.
66. Gupta, AK et al: Cyclosporin in the treatment of psoriatic arthritis. Arch Dermatol 125:507, 1989.
67. Drosos, AA et al: Cyclosporin A (CyA) in primary Sjögren's syndrome: A double blind study. Ann Rheum Dis 45:732, 1986.
68. Applebaum, T, and Itzkowitch, D: Cyclosporine in successful control of rapidly progressive scleroderma. Am J Med 82:866, 1987.
69. Levi, S, and Hodgson, HJ: Cyclosporin for dermatomyositis. Ann Rheum Dis 48:85, 1989.
70. Palestine, AG et al: Renal histopathologic alterations in patients treated with cyclosporin for uveitis. N Engl J Med 314:1293, 1986.
71. Starzl, TE et al: Reversibility of lymphomas and lymphoproliferative lesions developing under cyclosporin steroid therapy. Lancet i:583, 1984.
72. Csuka, ME, Carrera, GF, and McCarty, DJ: Treatment of intractable rheumatoid arthritis with combined cyclophosphamide, azathioprine and hydroxychloroquine. JAMA 255:2315, 1986.
73. Wallace, DJ, Metzger, AL, and White, KK: Combination immunosuppressive treatment of steroid-resistant dermatomyositis/polymyositis. Arthritis Rheum 28:590, 1985.

Chapter 14
Total Hip Replacement Arthroplasty in Patients with Inflammatory Arthritis

CHITRANJAN S. RANAWAT, M.D.
MICHAEL J. MAYNARD, M.D.
WILLIAM F. FLYNN, JR., M.D.

Inflammatory Hip Arthritis

Surgical treatment of inflammatory arthritis has advanced rapidly since the introduction of the "low friction arthroplasty" by Sir John Charnley in the early 1960s. Since that time, widespread adoption, investigation, and adaptation of Charnley's principles have fostered a rapid advancement of bioengineering technology and vastly improved understanding of the biomechanical principles germane to joint reconstruction. Patients with inflammatory arthritis have gained particular benefit from this revolution in surgical therapy as its application has expanded to include the hip, knee, shoulder, elbow, wrist, and other joints.

Total hip arthroplasty, in particular, has improved, over the course of a multitude of evolutionary changes, into a widely indicated surgical procedure with a high rate of predictable, durable success.

Hip pathologic states meeting the indications for surgical reconstruction may arise from numerous causes:

I. Degenerative Disease
   Osteoarthritis
   Post-traumatic arthritis
   Idiopathic avascular necrosis
   Preexisting condition, for example, congenitally dislocated hip, Legg-Calvé-Perthes disease, Charcot's joint, and slipped capital femoral epiphysis

II. Inflammatory Arthritis
   Rheumatoid arthritis (RA)
   Juvenile rheumatoid arthritis (Still's disease) (JRA)
   Seronegative spondyloarthropathy, for example, ankylosing spondylitis, psoriatic arthropathy
   Crystalline arthropathy (gout, calcium pyrophosphate deposition disease/[CPPD])
   Infectious arthritis

III. Connective tissue disease
   Systemic lupus erythematosus
   Mixed connective tissue disease

IV. Endocrine, Metabolic, Miscellaneous
   Ochronosis
   Hemochromatosis
   Pigmented villonodular synovitis (PVNS)
   Acromegaly

Rheumatoid Arthritis

Several reports have placed the incidence of symptomatic involvement of one or both hips, meeting appropriate criteria for surgical intervention, at 10 to 20 percent in patients with an established diagnosis of rheumatoid arthritis.[1-3] It is important to note, however, that a direct correlation between clinical findings and radiographic evidence of hip disease has been universally lacking. Hip disease may be significant on radiographic examination of RA patients with clinically normal hips. The converse of this situation is often true early in the course of the disease process when synovitis may cause severe hip pain and functional disability in the absence of any demonstrable radiographic changes. This variability of the presentation observed among patients underscores the fact that destruction of the hip should not be viewed as an inevitable event in the natural history of rheumatoid arthritis. Appropriate management of anti-inflammatory therapy, physical therapy, activity level, ambulatory aids, and nutrition can successfully avoid the need for hip surgery in the majority of patients.

Juvenile Rheumatoid Arthritis

The clinical disease entity known as juvenile rheumatoid arthritis encompasses several different subtypes that vary considerably in their initial presentation, clinical course, and ultimate prognosis. Overall, up to 10 percent of children diagnosed as having some form of JRA develop significant functional disability related to the hip.[4] However, in those patients presenting with the polyarthritis subtype of the disease, approximately 50 percent develop hip involvement that results in destruction of this joint.[5]

Early identification is crucial in JRA patients with hip disease. These patients are usually skeletally immature and, left untreated, may rapidly develop severe soft tissue contractures. If diagnosed early, physical therapy, occasionally augmented by surgical soft tissue release, can successfully delay or avoid arthroplasty. However, if significant contractures go untreated and are allowed to exert a persistent effect on an immature skeleton, severe bony deformity and/or ankylosis is an inevitable result. Increasing bony deformity correlates directly with increasing surgical technical difficulty and may, in and of itself, mandate extremely early surgical intervention in the interest of preserving some chance of surgical success. The worst case scenario—when joint implant arthroplasty becomes the only option for maintaining or regaining ambulatory capability—represents a clinical catastrophe, since the prospects for growth disturbance and/or failure of an arthroplasty implanted in a young child are significant.

Several considerations are unique to the treatment of arthritic children. Motivation and related psychosocial issues occupy a position of particular significance with respect to their ultimate functional outcome and must be considered in any therapeutic plan.[4] In addition, hip reconstruction in these patients nearly always presents significant surgical technical difficulties, a topic addressed more fully later in this discussion.

Other Inflammatory Arthritides

Patients carrying a diagnosis of ankylosing spondylitis demonstrate up to a 50 percent incidence of clinically significant hip arthritis,[6] often of bilateral involvement.[7,8] Hip pathologic findings may include the development of protrusion deformities and/or completely ankylosed hips. The frequent involvement of the spine and sacroiliac joints seen in ankylosing spondylitis may complicate the clinical evaluation of the hips. Heterotopic ossification of the soft tissues around the hip is a common occurrence postoperatively and, therefore, prophylaxis is indicated in these patients.[6,9,10]

Patients with psoriasis have a 10 percent incidence of associated hip arthritis. This may be as high as 40 percent in patients with juvenile onset disease.[11,12] If pain and functional disability become severe despite medical management, arthroplasty should be considered.

Reiter's disease, Crohn's disease, and ulcerative colitis may also present associated hip pathologic findings. Severe hip disease requiring arthroplasty is uncommon but not unknown.

Gout and calcium pyrophosphate deposition disease (CPPD, pseudogout) may cause hip arthritis. Joint space narrowing and subchondral cysts are seen radiographically and, in severe cases, joint arthroplasty may be indicated. The metabolic stress of surgery has been known to precipitate an acute flareup in patients with gout or pseudogout.

Systemic lupus erythematosus (SLE) and mixed connective tissue disease may rarely present with primary involvement of the hip joint. More commonly, the hip dysfunction seen in association with these disorders is secondary to the use of high-dose corticosteroids, in the control of the disease, which leads to avascular necrosis of the femoral head and subsequent femoral head collapse and painful arthritis of the hip joint. Osteoporosis and osteoarthritic changes including joint space narrowing and osteophyte formation are seen radiographically late in the disease process.

Ochronosis, hemachromatosis, pigmented villonodular synovitis, and acromegaly can cause destruction of the hip joint. The radiographic presentation of the hip pathologic states in these diseases is often similar to that seen in osteoarthritis. In ochronosis, homogentisic acid accumulates in the synovium and cartilage. Destruction of joint surfaces and a characteristic black staining are seen clinically. Hemachromatosis causes deposition of iron in the synovium, again leading to destruction of joint surfaces. The pathologic process seen in PVNS involves synovial pigmentation and hypertrophy of idiopathic etiology. Cartilage destruction, joint space narrowing, and cyst formation can be detected radiographically. Acromegaly involves the joints through hypertrophy, degeneration, and regeneration of cartilage and bone. Osteophytic changes are usually prominent and the large size of the bones may require the fabrication of custom implants.

Clinical and Radiographic Features of Rheumatoid Arthritis

Significant rheumatoid involvement of the hip may present with a variety of clinical symptoms, including pain, tenderness, gait disturbance, decreased range of motion (soft tissue contractures), leg length discrepancy, synovitis, and bursitis.

Adult patients usually present with pain, typically in the groin, as their chief complaint. The pain may persist at rest and may be present at night. Decreasing motion is commonly only a secondary complaint.

By contrast, the JRA patient seldom complains of pain in the hip but, rather, controls pain, over time, by decreasing voluntary motion.[4] As a direct result, they often develop a pronounced limp and advanced hip flexion and adduction contractures. Compensatory lumbar hyperlordosis and even scoliosis may appear. A resultant course of progressively diminishing ambulation is the late symptom that often precipitates their referral to the orthopedic surgeon.

Radiographs of hips affected by rheumatoid arthritis reveal osteopenic bone in the majority of patients. Loss of joint space due to destruction of the articular cartilage is common. Osteophyte formation is uncommon. The technical term for medial and/or superior displacement of the femoral head and acetabulum is *protrusion* or *protrusio deformity*. The appearance of this deformity represents significant bone loss in the pelvis and presents difficult technical problems to the reconstructive surgeon. Cyst formation, also signifying bone destruction, may also be apparent. Patients who have received corticosteroid therapy may demonstrate signs consistent with avascular necrosis and consequent collapse of the femoral head.[1]

Total Hip Replacement Arthroplasty

Indications

Over the years, various surgical techniques have been advocated in the treatment of the rheumatoid hip. The most commonly performed operative procedures are the following[13]:

Synovectomy
Soft tissue release
Fusion
Girdlestone pseudarthrosis
Arthroplasties
    Cup
    Femoral endoprosthesis
        Unipolar
        Bipolar
    Surface replacement
    Total hip replacement
Revision surgery

It is the authors' opinion and experience that, out of the above list, total hip arthroplasty is the surgical procedure with the most predictably satisfactory long-term performance in the rheumatoid arthritic hip. The fundamental indication for total hip arthroplasty in RA patients is severe pain and/or functional disability despite optimal medical management. This assumes that all other potential causes of hip pain such as spine or other joint involvement, tumor, synovitis, and other soft tissue inflammation have been ruled out or are not amenable to nonsurgical therapy. In addition, there should be objective radiographic evidence of hip disease.

Absolute contraindications include acute or chronic infection at any site in the patient and any medical condition that contraindicates anesthesia and surgery. Poor condition of the skin or vasculature of the involved extremity and previous sepsis in the involved joint are relative contraindications. Obesity, young age, and occupation requiring heavy labor are relative contraindications, commonly applicable to patients with osteoarthritis, but they usually do not apply to the RA patient population.

Finally, the summary condition of the patient, including other joint involvement, motivation, personal expectations, and overall ability to comply with postoperative rehabilitation should be taken into account. Patient, rheumatologist, and surgeon should all realize that the polyarticular nature of the disease may require the surgical treatment of several joints before any significant functional benefit is obtained. Furthermore, while pain relief is a consistently predictable outcome of joint replacement arthroplasty in rheumatoid arthritis, range of motion and overall functional improvement is much less so.

Postoperative rehabilitation can be made difficult and may not achieve optimal results in an uncooperative patient. Therefore, it is important to enlist the help of nurses, psychologists, social workers, and physical and occupational therapists prior to any surgical intervention. This type of team approach, while particularly applicable to young patients, is very beneficial for all patients with inflammatory arthritis. When the patient's toleration of multiple planned procedures is in doubt, it may be prudent to perform a relatively simple procedure first in order to assess the patient's ability to comply with the required postoperative protocol, before proceeding with surgery that entails more painful and arduous rehabilitation.[14]

Medical Considerations

The patient with inflammatory arthritis presents some unique considerations to the physician coordinating perioperative management. For this reason every patient should be managed by a medical consultant familiar with these considerations, preferably a rheumatologist, in the perioperative period.

The possibility of inflammatory involvement of the chest makes thorough preoperative assessment of each patient's cardiopulmonary status particularly critical in order to define which extra preparatory and precautionary measures may be warranted during anesthesia.

Patients who have been maintained on corticosteroid therapy are often adrenally suppressed. In these cases, perioperative medical management should include appropriate additional doses of corticosteroids to meet the requirements imposed by the metabolic stress of surgery.

A thorough preoperative search for potential sources of bacteremia and infection must be performed. This must include, as a minimum, evaluation of the lungs, heart, skin, teeth, and urinary tract. Patients with a history of gastrointestinal problems should be examined further for possible occult infection (e.g., gallbladder disease or diverticular abscess). Any preexisting source of infection must, of course, be erradicated prior to surgery. After surgical implantation of a prosthetic joint, periodic surveillance of potential sources of bacteremia should become part of routine medical management. Prophylactic antibiotics are mandatory prior to dental work and any invasive medical instrumentation (e.g., cystoscopy or colonoscopy) of these patients for the rest of their lives.

Surgical Considerations

Surgical technical difficulties arise secondary to osteoporosis and bony deformity, especially protrusion, which lead to a decrease in the amount of good-quality bone available for the support of an implanted prosthesis. Significant osteoporosis is present in most hips affected by rheumatoid arthritis. Up to 40 percent of RA patients presenting for total hip replacement arthroplasty may demonstrate protrusion of the femoral head and medial wall of the acetabulum into the pelvis.[15] Some patients, those with JRA in particular, present with subluxation and acetabular dysplasia, which is clinically quite similar to the presentation of congenital hip dysplasia. Coupled with severe deformity, the small bone size seen in JRA patients often requires the fabrication of custom implants and surgical tools.[16,17] All of the aforementioned considerations affect the choice of fixation and prosthetic implant, may lengthen the operative time, and may indicate the use of bone grafting and/or special prosthetic devices.[18-21]

Soft tissue contractures are frequently present in the rheumatoid hip and usually require the performance of extensive soft tissue releases, which may significantly reduce early postoperative hip muscle strength. If contractures are particularly severe, limb shortening may be necessary to achieve proper joint stability and motion.

Surgical Planning Considerations in Multiple Joint Involvement

Significant involvement of the cervical spine occurs in 30 to 40 percent of patients with rheumatoid arthritis.[22] Therefore, radiographic evaluation of the cervical spine for possible instability is mandatory prior to surgery. If cervical spine instability exists, it should be given first priority for surgical intervention. In addition to instability, deformity and/or loss of flexibility of the cervical spine are also commonly associated with rheumatoid arthritis, JRA, and ankylosing spondylitis. Additionally, patients with JRA may have temporomandibular joint involvement and micrognathia. These problems often mandate the use of special techniques such as bronchoscopy-guided intubation or tracheostomy, if general anesthesia is to be induced.[16] To avoid the pitfalls associated with these techniques, regional anesthesia is often the method of choice for the performance of lower extremity surgery in patients with rheumatoid arthritis.[4]

Many patients have significant involvement of both upper and lower extremity joints. If practical, surgical intervention should first address the lower extremities in order to avoid, if possible, imposing the weight-bearing demands of lower extremity rehabilitation upon upper extremity arthroplasties. However, adherence to this order of priorities would require that the patient's upper extremities be functional enough to assist weight bearing during lower extremity rehabilitation using canes, crutches, walker, or platform walker. If this is not the case, upper extremity arthroplasty may be required prior to lower extremity arthroplasty in order to achieve the ability to use the ambulatory aids required for lower extremity rehabilitation.

Lower extremity operative planning must take the status of both hips, both knees, both ankles, and both feet into account. First priority should be given to ensuring that the feet and ankles are stable and plantigrade and without any areas of skin breakdown or impending breakdown that could present a potential source of infection. Once the feet and ankles are satisfactory, the planning for hips and knees may then be addressed.

In a patient with ipsilateral hip and knee involvement, the hip operation should be performed first unless there is such severe flexion deformity or instability of the knee that it would effectively preclude adequate rehabilitation of the hip. This order of priority derives from the fact that hip rehabilitation generally requires less functional range of motion at the ipsilateral knee than knee rehabilitation requires at the ipsilateral hip. If both hips and/or both knees are involved, bilateral hip or knee arthroplasties can be carried out at a single operative event if the patient's medical status does not contraindicate.[1]

Typical Hospital Course and Rehabilitation

Total hip arthroplasty patients, especially those with inflammatory arthritis, should be admitted to the hospital no later than the night before surgery. This allows time for adequate last-minute patient instruction and physical preparation, and the assembly of all essential preoperative evaluations. Most standard protocols include the patient's taking a shower with pHisoHex or povidone-iodine (Betadine), and a bowel-cleansing enema on the night before surgery. In addition, most anesthesia protocols require that the patient ingest nothing by mouth after midnight of the night before surgery as a precaution against aspiration of stomach contents during anesthesia. Hospital admission on the day before surgery facilitates the accomplishment of these precautions.

Primary total hip arthroplasty generally requires from 1 to 3 hours of operative time to complete. Regional anesthesia has gained increasing popular support for use in the majority of lower extremity orthopedic surgical cases. In particular, epidural anesthesia used in combination with controlled hypotension, has been shown to be advantageous to the surgical outcome in total hip arthroplasty, resulting in reduced operative time, less blood loss, and radiographic evidence of improved implant fixation in cases in which cement fixation is employed.[23]

Surgical blood loss concomitant to a primary hip arthroplasty results in a requirement for 2 to 4 units of blood transfusion during and/or after surgery. Autologous predeposit of blood by the patient for his or her own use is available at many centers and often avoids nonautologous transfusion.

A suction drain is commonly placed in the hip at surgery to evacuate any potential early postoperative hematoma. This is usually removed after 24 to 48 hours. Abduction slings or an abduction pillow are also applied for a few days after surgery to protect the hip from dislocating forces while the patient is convalescing from surgery. Prophylactic antibiotics are begun before surgery and continued intravenously for 24 to 48 hours postoperatively. Anticoagulant therapy is begun either before, during, or immediately after surgery depending on the physician's preferred protocol. Most rehabilitation protocols call for the patient to begin standing up at the bedside by the second postoperative day. Progressive ambulation usually begins by the third postoperative day. When cement fixation has been used, full weight bearing can be allowed immediately after surgery. If a trochanteric osteotomy has been performed, special precautions and limited weight bearing on the hip are in order. When a noncemented device has been implanted, an extended period of minimal weight bearing is often prescribed.

Ambulatory assistive devices for rehabilitation are tailored to the patient's needs. Patients with rheumatoid involvement of the upper extremities may require a special walker with platforms, which avoids weight bearing on the hands and wrists. Most patients progress to discharge after a hospital stay of 7 to 10 days. Some patients with inflammatory arthritis may require further supervised rehabilitation and, based on individual needs, these patients are transferred, if possible, to a rehabilitation facility that is geared to accommodate their personal requirements. In most cases, an unsupervised program of ambulation at home is most often all that is necessary for a successful outcome after total hip arthroplasty.

Our long-term total hip arthroplasty rehabilitation protocol requires the use of some type of ambulatory aid for at least 2 months after surgery. A walker or two crutches is prescribed for the first month. This may progress to a single crutch for an additional month and then to a cane after that. Full benefit from the surgical intervention is usually realized by the end of 1 year.

Postoperatively, the performance of a total hip arthroplasty requires the observance of special precautions to avoid dislocation of the prosthetic joint. These are aimed at avoiding extremes of motion at the hip while the soft tissues violated by the surgery heal. After a posterior surgical approach, the technique commonly used at our hospital, acute flexion and internal rotation of the hip must be avoided. In this regard, the patient is carefully instructed in proper leg and body positioning as part of the rehabilitation protocol. He or she should use an elevated toilet seat and avoid soft or low chairs for several months after surgery. Instructions are given the patient not to lean forward from a sitting position and not to bend over from a standing position. Special assistive reachers and other devices are provided and should be used for dressing and other activities of daily living. A pillow held between the legs while sleeping is also prescribed for the first few months.

Intraoperative Complications

The overall intraoperative surgical complication rate in primary total hip arthroplasty is less than 5 percent.[13] The prevalence of neurologic complications related to total hip arthroplasty is approximately 1 to 3 percent[24-27] and the majority of these resolve within the first 6 months after surgery.[28] Although the exact prevalence of vascular complications is not known, they probably occur in less than 1 percent of cases.[28-30] Significant malpositioning of the prosthetic components manifesting as postoperative joint instability and dislocation occurs in less than 3 percent of cases.[13,28] The incidence of infection attributable to the surgical procedure itself after primary hip arthroplasty is less than 2 percent in the rheumatoid population.[13,31] Osteoporosis is commonly present in rheumatoid bone and makes gentle manipulation of the limb and careful utilization of bone-working tools a constant priority of the operating surgeon in order to avoid occasional bony complications such as femoral perforation or fracture, and perforation of the medial wall of the acetabulum.

Postoperative Complications

Deep Vein Thrombosis

Various reports in the literature have placed the incidence of deep vein thrombosis (all sites) following total hip arthroplasty in the range of 50 to 80 percent, although not all patients are symptomatic.[32-34] Based on clinical suspicion and V/Q scan, the incidence of related pulmonary embolism is estimated to be 6 to 19 percent. Fatal pulmonary embolism associated with total hip arthroplasty has been reported to be as high as 1 to 3 percent in patients without prophylaxis.[33,34] Thus, because of the obvious potential for significant morbidity and mortality in this regard, prophylaxis and surveillance are important components of perioperative and postoperative management.

Epidural anesthesia during the operative procedure, and aspirin therapy in the immediate postoperative period, are used for most patients according to our current prophylaxis protocol for deep vein thrombosis.[23] All patients receive venographic evaluation of the affected extremity on or about postoperative day 5. If thrombosis is demonstrated, warfarin therapy is started. All patients undergoing bilateral arthroplasty, and those with a prior history of pulmonary embolism, are begun on warfarin therapy, in lieu of aspirin therapy, on the night after surgery.

The incidence of deep vein thrombosis or pulmonary embolism may affect the function of the arthroplasty itself to the degree that the vascular event interferes with the course of postoperative rehabilitation. Otherwise, long-term effects on durability and function are neglible.

Infection

The incidence of early infection, defined as that appearing within 6 months of surgery, is similar for all diagnoses and is less than 1 percent.[13,28] The overall long-term infection rate for total hip arthroplasty performed using routine antibiotic prophylaxis and modern surgical technique is approximately 2 percent.[35] The long-term rate for various subgroups of patients varies significantly, however. The infection rate for osteoarthritic patients is approximately 0.3 percent, while rheumatoid arthritis patients have a risk of 1.2%.[31] The risk for psoriatic patients has been reported to be 5.5%,[31] and for diabetic patients 6.6%.[31] Patients in these groups also have a higher incidence of infection at other sites, such as lung, urinary tract, and skin, than do nonaffected patients. This is thought to be due to immune suppression caused by the disease processes themselves and related medications that degrade the effectiveness of the patient's immune response.

Established infection within a prosthetic joint is a devastating complication. The treatment of an established infection is removal of the implants and all associated fixation, and débridement of all locally infected soft tissue and bone. This is usually followed by a minimum of 6 weeks of appropriate intravenous antibiotic therapy.[28] Reimplantation of a new prosthesis may then be performed if the infectious source has been identified and removed and diagnostic testing demonstrates the eradication of the infectious organism. Occasionally, especially in a case of an infection involving a particularly virulent pathogen, it may be prudent to delay reimplantation until after a period of observation (sometimes up to a year), while the patient is kept off of antibiotic therapy.

Reimplantation after infection is technically more demanding than primary arthroplasty and always requires a surgeon experienced in its planning and execution who also has all of the necessary tools and implants available. Occasionally, it may require the fabrication of custom tools and implants, and bone grafting.

Dislocation

Dislocation of the prosthetic femoral head from within the prosthetic acetabulum averages 0.5 to 3 percent in most reports[13,26,28] and may occur at any time after total hip arthroplasty but is most common during the first several postoperative weeks. During this period, soft tissue and muscle weakness around the hip are least able to resist any dislocating forces that may be applied.

Poor surgical technique may be a factor in dislocation. However, the vast majority of dislocations occur as a result of patient error—usually noncompliance in the observance of prescribed precautions. As mentioned previously, appropriate precautions usually involve the avoidance of certain body positions and activities. These vary according to the details of the surgical technique as it relates to the weakening of various anatomic structures. Rehabilitation after total hip arthroplasty should always include thorough instruction in these precautions and should provide, if possible, various aids such as long shoe horns, hand-extension devices for putting on hosiery, elevated toilet seats, and other related devices that help the patient to avoid the extremes of hip motion in the early postoperative period.

If dislocation occurs, it should be considered a surgical emergency. Injury to neural and vascular structures may acutely accompany the dislocation or the relocation event.[35] A patient with suspected dislocation should be promptly transferred to a facility where radiographic evaluation and manipulative or operative treatment is available. The vast majority of dislocations are easily reducible after administering mild pain relief using muscle relaxation and gentle manipulation by an experienced physician. Severe dislocations may, however, require open reduction under anesthesia and sterile technique in an operating room.[35]

Trochanteric Complications

Trochanteric nonunion is reported to occur in 3 to 9.5 percent of cases in which a trochanteric osteotomy is performed as part of the surgical procedure.[36] The rate is increased in patients with repeat osteotomies and in those with osteoporosis or other conditions that are associated with poor bone healing. It has been reported to be as high as 24 percent in one series of patients with rheumatoid arthritis.[21] Nonunion may be painful but it is rarely disabling because a fibrous union usually develops. Approximately 50 percent of patients with nonunion or fibrous union demonstrate abductor weakness and a limp.[37] Complete trochanteric nonunion has a higher rate of dislocation and limp and may require surgical repair.

Heterotopic Ossification

Heterotopic ossification is a complication that may appear clinically with redness, low-grade fever, and aching pain around the affected hip. The diagnosis can be made radiographically when a hazy appearance can be seen in the soft tissue surrounding the hip. Males are affected two to three times more often than females, and the incidence in osteoarthritis is higher than in rheumatoid arthritis. Patients with ankylosing spondylitis, Paget's disease, and diffuse idiopathic skeletal hyperostosis (Forrestier's disease) carry a higher risk.[9,10] Although overall, heterotopic ossification of varying degree has been reported in up to 30 percent of patients after total hip arthroplasty,[35] the incidence of significant heterotopic ossification compromising function of the joint is probably less than 5 percent.[38]

For patients at particular risk, postoperative indomethacin has been shown to decrease the risk of heterotopic ossification.[9,39] Low-dose postoperative irradiation, 1000 rad given in five fractions of 200 rad each, has also been shown to be very effective.[40] If severe heterotopic ossification does occur, it can significantly compromise joint function and may require surgical excision.

Leg Length Discrepancy

Leg length discrepancy is an occasional complication of hip reconstruction that may be quite annoying to the patient. Excessive lengthening is most often associated with a posterior surgical approach to the hip joint, since lengthening may be required to achieve proper joint stability after this exposure.[28] On the other hand, limb shortening may be required to achieve joint stability in cases in which severe soft tissue contractures are present. In most cases, leg length discrepancy that is deemed clinically significant postoperatively can be satisfactorily treated with the use of a shoe lift. Revision surgery is rarely indicated.

Metal Toxicity

Metal sensitization has not yet been shown to occur to any significant degree after implantation of cemented metal-on-plastic articulations.[35,41] However, it is too early to assume that the same will be true of cementless components which, if they incorporate a metallic microstructured design for bone-ingrowth fixation, present a much larger surface area for the processes of local corrosion and ion leaching to take place.

Nickel and cobalt are two suspected human carcinogens routinely present in the most popular alloys used for implant fabrication.[35] Yet, the observed incidence of primary malignant tumors arising in the vicinity of total hip arthroplasties has been vanishingly rare.[42,43]

Long-Term Results

General Considerations

Nearly 100 percent of RA patients experience dramatic immediate and complete relief of their hip pain after cemented total hip arthroplasty.[15,44] Functional improvement is also apparent in the vast majority of patients but, due to the polyarticular nature of the disease, the degree of ultimate improvement seen over the long term is not as complete or predictable.

Cemented Fixation

The long-term performance of cemented total hip arthroplasty in rheumatoid arthritis, implanted prior to the advent of improved cementing techniques that came into widespread use in the late 1970s, has been reported in the orthopedic literature by many authors.[1,13,15-19,21,25-27,45-50] Review of a representative series of such patients treated at the Hospital for Special Surgery in New York City revealed a greater than 80 percent survivorship of the arthroplasty longer than 12 years using the endpoint of revision surgery for actuarial analysis.[44] Aseptic loosening is uniformly reported in all series as the most frequent long-term complication associated with cemented total hip arthroplasty for rheumatoid arthritis and it is the leading cause for revision arthroplasty. The main conclusion to be derived from the long-term experiences reported in the series just cited is that longevity of fixation of a cemented implant is directly related to the quality of the initial surgical technique, the quality and quantity of bone available to support the prosthesis, and patient-related variables such as age, activity level, and body weight.

Surgical technique is perhaps the single most important determinant. Current standards require thorough bone preparation and careful cement handling and pressurization to achieve satisfactory cement-bone microinterlock. Improvements in prosthetic design have made durable cement-prosthesis bonding relatively easy to achieve. Actuarial curves derived for a more recent series of patients, treated using the improved cementing techniques and materials, projects significant improvement of long term durability over the previous series. At present, a 90 percent success rate at 10 years can be predicted for the average patient receiving a cemented total hip replacement for rheumatoid arthritis.[51]

Alternatives to Cemented Fixation

Currently, much attention is focused on the development of suitable alternatives to cement fixation in an effort to provide a satisfactory solution to the problem of long-term implant fixation. The alternatives presently receiving the most scrutiny are "press-fit," "microstructured," and "hydroxyapatite osteoconductive" designs. The press-fit prostheses rely on intimate contact "interference" fit between prosthesis and bone for fixation. Microstructured prostheses have specially engineered surfaces designed to allow bone ingrowth into the pores of the surface for fixation by interdigitation of bone and implant. Hydroxyapatite osteoconduction prostheses are coated with hydroxyapatite ceramic on a microstructured surface. This substance is the main inorganic component of human bone matrix and is expected to facilitate the conduction of living bone ingrowth and interdigitation with the prosthesis.

Microstructured or porous-ingrowth prostheses have, to date, received the most extensive use. Controversy abounds concerning how much and what type of surface provides optimal fixation. Most surgeons agree, however, that good bone quality and proper prosthetic fit are prerequisites for success of these implants, since the growth of bony interdigitation appears to require intimate contact without motion at the interface.

Patients meeting current indications for use of an uncemented implant include those at high risk for loosening of a cemented implant (i.e., young, active, or heavy patients) who have good bone quality regardless of arthritic etiology.

The performance of uncemented acetabular fixation has thus far been excellent in a wide range of patients. Uncemented fixation of the femoral component has remained problematic, however, with persistent thigh pain presenting in 15 to 30 percent of patients.[52,53] Based on the assumption that the performance of uncemented sockets will remain good in the long term and the knowledge that modern cementing technique has significantly improved the durability of cemented stem fixation, the use of a "hybrid" arthroplasty consisting of an uncemented acetabular component and a cemented femoral component has become popular.

References

1. Ranawat, CS: Surgery for rheumatoid arthritis: Lower limb, surgery of the hip. Curr Orthop 3:146, 1989.
2. Lehtimäki, MY, Kaarela, K, and Hämäläinen, MMJ: Incidence of hip involvement and need for total hip replacement in rheumatoid arthritis: An eight-year-follow-up study. Scand J Rheumatol 15:387, 1986.
3. Gschwend, N: Surgical Treatment of Rheumatoid Arthritis. Philadelphia, WB Saunders, 1980.
4. Scott, RD, and Sledge, CB: Juvenile rheumatoid arthritis. In Steinberg, ME (ed): The Hip and Its Disorders. Philadelphia, WB Saunders, 1991, p. 470.
5. Cassidy, JT, and Petty, RE: Textbook of Pediatric Rheumatology, ed. 2. New York, Churchill Livingstone, 1990, p. 182.
6. Bisla, RS, Ranawat, CS, and Inglis, AE: Total hip replacement in ankylosing spondylitis with involvement of the hip. J Bone Joint Surg (Am) 58:233, 1976.
7. Wilkinson, M, and Bywaters, EGL: Clinical features and the course of ankylosing spondylitis as seen in followup of 222 hospital referred cases. Ann Rheum Dis 17:209, 1958.
8. Julkunen, H: Rheumatoid spondylitis. Clinical and laboratory study of 149 cases compared with 182 cases of rheumatoid arthritis. Acta Rheumatol Scand (Suppl 4), 1962.
9. Ritter, MA, and Gioe, T: The effect of indomethacin on paraarticular ossification following total hip arthroplasty. Clin Orthop 167:113, 1982.
10. Parkinson, JB, Evarts, CM, and Hubbard, LF: Radiation therapy in the prevention of heterotopic ossification after total hip arthroplasty. In Nelson, JP (ed): The Hip: Proceedings of the Tenth Open Scientific Meeting of the Hip Society, 1982. St. Louis, CV Mosby, 1982, p. 211.
11. Leonard, DG, O'Duffy, JD, and Rogers, RS, III: A prospective evaluation of psoriatic arthritis in patients hospitalized for psoriasis. Mayo Clin Proc 53:511, 1978.
12. Shore, A, and Ansell, BM: Juvenile psoriatic arthritis: An analysis of 60 cases. J Pediatr 100:529, 1982.
13. Steinberg, M: Hip surgery. In Utsinger, PD, Zvaifler, NJ, and Ehrlich, GE (eds): Rheumatoid Arthritis. Philadelphia, JB Lippincott, 1985, p. 767.
14. Sledge, CB: Surgery for rheumatoid arthritis. Curr Orthop 3:1, 1989.
15. Poss, R et al: Six to 11-year results of total hip arthroplasty in rheumatoid arthritis. Clin Orthop 182:109, 1984.
16. Ruddlesdin, C et al: Total hip replacement in children with juvenile chronic arthritis. J Bone Joint Surg (Br) 68:218, 1986.
17. Bisla, RS, Inglis, AE, and Ranawat, CS: Joint replacement surgery in patients under thirty. J Bone Joint Surg (Am) 58:1098, 1976.
18. Lachiewicz, PF et al: Total hip arthroplasty in juvenile rheumatoid arthritis: Two- to eleven-year results. J Bone Joint Surg (Am) 68:502, 1986.
19. Ranawat, CS, and Zahn, MG: Role of bone grafting in correction of protrusio acetabuli by total hip arthroplasty. J Arthroplasty 1:131, 1986.
20. McCollum, DE, Nunley, JA, and Harrelson, JM: Bone-grafting in total hip replacement for acetabular protrusion. J Bone Joint Surg (Am) 62:1065, 1980.
21. Ranawat, CS, Dorr, LD, and Inglis, AE: Total hip arthroplasty in protrusio acetabuli of rheumatoid arthritis. J Bone Joint Surg (Am) 6:1059, 1980.
22. Ranawat, CS: Rheumatoid arthritis of the cervical spine. J Neurosurg 3340, 1984.
23. Ranawat, CS et al: Effect of hypotensive epidural anesthesia on acetabular cement-bone fixation in total hip arthroplasty. J Bone Joint Surg (Br) (accepted for publication) 1991.

24. Silski, JM, and Scott, RD: Obturator nerve palsy resulting from intrapelvic extrusion of cement during total hip arthroplasty. J Bone Joint Surg (Am) 67:1225, 1985.
25. Beckenbaugh, RD, and Ilstrup, DM: Total hip arthroplasty: A review of three hundred and thirty-three cases with long follow-up. J Bone Joint Surg (Am) 60:306, 1978.
26. Charnley, J, and Cupic, Z: Nine and 10 year results of low friction arthroplasty of the hip. Clin Orthop 95:9, 1973.
27. Eftekhar, NS, and Stinchfield, FE: Experience with low friction arthroplasty: A statistical review of early results and complications. Clin Orthop 95:60, 1973.
28. Ranawat, CS, and Figgie, MP: Early complications of total hip replacement. In Steinberg, ME (ed): The Hip and Its Disorders. Philadelphia, WB Saunders, 1991, p. 1042.
29. Berquist, D, Carlsson, AS, and Ericsson, BF: Vascular complications after total hip arthroplasty. Acta Orthop Scand 54:157, 1983.
30. Nachbur, B et al: The moechanisms of severe arterial injury in surgery of the hip joint. Clin Orthop 141:122, 1979.
31. Wroblewski, BM, and Del Sel, HJ: Urethral instrumentation and deep sepsis in total hip replacement. Clin Orthop 146:209, 1980.
32. Paiement, G et al: Low dose warfarin versus external pneumatic compression for prophylaxis against venous thromboembolism following total hip replacement. J Orthop 2:23, 1987.
33. Paiement, GD et al: Advances in the prevention of venous thromboembolic disease after hip and knee surgery. Orthop Rev 18, (Suppl):1, 1989.
34. Kakkar, VV et al: Heparin and dihydroergotamine prophylaxis against thromboembolism after hip arthroplasty. J Bone Joint Surg (Br) 67:538, 1985.
35. Bierbaum, BE, Pomeroy, DL, and Berklacich, FM: Late complications of total hip replacement. In Steinberg, ME (ed): The Hip and Its Disorders. Philadelphia, WB Saunders, 1991, p. 1061.
36. Boardman, KP, Bocco, F, and Charnley, J: An evaluation of methods of trochanteric fixation using 3 wires in the Charnley low friction arthroplasty. Clin Orthop 132:31, 1978.
37. Ritter, MA, Gioe, TJ, and Stringer, EA: Functional significance of non-union of the greater trochanter. Clin Orthop 159:177, 1982.
38. Charnley, J: The long term results of low-friction arthroplasty of the hip performed as a primary intervention. J Bone Joint Surg (Br) 54:61, 1972.
39. Almasbakk, K, and Rosyland, P: Does indomethacin (IMC) prevent postoperative ectopic ossification in total hip replacement? Acta Orthop Scand 48:556, 1977.
40. Ayers, DC, Evarts, CM, and Parkinson, JR: The prevention of heterotopic ossification in high risk patients by low dose radiation therapy following total hip arthroplasty. J Bone Joint Surg (Am) 68:1423, 1986.
41. Rooker, GD, and Wilkinson, JD: Metal sensitivity in patients undergoing hip replacement. J Bone Joint Surg (Br) 62:502, 1980.
42. Penman, HG, and Ring, PA: Osteosarcoma in association with total hip replacement. J Bone Joint Surg (Br) 66:632, 1984.
43. Swann, M: Malignant soft tissue tumor at the site of a total hip replacement. J Bone Joint Surg (Br) 66:629, 1984.
44. Unger, AS et al: Total hip arthroplasty in rheumatoid arthritis. J Arthroplasty 2:191, 1987.
45. Charnley, J: Low Friction Arthroplasty of the Hip: Theory and Practice. Berlin, Springer-Verlag, 1979.
46. Charnley, J: Long term results of low friction arthroplasty. In Nelson, JP (ed): The Hip: Proceedings of the Tenth Open Scientific Meeting of the Hip Society, 1982. St. Louis, CV Mosby, 1982, p. 42.
47. Collis, DK: Long-term radiographic follow-up of total hip replacements. In Nelson, JP (ed): The Hip: Proceedings of the Tenth Open Scientific Meeting of the Hip Society, 1982. St. Louis, CV Mosby, 1982, p. 1.
48. Colville, J, and Raunio, P: Total hip replacement in juvenile rheumatoid arthritis. Acta Orthop Scand 50:197, 1979.
49. Coventry, MB, and Stauffer, RN: Long-term results of total hip arthroplasty. In Nelson, JP (ed): The Hip: Proceedings of the Tenth Open Scientific Meeting of the Hip Society, 1982. St. Louis, CV Mosby, 1982, p. 34.
50. Gustilo, RB, and Burnham, WH: Long-term results of total hip arthroplasty in young patients. In Nelson, JP (ed): The Hip: Proceedings of the Tenth Open Scientific Meeting of the Hip Society, 1982. St. Louis, CV Mosby, 1982, p. 27.
51. Ranawat, CS, and Cornell, CN: The effect of improved cement technique.
52. Engh, CA, and Bobyn, JD: Results of porous-coated hip replacement using the AML prosthesis. In Fitzgerald, R, Jr (ed): Non-Cemented Total Hip Arthroplasty. New York, Raven Press, 1988, p. 393.
53. Galante, JO: Clinical results with the HGP cementless total hip prosthesis. In Fitzgerald, R, Jr (ed): Non-Cemented Total Hip Arthroplasty. New York, Raven Press, 1988, p. 427.

Chapter 15
Nonoperative Orthopedics

NORMAN A. JOHANSON, M.D.

Introduction

The musculoskeletal disorders mentioned in this chapter are frequently encountered in the office practices of many different types of primary care physicians. They are conditions that often lead to the referral of the patient to an orthopedic surgeon or to a rheumatologist. Situations that are directly related to trauma are more frequently referred to an orthopedist, either to rule out a fracture or dislocation, or in anticipation of possible surgical intervention. However, most of the disorders described here do not require surgery. Many are "overuse syndromes" that are best treated with rest of the appropriate body part, anti-inflammatory medications, and physical therapy.

Neck

Acute Muscle Spasm

Irritability of paracervical muscles may arise as a result of an injury, most commonly in a rapid acceleration/deceleration such as a rear-end motor vehicle collision (whiplash). In response to ligamentous injury to the facet joints of the cervical spine the cervical muscles contract, preventing excessive joint motion.

Cervical muscle spasm occurs in response to prolonged postural positions that tend to place excessive mechanical strain on the muscles. This is commonly found in patients who have spent long hours studying. This may be exacerbated by underlying emotional stress. Acute neck pain may be seen in fibromyalgia, in which multiple trigger points are identified.

Patients with acute muscle spasm of the neck present with posterior neck pain that may radiate to the interscapular region as well as to the shoulders. Occipital headaches may be an associated complaint. The patient holds the neck in a flexed and sometimes rotated position and resists any kind of passive motion. Palpable muscle spasm is often present. Neurologic examination is usually normal. X-ray studies of the cervical spine are either normal or reveal a straightening of the normal cervical lordosis.

Acute neck spasm must be distinguished from referred neck pain associated with disorders such as myocardial infarction or apical pulmonary lesions (Pancoast's tumor). Systemic disorders such as rheumatoid arthritis or ankylosing spondylitis can present with neck pain and spasm.

Treatment of acute neck spasm is directed at resting of the muscles using a hard plastic cervical collar, and local heat. Nonsteroidal anti-inflammatory medication and muscle relaxants are useful for symptomatic control. A cervical collar worn for 3 days substantially relieves symptoms, permitting the patient to be weaned from the collar over a period of 2 to 3 weeks. In the instance of whiplash injuries the time a collar is required may be much more protracted.

Cervical Radiculopathy

Cervical radiculopathy may arise in the setting of an acute disk herniation in which the nucleus pulposus impinges upon one of the cervical nerve roots as it exits through the neural foramen; in degenerative disk disease an osteophyte from the posterolateral corner of the vertebral body is capable of producing similar symptoms. In a severe situation a herniated disk or large osteophyte may be capable of causing spinal cord compression; therefore the patient should always be evaluated for evidence of myelopathy.

The clinical course of cervical radiculopathy may be more varied and more insidious in its onset than that of acute neck muscle spasm, although symptoms of radiculopathy may be accompanied by severe neck pain and reflex muscle spasm. The prominent feature of radiculopathy is pain and/or paresthesias in the dermatomal distribution of one of the cervical segments, most commonly in the C-6 distribution. Examination may reveal decreased sensation, muscle weakness, and loss of a reflex (biceps, triceps, or brachioradialis muscles). Occasionally symptoms of carpal tunnel syndrome (see later section) may overlap with cervical radiculopathy in the so-called double crush syndrome.

Plain lateral cervical spine x-ray films are often normal in the setting of an acute cervical disk herniation and either a computed tomography (CT) scan or magnetic resonance imaging (MRI) scan of the cervical spine is required to demonstrate the lesion. Degenerative disk disease is often accompanied by radiographic changes that are easily recognized as disk space narrowing and posterior osteophyte formation, most commonly at the level of C5-6.

Cervical radiculopathy is treated with immobilization of the cervical spine using a hard cervical collar, in conjunction with nonsteroidal anti-inflammatory medications and muscle relaxants as needed. In the case of acute disk herniation intermittent cervical traction using 10 to 20 pounds for 20 to 30 minutes each session may be of benefit. The duration of traction is guided by the clinical response.

Symptoms of cervical radiculopathy are frequently self-limiting, although they may be recurrent. Unremitting pain because of a herniated disk or impinging osteophyte secondary to degenerative disk disease may be treated with disk and/or osteophyte excision through the anterior approach in conjunction with an anterior interbody cervical fusion. It must be noted, however, that only rarely do patients with cervical spine degenerative disk/joint disease need surgical intervention. Most cases respond to the conservative approach outlined above.

Shoulder

Impingement Syndrome

Impingement syndrome is caused by a spectrum of pathologic changes occurring in the rotator cuff, the subacromial bursa, and the undersurface of the acromion. With inflammation of the bursal tissues separating the rotator cuff and the undersurface of the acromion the tissues become edematous, and the mechanical pressure in the subacromial space increases. This can be further exacerbated by continued attempts by the patient to perform overhead work or heavy lifting.

As the inflammatory condition becomes chronic the rotator cuff begins to degenerate and small degenerative tears may appear in the substance of the tendon, usually near the insertion of the rotator cuff on the greater tuberosity of the humerus. With attrition of the rotator cuff the humeral head begins to migrate superiorly and moves closer to the undersurface of the acromion.

The patient may present with progressive pain in the shoulder following a relatively minor injury or there may be no history of injury, the pain arising insidiously. It is most affected by attempting to perform overhead work or heavy lifting activities, and often interferes with sleep.

The physical findings of the impingement syndrome include varying degrees of limitation of active abduction of the shoulder, painful passive rotation with the shoulder in 90° of abduction, and pain during the final 15° to 20° of passive forward flexion (impingement sign).

In the early stages of the impingement syndrome x-ray studies of the shoulder are normal. In chronic impingement there is a characteristic superior migration of the humeral head and sclerosis of the undersurface of the acromion. This is indicative of a degenerative rotator cuff tear (cuff arthropathy).

The initial treatment of acute impingement syndrome is rest, nonsteroidal anti-inflammatory medication, and local heat. When pain is excruciating or other conservative means have failed, an injection of a steroid preparation into the subacromial space is necessary (40 mg methylprednisolone acetate). Multiple injections may be required, but no more than two or three injections should be given within the course of 1 year. If pain continues despite conservative therapy, magnetic resonance imaging (MRI) of the shoulder should be performed to rule out a rotator cuff tear. If pain persists for 6 months, resection of the undersurface of the acromion (acromioplasty) with or without a rotator cuff repair should be strongly considered.

Most pain associated with the impingement syndrome is self-limiting and should be followed by a program of gentle strengthening of the musculature around the shoulder, and by using care to avoid those daily activities that lead to exacerbation of symptoms.

Calcific Tendinitis

Acute and excruciating shoulder pain may be accompanied by mineralization of the substance of the rotator cuff tendon. As the volume of this chalky substance increases there is a tendency for further degeneration and mechanical weakness of the rotator cuff.

The physical findings in calcific tendinitis are similar to those in impingement, although they tend to be more dramatic. The patient frequently guards against any shoulder motion because of severe pain.

X-ray studies demonstrate a calcific density in the subacromial space, usually near the insertion of the rotator cuff on the greater tuberosity. This density is variable in size from a few flecks to a massive collection of mineralized material.

Although symptoms in this condition may improve spontaneously, the majority of cases require at least one injection of 40 mg of methylprednisolone into the subacromial space. An attempt is made to mechanically disrupt the calcification and enhance its reabsorption. For refractory cases acromioplasty and surgical débridement of the rotator cuff may be necessary.

Adhesive Capsulitis

Although the term *adhesive capsulitis* implies an inflammatory condition that involves the capsular structures of the shoulder, its etiology and underlying pathologic basis remain obscure. It is thought that disuse of the shoulder leads to tightening of the capsular structures and therefore to a cycle of painful movement, further disuse, and increasing contracture. The patient presents with pain and progressive loss of motion of the involved shoulder. This condition is sometimes associated with other disorders such as diabetes, cervical spondylosis, or psychiatric conditions associated with movement disorders. It may also be associated with inadequately treated impingement syndrome. X-ray films of the shoulder are frequently normal.

Aggressive physical therapy is required at least three times a week to reestablish a functional range of glenohumeral motion. Nonsteroidal anti-inflammatory medications are usually ineffective in this condition. At least 3 months of physical therapy is required to reestablish a normal range of motion in severely affected patients. If no improvement is noted, arthroscopic inspection of the shoulder and/or manipulation should be considered.

Reflex Sympathetic Dystrophy

Reflex sympathetic dystrophy of the upper extremity is a condition that is characterized by pain, diffuse tenderness, and vasomotor changes that include swelling and trophic skin changes. It has been found in association with upper extremity trauma, neurologic disease, cardiovascular disease, osteoarthritis, and pulmonary tuberculosis. Its pathogenesis is poorly understood, but the process appears to be driven by a localized overactivity of the sympathetic nervous system.

Physical examination reveals poor mobility in an edematous upper extremity, accompanied by hypersensitivity to touch, coolness of the skin, and hair loss. Stiffness is usually present in the hand, wrist, and elbow.

Radiographic changes include diffuse or juxtaarticular osteopenia on plain x-ray films and a diffusely high intake in the affected extremity found on a technetium bone scan.

The treatment of reflex sympathetic dystrophy consists of aggressive physical therapy for mobilization of the entire upper extremity with active, active assisted, and passive range of motion exercises at least three times a week. This may be performed in conjunction with sympathetic nerve blocks administered by an experienced anesthesiologist. Manipulation under regional anesthesia may be required for refractory stiffness.

Elbow

Olecranon Bursitis

The olecranon bursa is one of 160 bursae throughout the body; these contain a small amount of synovial fluid and are lined with a cellular membrane similar to that seen in the lining of joints. The olecranon bursa is located in the subcutaneous tissue overlying the olecranon process of the proximal ulna. It allows the skin to glide smoothly over the underlying bone during elbow flexion and extension. During inflammatory conditions the bursa fills with fluid and becomes prominent on the posterior aspect of the elbow. This prominence predisposes the bursa to becoming further inflamed by repeated trauma. The condition may or may not be painful, but if a chronic condition develops the constant irritation becomes bothersome and the patient usually seeks attention for this problem.

On physical examination there is a prominent fluid-filled mass over the olecranon process. This is usually a bland condition but can be associated with erythema and induration when due to an acute attack of gout or an infectious process. Elbow range of motion is usually normal, but may be uncomfortable in flexion.

X-ray studies of the elbow define the soft tissue mass and possibly demonstrate a prominence on the underlying olecranon that may have been a predisposing factor to developing this condition.

The treatment of noninfectious olecranon bursitis is conservative, with observation and the use of nonsteroidal anti-inflammatory medications and mechanical protection from further trauma. If a septic process is suspected the bursa should be aspirated and the fluid cultured. While awaiting the culture results an anti-Staphylococcus aureus antibiotic should be started. If there is significant induration and evidence of spreading cellulitis into the forearm, the patient should be placed on intravenous antibiotics until control is established. This represents a medical emergency because necrotizing fasciitis is a potential complication. If an aseptic bursitis does not resolve over a 10-day to 2-week period an aspiration of the bursa is indicated. If there is another recurrence, 40 mg of methylprednisolone may be injected after reaspiration. In general, aspiration should be avoided because of the potential complication of infection introduced through the shallow needle track. A chronically infected olecranon bursa is extremely difficult to treat and may require surgical excision.

Epicondylitis

The medial and lateral epicondyles of the distal humerus are sites of attachment of the common flexor and common extensor origins of the musculature of the forearm. These muscles give rise to broad tendinous bands prior to inserting on ridges that define the flare of the distal humerus. The most common inflammatory condition of these tendons is lateral epicondylitis, commonly referred to as tennis elbow. The repeated bracing of wrist extensors during the backhand stroke combined with the impact of the ball on the racquet causes small tendon fibers to pull free of the bone, causing an inflammatory process. This can occur in non-tennis players through repeated dorsiflexion of the wrist against resistance. A similar condition, although less common, may occur on the medial epicondyle through repeated use of the flexor musculature.

The patient with epicondylitis presents with severe, well-localized pain that is exacerbated by activities, especially those that involve bracing of the wrist against resistance or during a power grasp. Pain occasionally radiates above and below the elbow.

On physical examination there is point tenderness over the epicondyle, with some tenderness along the common flexor or extensor tendon. This tenderness is exacerbated by resisted wrist extension or flexion and by extension.

The treatment of epicondylitis is at first conservative, using nonsteroidal anti-inflammatory medications and a forearm strap that is thought to be helpful in redistributing muscle forces across the tendons and into the bone. A wide variety of straps and splints are available for this purpose. If pain does not subside, an injection of 40 mg of methylprednisolone may be delivered to the extensor or flexor origin. In refractory cases a surgical procedure may be performed to débride the area of degenerated tendon and to refasten the tendon to the bone using suture material tied through drill holes in the epicondyle.

Hand and Wrist

Carpal Tunnel Syndrome

The boundaries of the carpal tunnel in the wrist are defined dorsally, medially, and laterally by the carpal bones and volarly by the flexor retinaculum. A retinaculum is a thick, fibrous ligament that crosses the wrist transversely. The carpal tunnel contains the flexor tendons of the hand and the median nerve. Inflammation of the tenosynovium surrounding the flexor tendons may lead to increased swelling and tissue bulk causing compression of the median nerve. This gives rise to the characteristic symptoms of carpal tunnel syndrome. This condition may arise in association with rheumatoid arthritis, myxedema, acromegaly or amyloidosis, and therefore attention should be given to the diagnosis of systemic disease along with the local phenomenon.

The patient with carpal tunnel syndrome presents with wrist pain and paresthesias of the hand, particularly in the thumb, index, and long fingers. The occurrence of symptoms is more intense at night, and the patient may report awakening with pain and paresthesias that require shaking or rubbing of the hand for relief.

Physical examination may reveal a completely normal neurologic examination, or varying degrees of sensory loss in the thumb, index, as well as long and radial side of the ring finger. Motor dysfunction is uncommon, but in advanced cases thenar muscle atrophy may be observed. This may be accompanied by difficulty with thumb opposition. Often paresthesias may be elicited by flexing the wrist for 30 to 60 seconds (Phalen's sign). Tapping the median nerve at the wrist may elicit similar symptoms (Tinel's sign).

Electrophysiolgic studies may confirm the presence of carpal tunnel syndrome. Plain x-ray evaluation is often not helpful unless carpal tunnel syndrome has arisen as a result of a post-traumatic fracture deformity or secondary to an inflammatory joint disorder. Computed tomography scanning of the wrist is an effective method of visualizing soft tissue structures in the carpal tunnel that may be responsible for causing symptoms.

Treatment of carpal tunnel syndrome is conservative, using resting splints or nonsteroidal anti-inflammatory medication. Injection of 40 mg of methylprednisolone into the carpal tunnel may provide transient relief of symptoms. Relief is not frequently long-lasting, and there is a potential for injuring the median nerve during such an injection. In refractory cases of carpal tunnel syndrome surgical release of the flexor retinaculum is indicated. This provides reliable and long-lasting relief of symptoms. During this procedure an exploration of the carpal tunnel, biopsy of the tenosynovium, and exploration of the motor branch of the median nerve may be performed.

DeQuervain's Stenosing Tenosynovitis

The extensor tendons of the hand and wrist are contained in six separate compartments defined by fibrous sheaths attached to the dorsum of the wrist. The first compartment contains the tendons of the abductor pollicis longus and extensor pollicis brevis muscles. With repetitive movements of the thumb and wrist these tendons may become inflamed, with the tenosynovium surrounding the tendons swelling and causing a relative stenosis of the extensor compartment.

The patient complains of dorsoradial wrist pain, particularly with ulnar deviation (lifting with the wrist in neutral position). Physical examination reveals pain on flexion of the thumb and ulnar deviation of the wrist (Finkelstein test). DeQuervain's disease can be distinguished radiographically from arthritis of the base of the thumb and wrist arthritis.

Treatment of DeQuervain's tenosynovitis is initially conservative, using a splint to immobilize the thumb and wrist. The first extensor compartment may be injected with 2 to 4 mg of dexamethasone. If no resolution of symptoms occurs with this treatment, surgical release of the extensor compartment may be performed with the expectation of an excellent result.

Trigger Finger or Thumb

The flexor tendons of the fingers pass through a complex arrangement of fibrous pulleys beginning at the level of the metacarpophalangeal joints and extending out into the finger. The close tolerances of this system predispose to the development of stenosing tenosynovitis when the tenosynovium surrounding the tendon becomes inflamed. Initially swelling begins to obstruct the normal gliding mechanism of the tendon through the pulley system. As chronic changes occur the tendon itself becomes swollen and edematous, and a nodule develops that may become large enough to obstruct the passage of the tendon through the pulley. In this situation the nodule prevents flexion or extension of the finger until sufficient force is exerted to pull the nodule through the pulley. This causes a "triggering" phenomenon that is characteristic of this condition.

On physical examination a nodule associated with the flexor tendon is usually palpable, and the snapping sensation as the finger flexes and extends localizes the area of relative stenosis. Most of the time this is at the most proximal end of the pulley system, at the level of the metacarpophalangeal joint.

Trigger fingers may be treated with a 7- to 10-day course of nonsteroidal anti-inflammatory medication. If no improvement is noted, an injection of dexamethasone 2 to 4 mg is given into the flexor tendon sheath and the finger is actively and passively flexed and extended to distribute the medication. If a large nodule is palpable within the substance of the tendon it is likely that surgical release of the most proximal pulley (A-1 pulley) is required.

Lumbar Spine

Muscular and Ligamentous Strain

The segments of the lumbar spine are held together by a complex arrangement of ligaments connecting the vertebral bodies, the posterior elements (laminae and spinous processes), and the articular facets. These ligaments are arranged so that limited amounts of motion are permitted. With excessive motion, however, as seen in certain types of flexion or torsional injuries, the ligaments may become stretched or partially torn. This type of injury incites a localized inflammatory response and results in a generalized reactive paraspinal muscle spasm.

The paraspinal musculature attaches to each vertebral segment and runs along the length of the spinal column. This musculature is composed primarily of slow-twitch muscle fibers that are designed for prolonged aerobic contractile activity that is well suited for maintenance of the upright posture. When irritated either by direct injury or in response to local injury to the bony or soft tissue elements of the spinal column, these muscles are prone to develop painful spastic contractions that may produce significant disability.

The vast majority of complaints of low back pain arise from disorders of the musculoligamentous complex around the lumbar spine. Pinpointing the actual underlying cause, however, is problematic, and has been the source of considerable controversy. This topic remains an area of active research because of its high cost in terms of direct medical expense as well as the loss of productivity encountered by persons affected with low back disorders.

A patient with acute, well-localized low back pain is usually in the fourth or fifth decade and otherwise healthy, presenting with a history of a relatively trivial traumatic event that may have been precipitated by a bending, lifting, or twisting activity. Often this is associated with some recreational activity that may not cause immediate pain, but over a 24-hour period discomfort may progress to stiffness and ultimately to acute pain that is unrelieved. Work-related injuries are somewhat more difficult to evaluate because of the patient's perceptions regarding the causative factors at work in relation to unreported outside events. It is necessary, however, to record carefully the date and circumstance surrounding the reported injury, to evaluate the physical and radiographic findings, and to make a determination whether the reported injury is the actual cause of the clinical syndrome under consideration. This is often a difficult task, and partially explains the reluctance of many physicians to deal with work-related injuries.

Physical examination of a patient with acute low back strain reveals a patient who is anxious and sometimes frightened. There is inability to stand completely erect because of the loss of the normal lumbar lordotic curve. The patient therefore appears to be bent forward at the waist and may have a lateral list as well. The patient is usually uncomfortable sitting or lying in the supine or prone position, and is usually most comfortable in the lateral decubitus position with the knees and hips flexed and a pillow placed between the legs. A full physical examination is therefore often difficult, if not impossible. On palpation the paraspinal musculature is in spasm and tender. Motion of the lumbar spinal segments is severely restricted by muscle spasm. Neurologic examination of the lower extremities is normal, and range of motion of the hips and knees when performed in a gentle fashion is usually found to be normal. In the acute situation the straight leg raising test used to determine the extent of nerve root irritation may be falsely positive and a followup evaluation when the patient is less symptomatic is necessary to evaluate the presence or absence of radiculopathy.

Radiographic evaluation of the lumbosacral spine in acute lumbar strain is usually normal with the exception of straightening of the normal lumbar lordosis seen on the lateral projection. The necessity of obtaining radiographs on all patients with this condition is controversial and is probably not cost-effective in identifying serious conditions that would require immediate and specific treatment.

The treatment of acute lumbar strain is reassurance, rest, and analgesia as necessary. Within 2 to 7 days the patient usually improves and is ready to return to productive activities. In some cases the patient may require additional treatment with physical therapy that may include pelvic traction, ultrasound to the paraspinal muscles, and treatment with nonsteroidal anti-inflammatory medication and muscle relaxants. In these situations it becomes necessary to evaluate more closely the patient's psychosocial status and working environment. There is considerable interplay between high emotional stress states and low back conditions.

Following recovery from low back strain the patient should be placed on a preventive exercise program that includes lower extremity and abdominal muscle strengthening using flexion techniques that do not overstretch the musculoligamentous complex of the lower back. Exercises such as straight leg raises, half sit-ups, and pelvic tilts are appropriate for patients suffering low back problems. More aggressive stretching and strengthening programs should be undertaken under the close supervision of a qualified trainer or physical therapist. Often a comprehensive approach to back problems in a back treatment and learning center is helpful for a patient who needs support and motivation from others to undertake such a preventive exercise regimen.

Chronic Low Back Pain

The patient who develops chronic, persistent, or intermittent low back pain requires a thorough medical and radiographic evaluation to rule out serious musculoskeletal disorders (spondylolisthesis, congenital spine problems, metastatic disease), and to rule out medical problems associated with pain referred to the lower back (aortic aneurysm, pelvic masses, renal stones or infection, prostate disorders, pancreatic disease, retroperitoneal infections, or neoplastic disorders). Plain radiographs, technetium bone scan, and if necessary, MRI of the abdomen and lumbar spine may be required. If significant medical or orthopedic problems have been ruled out, attention should be focused primarily on the patient's behavior in relationship to the low back condition. If the patient is overweight a plan for weight reduction should be considered. All aspects of the patient's daily activities should be investigated to identify potential offending activities or postural positions that may be targets for alteration. There are numerous philosophies and approaches to chronic low back disorders, but it is not within the scope of this discussion to review them. The patient's personality must be taken into account when selecting the most appropriate treatment regimen.

Herniated Disk

The vertebral bodies are separated by a gelatinous material (nucleus pulposus) that is encased in a dense, fibrous envelope (annulus fibrosus) that is attached to the margins of the vertebral bodies. In its normal state the intervertebral disk is well designed to provide adequate support of the posture and movement of the spinal column. The fibrous envelope, however, is not uniform in its mechanical strength and may develop bulging near the lateral recess adjacent to the nerve roots of the cauda equina as they exit the spinal canal. A rupture of the annulus fibrosus and extrusion of the nucleus pulposus is an extreme example of a disk herniation. Milder forms of disk bulging are capable of producing radicular symptoms.

A patient with lumbar disk herniation presents with pain that radiates into the buttock and down the posterior aspect of the leg, most commonly in the dermatomal distribution of S-1 or L-5. Actual low back pain is variable and may be absent. The patient may have intense paraspinal muscle spasm causing a severe list. Symptoms of numbness in the perianal region and reported dysfunction of the bowel or bladder suggest the presence of cauda equina syndrome. This represents a surgical emergency, and decompression laminectomy and disk removal should be performed as soon as possible.

The physical examination may be much the same as that seen in lumbar strain. The straight leg raising test, however, is usually positive. Eliciting contralateral symptoms by straight leg raising of the unaffected leg (crossed straight leg raising response) is strongly indicative of diskogenic pain. The neurologic examination in disk herniation is variable, and is determined by the level at which the disk herniation has occurred. In an L-5 to S-1 disk herniation the ankle jerk may be absent and sensation on the plantar surface of the foot may be reduced. Weakness of plantar flexion and eversion are also characteristics of S-1 nerve root dysfunction. In a herniation of L4-5, sensation is diminished in the first web space of the dorsum of the foot, and weakness of dorsiflexion of the foot and toes may be present.

Radiographs of the lumbar spine may be normal with a herniated disk, but may show straightening of the normal lumbar lordosis, degeneration and narrowing of the involved disk space, and possibly a nonstructural scoliosis. The diagnosis of disk herniation is confirmed by either myelography with or without CT scanning, or MRI.

The primary treatment of disk herniation is rest until the symptoms subside. Nonsteroidal anti-inflammatory medications may have a place in reducing the swelling around the disk thereby relieving the nerve root irritation. Complete bed rest is recommended for 2 to 7 days, but it has been shown that the length of time in bed has little or no relation to the ultimate outcome. More modern approaches to this problem, therefore, have been directed at earlier mobilization of the patient and his or her involvement in behavior modification and preventive exercise programs. The majority of disk herniations resolve spontaneously, leaving few residual effects.

Lumbar Spinal Stenosis

Spinal stenosis characteristically occurs in patients in their seventh and eighth decades and most commonly occurs at the L4-5 level. Multilevel disease, however, is common. The etiology of spinal stenosis is multifactoral with both bony deformity and soft tissue hypertrophy within the spinal canal contributing to symptoms. As degenerative changes develop in the lumbar spine, hypertrophic osteophytes may form and project into the lateral recess through which passes the spinal nerve root on its way out of the spinal canal. Degenerative disk disease may contribute to nerve root impingement and cause symptoms of lateral recess stenosis, not unlike radicular symptoms seen in disk herniation. Central spinal stenosis is caused primarily by a thickened ligamentum flavum that passes beneath the laminae on either side of the midline. Symptoms may be exacerbated by slippage of one vertebral segment on another because of instability in the facet joints, a condition known as degenerative spondylolisthesis. Most cases of lumbar spinal stenosis are due to a combination of central and lateral recess stenosis; hence there are a variety of symptoms and unpredictability of physical findings associated with this disorder.

Presenting complaints in spinal stenosis are variable. Low back pain is usually present, but leg symptoms are predominant. They may occur with exercise and therefore may mimic vascular claudication. This point needs to be kept in mind, since peripheral vascular disease and spinal stenosis occur primarily in the same age group. Compared with lumbar strain and herniated disk in younger patients, the patient's ability to sit, stand, and walk is not as predictable. A history of bowel or bladder problems is less specific for severe neurologic involvement because of the overlap with various forms of incontinence that occur in an elderly population. Likewise, the physical examination of a patient with spinal stenosis may be surprisingly benign, with the patient's spinal flexibility not apparently hampered and radicular signs such as straight leg raising being negative in many cases.

Plain radiographs of the lumbar spine may demonstrate severe degenerative change in the facet joints and degenerative L4-5 spondylolisthesis. The CT scan of the lumbar spine confirms the diagnosis of spinal stenosis and demonstrates the levels of involvement. Myelography may demonstrate a complete block at the involved level.

Lumbar spinal stenosis is best treated conservatively using a spinal orthosis such as a Knight spinal brace. The stability gained by using an orthosis may be enough to control the nerve root inflammation. A brace is usually poorly tolerated by obese persons or patients who are cachectic and have bony prominences around the trunk and iliac region. A custom-made polyethylene brace may be required for these situations. There is controversy on the efficacy of epidural steroid injections in controlling back pain. This technique may be tried in elderly patients who are not surgical candidates. In refractory cases surgical decompression of the involved spinal segments with or without fusion or instrumentation is indicated. This often gives dramatic relief of pain to patients and should be considered even in elderly persons.

Osteoporotic Compression Fractures

Senile osteoporosis of the axial skeleton is often accompanied by progressive thoracic kyphotic deformity and pain localized to the midportion of the back, with occasional radiation in a bandlike distribution around the rib cage. As the cancellous bone in the vertebral bodies becomes less dense, the bone is at risk for compression fracture. This phenomenon is manifest on a lateral thoracic x-ray study as a loss of anterior height of the vertebral body (wedge deformity). Wedge deformities are most commonly seen in the lower thoracic and upper lumbar spine. They may occur acutely, causing a severe pain syndrome, or gradually, causing less severe, intermittent pain. It is very difficult to distinguish new fractures from old fractures without a technetium bone scan. A bone scan also helps to evaluate the patient for possible metastatic disease. In severe cases, a compression fracture may result in retropulsion of a fragment of vertebral body into the spinal canal, causing compression of the spinal cord.

Patients with osteoporotic compression fractures should be treated symptomatically. Acute pain, at times lasting as long as 4 to 6 weeks, may be treated with bed rest followed by mobilization as soon as the patient becomes less symptomatic. Pool therapy is often helpful in regaining the patient's confidence and mobility. Prolonged periods of bed rest are contraindicated because of the risk of further bone loss during the inactive period. Spinal braces may be of benefit for upper lumbar and mid to lower thoracic compression fractures; however, these are poorly tolerated by most elderly patients.

While osteoporosis may be due to hormonal factors related to the postmenopausal state, other causes of osteopenia must be sought, including neoplasms (e.g., multiple myeloma), hormonal disorders (e.g., Cushing's syndrome or exogenous steroid therapy, hyperparathyroidism, or hyperthyroidism), nutritional factors, or medications (e.g., phenobarbitol or phenytoin [Dilantin]). A full medical workup is indicated, and therapy with calcium, vitamin D, calcitonin, or estrogen may be appropriate.

Hip

Trochanteric Bursitis

The trochanteric bursa is located adjacent to the greater trochanter of the proximal femur. It is interposed between the thick tendinous iliotibial band in the lateral thigh and the greater trochanter, a prominence that provides attachment for the abductor muscles of the hip. During the gait cycle, with hip flexion and extension the iliotibial band passes anterior and posterior to the greater trochanter. When the bursa becomes inflamed the gliding mechanism between the bone and the tendon is disrupted, leading to a painful condition in which the patient complains of a snapping sensation over the outer aspect of the proximal thigh, exacerbated by walking.

Physical examination usually reveals tenderness over the greater trochanter, and often snapping of the iliotibial band over the trachanter can be elicited with the patient in the lateral decubitus position and the hip adducted, bringing the hip from flexion into extension.

Trochanteric bursitis may be treated using nonsteroidal anti-inflammatory medication. Some restriction of activities is often necessary for relief of symptoms, particularly if the patient is engaging in vigorous activities. Refractory symptoms of trochanteric bursitis may be treated with injections of 40 mg of methylprednisolone directly into the trochanteric bursa. This treatment usually produces long-lasting relief of symptoms, but may need to be repeated several times. As a last resort surgical removal of the trochanteric bursa may be performed for pain that does not resolve with conservative treatment.

Tendinitis

The tendons of the flexors, adductors, and extensors of the hip pass through the groin region in close proximity to the hip joint itself. Consequently, inflammation in or around these tendons may simulate hip pain and need to be distinguished from symptoms of early hip arthritis. Tendinitis around the hip usually occurs in a younger patient who is involved in vigorous activities. The etiology of the tendinitis is most likely microtrauma to the tendinous insertions because of overuse. In athletes this has been referred to as a "pulled groin."

On physical examination the patient walks guarding against motion of the hip. The pelvis therefore tends to rotate around the relatively fixed hip in what is called a stiff hip gait. On palpation the groin region is usually tender, and motion that tends to stretch the affected muscle tendons is painful (abduction and flexion for the hamstrings and extension and internal rotation for the iliopsoas tendon). X-ray films of the hip are usually normal. Rarely, calcific deposits may be present around the insertion of the affected tendons into the ischium, ilium, or lesser trochanter.

Tendinitis around the hip often requires prolonged rest from those activities that are responsible for causing the condition. The length of time for healing is variable and must be individualized. Nonsteroidal anti-inflammatory medication may improve symptoms. Whirlpool therapy and other physical therapy modalities may be useful.

Synovitis

Intra-articular inflammation of the hip joint can occur as a result of an infectious or noninfectious etiology. This discussion is confined to the causes and treatment of noninfectious synovitis of the hip. Spontaneous synovitis of the hip may occur as an initial phase of any arthritic process and therefore it is initially nonspecific. Followup over time is required for definitive diagnosis. The clinical presentation of hip synovitis is not unlike that of tendinitis. The patient complains of pain in the groin exacerbated by activities. Night pain may be present, as well as morning stiffness.

On physical examination the patient walks with a stiff hip gait. Range of motion of the hip is painful, particularly in extension and internal rotation. In this position the hip capsule is tightened against the femoral neck, causing increased intra-articular pressure.

Hip x-ray studies in synovitis often yield negative results unless intra-articular calcified loose bodies are identified or chronic changes begin to occur on the femoral neck. Evidence of erosion of articular cartilage suggests that a chronic arthritis is developing.

If the x-ray evaluation is normal and the pain has persisted for more than 2 to 3 weeks, an aspiration arthrogram of the hip should be ordered. If fever, chills, or night sweats are elicited, hip arthrocentesis should be done immediately to rule out a pyogenic hip joint infection. Under fluoroscopic control fluid should be aspirated from the hip and sent for culture, cell count, and crystal examination. Radiopaque dye delineates the extent of synovial hypertrophy and capsular tightness. During the arthrogram an intra-articular injection of 1 percent lidocaine (Xylocaine) may be given and its effect on hip pain noted. This is of diagnostic value.

A noninfectious synovitis of the hip is best treated with nonsteroidal anti-inflammatory medications and rest. Intra-articular injections of methylprednisolone require radiographic assistance, but may provide effective pain relief. If symptoms of synovitis persist despite conservative treatment, arthroscopic débridement of the hip should be considered along with a synovial biopsy to establish the diagnosis. Medical evaluation is required to rule out systemic rheumatic diseases. Although monoarticular hip synovitis may be due to disorders such as rheumatoid arthritis, or seronegative spondyloarthropathies, infection (primarily with tuberculosis) must always be ruled out. Other alternatives include osteonecrosis, pigmented villonodular synovitis, or transient regional osteoporosis of the hip.

Osteoarthritis

Osteoarthritis of the hip is a common cause of pain and disability in the sixth, seventh, and eighth decades of life. This condition is associated with changes in the articular cartilage, subchondral bone, and the synovial lining of the joint. It is commonly thought to be a noninflammatory condition, but a significant number of cases have a highly inflammatory component. The etiology of osteoarthritis is unknown, but many different causes are probably involved in leading to a common end-stage pathologic state that is characterized by the following: (1) erosion of articular cartilage, particularly on the weight-bearing surface; (2) sclerosis of subchondral bone with osteophytes developing as a result of cartilage and bone remodeling at the articular margins; (3) subchondral bone cysts; and (4) synovial hypertrophy and hyperplasia.

Patients with osteoarthritis complain of groin and thigh pain that occasionally radiates to the knee and to the buttock. The patient often complains of functional disturbances in walking, stair climbing, and putting on shoes and socks.

Physical examination may reveal a patient who walks with a lurching gait in an effort to bring the center of gravity over the hip joint and to reduce the forces acting across the joint. Range of motion of the hip is usually restricted, especially in rotation and abduction. A flexion contracture of the hip may be present.

Nonsteroidal anti-inflammatory medications are often used to treat osteoarthritis, but their success is less predictable than in more consistently inflammatory conditions. Rest probably provides only transient symptomatic relief, and return to activities increases the level of pain. A cane held in the contralateral hand may be of some benefit. If conservative measures fail over a 3- to 6-month period and symptoms are progressively increasing in both intensity and frequency, total hip replacement is recommended for pain relief and restoration of function.

Rheumatoid Arthritis

Rheumatoid arthritis frequently affects the hip, with involvement often being bilateral. In contrast to osteoarthritis, joint space narrowing seen radiographically is often concentric and the subchondral bone is osteopenic and demonstrates erosive rather than sclerotic changes.

On physical examination patients often have polyarticular involvement and therefore the diagnosis of rheumatoid arthritis may already have been established. Range of hip motion is variable, and even in markedly affected hips range of motion may be painful but nearly normal.

The first line of treatment for rheumatoid arthritis is medical, and varies according to the "activity" of the arthritis. If pain and disability progress despite adequate conservative management, total hip replacement is the treatment of choice.

Osteonecrosis

Osteonecrosis occurs in the femoral head as a result of the ischemic death of a segment of the subchondal bone. Many etiologic agents have been cited, including high intake of ethanol or steroid use. Most cases, however, are idiopathic. After ischemia and death of osteocytes in a given segment of the femoral head, bone reabsorption at the margins of the necrotic area begins. The reabsorption of bone is accompanied by new bone growing in from the margins, a process called creeping substitution. In many cases, however, reabsorption outpaces substitution, and there is structural weakening of the subchondral bone. Ultimately the articular surface of the femoral head may collapse, leading to arthritic symptoms.

A commonly used staging system for osteonecrosis has four radiographic stages that often parallel clinical symptoms: Stage 1, mild or absent symptoms; radiographs are normal; bone scan or MRI is positive. Stage 2: mild pain; radiographs demonstrate relative density surrounded by irregular lucency, producing a mottling of the femoral head. Stage 3: moderate to severe pain; there is evidence of subchondral bone collapse leading to a flattening of the articular surface. Stage 4: severe arthritic symptoms with evidence of advanced arthritis on x-ray study.

The treatment of stage 1 and stage 2 osteonecrosis is controversial. Some orthopedists recommend a core decompression of the femoral head, aimed at decreasing the intraosseous pressure leading to osteonecrosis. Others favor conservative management. This involves varying degrees of protected weight bearing, the use of nonsteroidal anti-inflammatory medications, and in refractory cases, aspiration of the hip and injection of methylprednisolone. Stage 3 and stage 4 osteonecrosis are also treated conservatively, using protected weight bearing as necessary, and nonsteroidal anti-inflammatory medication. If symptoms become intolerable total hip replacement is considered, but this is usually weighed against the risk of surgical intervention in a relatively young population. Patients in their second, third, and fourth decades should be informed of the significant risk of mechanical failure during their lifetime and the need for possible revision surgery.

Stress Fracture

Stress fractures of the femoral neck are the result of multiple repetitive loads across the hip, applied within a short span of time, leading to a nondisplaced fracture. Another mechanism of stress fracture is by normal loads in bone that is significantly compromised in its mechanical strength (e.g., osteoporosis). In either case the bone has insufficient time to repair itself.

The patient usually presents with groin or thigh pain that is insidious in its onset but progressive. A limp may be present and motion is painful.

X-ray films of the hip are frequently normal and a technetium bone scan is required to confirm the diagnosis.

Stress fractures in young persons may be treated conservatively with crutch walking until symptoms subside. In an older patient with osteoporosis it is advisable to perform a pinning of the hip to avoid displacement of the fracture.

Knee

Patellofemoral Pain Syndrome (Chondromalacia)

The patella articulates with the end of the femur by tracking in a cleft between the medial and lateral femoral condyles. Because of the diversity of patellar configurations and varying depths of the femoral articulation, the patellofemoral joint is not usually a congruent articulation. This, combined with the fact that various soft tissue constraints cause a differing pattern of patellar tracking, predisposes the patellofemoral joint to overloading and underloading of certain regions. It is thought that such unphysiologic mechanical environments cause this commonly encountered knee pain syndrome.

A patient with patellofemoral pain complains of anterior knee pain that is exacerbated by activities such as going up and down stairs, sitting for long periods of time, and occasionally jogging. Sometimes the pain arises spontaneously with no known associated activity.

On physical examination in severe cases, a knee effusion may be present. Tenderness may be observed anteromedially or anterolaterally. Joint line tenderness may also be present. Patellofemoral crepitus is usually noted throughout the range of motion. Laxity of the patellar retinaculum leading to hypermobility of the patella may be an associated finding. Occasionally the tibial tubercle where the patellar tendon inserts may be unusually lateral in its location. This is a cause of abnormal patellar tracking.

Anteroposterior and lateral x-ray films of the knee are usually normal in the patellofemoral pain syndrome. A Merchant view may show a tilting or a subluxation of the patella laterally, suggesting an unequal distribution of forces across the patella.

Treatment of patellofemoral pain syndrome is conservative and indicates knee extension exercises in an arc of motion of 90° to 30°. Three or four sets of ten repetitions should be performed using weights that cause fatigue to the quadriceps muscles after the exercise, but not knee pain. It must be stressed to the patient that at least 4 to 6 weeks of this exercise regimen 3 to 5 days a week is necessary to combat the symptoms of knee pain. Arthroscopic surgery is rarely needed for this condition, and in a small number of cases arthroscopy may actually exacerbate the symptoms. If significant malalignment in the quadriceps and patellar mechanism is present, realignment of the quadriceps musculature and/or placement of the tibial tubercle in a more medial location may be indicated. In far advanced cases in which actual patellofemoral arthritis is present, elevation of the tibial tubercle may be performed to enhance the mechanical environment of the patellofemoral articulation.

Meniscal Tears

The medial and lateral menisci are crescent-shaped fibrocartilaginous structures that rim the knee joint and connect anteriorly and posteriorly to the cruciate ligaments. They act to distribute load more equitably across the knee joint and are connected to peripheral structures in a manner that renders them partially mobile and under normal circumstances able to translate according to knee flexion/extension and tibial rotation. A sudden traumatic twisting and angular force applied to the knee can exert forces on the meniscus that will cause a tear in its substance. With aging the fibrocartilaginous matrix gradually degenerates and fibrillated areas may develop that lead ultimately to a degenerative tear.

Patients with meniscal tears present with well-localized pain on the medial or lateral joint line. A knee effusion may be present in both acute trauma and in a degenerative tear. The patient may report a locking of the knee in a certain position that unlocks only after rotation of the lower leg and gradual extension of the knee.

X-ray studies of the knee may be normal or may display narrowing of the joint compartment involved by the meniscal tear. This is especially true with degenerative tears. It is important to obtain x-ray films with the patient standing for the purposes of diagnosis. Arthrography is helpful to make the diagnosis of meniscal tear. Magnetic resonance imaging has been found to be useful, but may lead to a false-positive diagnosis.

Meniscal tears are often tolerated by the patient, and in fact remain asymptomatic for many years. A symptomatic meniscal tear should be evaluated with arthroscopy, and if necessary a partial meniscectomy should be performed. In a degenerative meniscal tear arthroscopic débridement of the meniscus and inflamed synovium is helpful in providing temporary relief of symptoms. There is, however, in a degenerative tear a higher probability of recurrence of symptoms than with an acute tear in a younger person.

Synovitis

Inflammation of the joint lining of the knee results in a knee effusion and some degree of loss of function. Chronic synovial thickening and effusion are commonly seen in rheumatoid and osteoarthritis. Other conditions such as gouty arthritis or calcium pyrophosphate deposition disease are associated with an acute inflammatory reaction in the joint lining. A septic knee presents with a large painful effusion in the knee and may represent a surgical emergency. A persistent or recurring monoarticular knee synovitis should alert the physician to consider tuberculosis, and Lyme disease.

X-ray findings in synovitis may be normal except for the demonstration of an effusion on the lateral projection. Aspiration of joint fluid is helpful in establishing the diagnosis with culture, cell analysis, and crystal analysis. Aspiration is also therapeutic in that substantial pain relief may be achieved.

Synovitis is treated using nonsteroidal anti-inflammatory medication and if infection is ruled out, an injection of 40 mg of methylprednisolone may be performed. If knee x-ray studies are normal and the synovitis is acute, aspiration alone may suffice. Intra-articular steroids in general should only be used when more advanced degenerative changes are documented. Septic arthritis is usually best treated with arthroscopic débridement in conjunction with intravenous antibiotics. Arthroscopic synovectomy has proved to be of substantial benefit in refractory cases of aseptic knee synovitis.

Ligament Injury

Because of the high degree of mobility of the knee and its accommodation to a wide variety of bodily movements and functions, the ligaments of the knee are of real importance in providing extrinsic stability to the joint. In contrast to the inherent stability of the hip joint, which under normal load bearing does not require ligamentous support, the knee is a much less stable joint. Consequently, four major ligaments along with other capsular constraints are required for stable knee function. The medial and lateral collateral ligaments provide resistance against valgus and varus forces, whereas the anterior and posterior cruciate ligaments stabilize the knee against anterior and posterior translation. These four ligaments in combination provide for a smoothly functioning knee that is stable in all ranges of motion.

An isolated tear of the medial collateral ligament usually occurs when a valgus stress of mild to moderate force is applied to the knee. If the other three ligaments are preserved a good result would be expected after the ligament heals. Conservative treatment, using a splint followed by early mobilization of the knee to prevent stiffness, is recommended. More severe stress to the knee usually results in tears of the medial collateral and anterior cruciate ligaments with a possible medial meniscal tear. This is a serious injury that requires ligamentous and meniscal repair. Isolated injury to the anterior cruciate ligament, usually through a hyperextension type of mechanism, may be treated conservatively or surgically depending on several patient-specific factors, such as age, athletic history and goals, and degree of knee degeneration. A highly competitive athlete who wishes to return to this activity should be treated with anterior cruciate ligament repair and augmentation using the semitendinosus tendon. The treatment of a recreational athlete or sedentary person with an isolated anterior cruciate ligament tear is more controversial, and related to the individual surgeon's philosophy and experience. A conservative approach would use temporary immobilization followed by rehabilitation of the quadriceps and hamstrings, combined with bracing for athletic activities. If instability becomes intolerable, a late reconstruction of the anterior cruciate ligament can be performed.

Foot and Ankle

Achilles Tendinitis

The achilles tendon connects the large muscles of the calf (gastrocnemius and soleus) to the calcaneus. Contraction of these muscles results in significant forces across the ankle in producing plantar flexion. The achilles tendon is covered with tenosynovium and located in a subcutaneous position just before its insertion. With repetitive loading produced by forceful contraction of the gastrocnemius/soleus complex, the achilles tendon is subjected to stresses that may cause focal tearing and degeneration. This may result in an inflammatory condition that can be associated with significant disability. This often occurs in joggers, basketball players, and aerobic dancers.

The patient complains of activity-related pain that usually subsides with rest. A long distance runner who does not adequately stretch is predisposed to this condition. Physical examination may reveal tightness of the gastrocnemius/soleus muscles when the knee is in extension. Point tenderness and swelling are noted around the achilles tendon insertion.

The treatment of achilles tendinitis is rest, ice, elevation, and nonsteroidal anti-inflammatory medication. Total abstinence from activities that cause pain is recommended. Several weeks may be required for the pain to subside enough so that the patient may fully recover. Part of the rehabilitation program should include a stretching protocol for rendering the gastrocnemius/soleus more flexible. This should be performed with the knee in full extension, since maximal stretching can be obtained when the ankle is dorsiflexed. Local injections of steroids may lead to weakening of the tendon, and possible rupture.

In an older patient care should be taken in the treatment of achilles tendinitis. The tendon may become infiltrated with cholesterol deposits in persons with hypercholesterolemia. Vigorous activities in this case may lead to rupture of the weakened tendon. A heel lift is often useful to reduce the stress across the tendon during the period of recovery.

Heel Pain

During the gait cycle the heel receives the initial floor impact in the phase known as the heel strike. As the heel strikes the ground considerable load is transmitted through the subcutaneous tissue to the calcaneus and up through the ankle and tibial shaft. The tissue between the skin and calcaneus is made up of a complex network of fat and fibrous tissue that provides an insulation to dampen the shock waves that would otherwise be generated by heel strike. This well-designed system of shock absorption is prone to degeneration with age. The normal hydrostatic pressure required within the fatty tissue of the heel probably deteriorates, leaving the plantar fat pad less able to perform its function.

Heel pain in elderly patients causes excruciating and disabling problems. It is especially severe during the first few weight-bearing cycles in the morning when the hydrostatic pressure of the plantar fat pad is probably at its lowest. Inflammatory changes in the fascia may also contribute to the pain syndrome. Very little is known about the actual pathologic changes in the soft tissue of the plantar fat pad that lead to the painful heel. It is assumed to be a nonspecific inflammatory reaction. Heel pain with plantar fasciitis may be seen in disorders such as Reiter's syndrome, and other seronegative spondyloarthropathies.

The treatment of heel pain is improved mechanical padding with a honeycombed plastic or rubber heel cup. Alternatively, and less expensively, a thick felt heel insert may be cut out with stress relief beneath the point of maximal tenderness. It may be helpful to advise the patient to keep a well-padded pair of slippers by the bedside so that on awakening to use the bathroom he or she will not have to walk barefoot. For severe cases a local injection of methylprednisolone may give significant relief.

Metatarsalgia

Pain underneath the metatarsal heads usually arises from an overuse syndrome associated with an inadequate fat pad beneath the metatarsal heads. This problem is frequently seen in rheumatoid arthritis or other conditions leading to atrophy of the plantar fat pad. In rheumatoid arthritis the toes often become clawed, causing a hyperextension deformity of the metatarsophalangeal joints. This further uncovers and concentrates load across the distal metatarsal. A high medial longitudinal arch exacerbates this problem by causing the load bearing of the metatarsals to be concentrated primarily at the metatarsal heads.

The patient complains of well-localized pain underneath the metatarsal heads. This is often accompanied by callus formation, usually in the region of the second or third metatarsal head. Point tenderness on the plantar surface of the forefoot is often present, along with clawing of the toes and a high medial longitudinal arch. Planovalgus foot deformities can also be associated with metatarsalgia, but in this condition the first metatarsal is frequently the most painful.

The treatment of metatarsalgia is conservative, using custom-made orthotics that contain stress relief and buildup to relieve the metatarsal heads of load and transfer it proximally to the midfoot. The medial longitudinal arch should be supported in an effort to redistribute the patient's weight. In severe cases of metatarsalgia, usually associated with rheumatoid arthritis, surgery may be required to the second to fifth metatarsal heads (Hoffman procedure). This is a reliable technique that provides relief of pain for severely affected rheumatoid feet.

Interdigital Neuroma

The common digital nerves pass distally between the metatarsals and bifurcate underneath the transverse intermetatarsal ligaments to supply sensation to the opposing surfaces of two adjacent toes. With repetitive loading of the metatarsal heads the bifurcation of the nerve is subjected to multiple minor traumatic events that may lead to fibrosis of the nerve and enlargement. Enlargement of the nerve in turn makes the nerve more prominent and prone to mechanical trauma. This enlargement is referred to as a neuroma.

The patient presents with burning pain that radiates onto the dorsum of the foot and complicates shoe wearing, sometimes to the point of having to repeatedly remove the shoe to obtain comfort.

The treatment of interdigital neuroma includes padding of the forefoot using a molded orthotic or in severe cases, an injection of the neuroma with 2 to 4 mg of dexamethasone and 1% Xylocaine. If pain is relieved by injection and then reoccurs it is advisable to resect the neuroma along with its nerve branches.

Bunions

The first metatarsophalangeal joint, particularly in women, is chronically stressed by fashionable footwear. A pointed-toe shoe forces the great toe laterally and exerts marked pressure on the first metatarsal head. This may cause a reactive inflammation and enlargement of the soft tissues around the fist metatarsophalangeal joint. With chronic pressure the soft tissue thickens making comfortable footwear more difficult to find. At the same time reactive bone changes in the metatarsal head medially leads to enlargement of the metatarsal head and thickening of adjacent soft tissue. As the bunion grows and the medial capsule stretches, the great toe drifts laterally, often causing dorsal or plantar displacement of the second toe. Pain may be the result of such a process, but the existence of pain with even severe forefoot deformities is variable.

The lateral displacement of the great toe (hallux valgus) and the bunion deformity are best treated with accommodating footwear. A painful bunion or one that causes great difficulty in finding proper footwear should be treated with excision. A soft tissue realignment of the great toe (McBride procedure) may be performed as part of the same procedure. If degenerative arthritis affects the first metatarsophalangeal joint, a partial resection of the proximal phalanx of the great toe can be performed with capsular realignment and pin fixation (Keller procedure). Surgery for bunions should be reserved for only the most symptomatic patients.

Because the hallux valgus deformity often affects the second toe (claw toe deformity), surgical correction of the second toe should be performed at the same time as bunion surgery.

Corns

Hard dorsal corns usually form on the proximal interphalangeal joints of the lesser toes. These are frequently associated with claw toe deformities. This deformity is the result of a hyperextension of the metatarsophalangeal joint and flexion deformity of the proximal interphalangeal joint. The cause of the corn is chronic rubbing and pressure of the toe on the toe box of the shoe. It is actually a callus or hyperkeratosis of the skin that forms in reaction to chronic pressure. Soft corns arise between the toes in areas of maceration when two toes are pressed together with an underlying prominence in one of the toes. This is commonly seen on the medial aspect of the fifth toe, which may receive pressure from prominences on the proximal phalanx. The corn is soft rather than hard because of the chronic exposure to moisture in areas of poor ventilation.

Patients may or may not complain of painful corns and treatment should be individualized according to symptoms and not necessarily according to deformity. In a severely painful corn that has not responded to conservative management (corn pads), a surgical resection of the proximal interphalangeal joint, with correction of the flexion deformity and pinning, is indicated. A release of the dorsal capsule of the metatarsophalangeal joint and lengthening of the extensor tendon is often necessary to correct the hyperextension deformity of the matatarsophalangeal joint.

The treatment of soft corns is interposition of lamb's wool between the toes. Lamb's wool contains oils that prevent the wool from becoming macerated and matted as would a piece of cotton. Soft corns are treated by removing the offending bony prominence on the adjacent toe. For a chronic soft corn of the fifth toe it is often preferable to remove the proximal phalanx of the fifth toe (Ruiz procedure).

Bibliography

Beary, JF, Christian, CL, and Johanson, NA: Manual of Rheumatology and Outpatient Orthopedic Disorders, ed 2. Boston, Little, Brown, 1987.

D'Ambrosia, RD: Musculoskeletal Disorders: Regional Examination and Differential Diagnosis, ed 2. Philadelphia, JB Lippincott, 1986.

Greenspan, A: Orthopaedic Radiology: A Practical Approach. Philadelphia, JB Lippincott, 1988.

Hoppenfeld, S: Physical Examination of the Spine and Extremities. New York, Appleton-Century-Crofts, 1976.

Levine, DB: The Painful Low Back. New York, P W Communications, Inc., 1979.

Ramamurti, CP: Orthopaedics in Primary Care. Baltimore, Williams & Wilkins, 1979.

Sculco, TP: Orthopaedic Care of the Geriatric Patient. St. Louis, CV Mosby, 1985.

Index

Page numbers followed by t and f indicate tables and figures, respectively.

Achilles tendinitis, 235
Acrodermatitis chronica atrophicans, 85
Acromegaly
  hip arthritis with, 214–215
  osteoarthritis with, 94t, 104
Activities of daily living assessment, for rheumatoid arthritis patient, 45
Acute rheumatic fever, 1
  differential diagnosis of, laboratory studies for, 4t
Adhesive capsulitis, shoulder, 225
Adrenocorticotropic hormone, for acute gout, 143
Adult Still's disease, 32–33
Advil. See Ibuprofen
Aging, cartilage features in, 96t, 96
Alkaline phosphatase, 4t
  elevated, 39
Allergic myositis, experimental, 165
Allergic vasculitis
  diagnosis of, 119
  differential diagnosis of, 119t
Allopurinol
  dosage and administration of, 145
  for gout, indications for, 144, 145t
  prophylaxis, for gout, 144–145
  side effects of, 145
Allopurinol hypersensitivity syndrome, 145
Alveolitis, fibrosing, diagnosis of, 179–180
Ambulatory assistive devices, 217
Amethopterin. See Methotrexate
Amoxicillin, for Lyme disease, 85–86
Ampicillin, for Lyme disease, 85
Amyloidosis
  differential diagnosis of, 188
  laboratory studies for, 4t–5t
  with rheumatoid arthritis, 37f, 37

Anemia, 31
  autoimmune hemolytic, with systemic lupus erythematosus, 156
    treatment of, 159
  of chronic disease
    differential diagnosis of, laboratory studies for, 5t
    with systemic lupus erythematosus, 156
  cold hemolytic, autoantibodies with high degree of diagnostic specificity for, 9t
  hemolytic, differential diagnosis of, laboratory studies for, 5t
  iron deficiency, differential diagnosis of, laboratory studies for, 5t
  pernicious, 38
  with rheumatoid arthritis, 37f, 38
Angiitis, acute necrotizing, 190
Angiography, diagnostic, indications for, 126
Ankle
  with gout, 142f
  musculoskeletal disorders of, nonoperative treatment of, 235–237
Ankylosing spondylitis, 111
  demographic characteristics of, 2
  differential diagnosis of, 41
  hip arthritis with, 214
Ankylosis, with rheumatoid arthritis, 40
Anterior cruciate ligament
  injury to, 234–235
  transection of, osteoarthritis after, 94t
Anthranilic acids, for rheumatoid arthritis, 64t
Anti-acetylcholine receptor antibody
  diagnostic specificity of, 9t
  pathogenic effects of, 12
  and tissue injury, 10

Antibiotic therapy. *See also specific drug*
  for joint prosthesis infection, 90
Antibodies. *See also specific antibody*
  lymphocytotoxic, and tissue injury, 10
  natural, 7
  polyclonal, 7
Antibody-dependent cellular cytotoxicity, 12
Anticardiolipin antibody
  prognostic value of, 10
  in systemic lupus erythematosus, 153t
Anticentromere antibodies, 1
  diagnostic specificity of, 9t
  diagnostic value of, 14
  measurement of, indications for, 4t
  prognostic value of, 10
  with scleroderma, 177t
Anticoagulants, 2
Anti-collagen type IV antibody, with scleroderma, 177t
Anti-DNA antibody
  cross-reaction with LAMP antigen, 12
  specificity of, 8
Anti-dsDNA antibody
  diagnostic specificity, 9t
  in systemic lupus erythematosus, 153t
Anti-dsDNA antibody test, 3
  indications for, 4t
Antierythrocyte antibody, 153
  in systemic lupus erythematosus, 153t
Antihistone antibody, in systemic lupus erythematosus, 153t
Anti-Hsp73 antibody, in systemic lupus erythematosus, 153t
Anti-Hsp90 antibody, in systemic lupus erythematosus, 153t

239

Anti-I autoantibody
  diagnostic specificity of, 9t
  production of, 12
Anti-Jo-1 antibody
  with interstitial lung disease, 163
  with myositis, 165
  with polymyositis, 163
Anti-Jo-1 antibody test, indications for, 4t
Anti-La antibodies, prognostic value of, 10
Antilaminin autoantibody, with scleroderma, 177t
Antilamins autoantibody, in systemic lupus erythematosus, 153t
Anti-La/SS-B antibody
  prognostic value of, 10
  in Sjögren's syndrome patients, 193
  in systemic lupus erythematosus, 153t
Antilymphocyte antibody, 153
  in systemic lupus erythematosus, 153t
Antimalarial agents, 47
  and retinal disease, 36
  side effects of, 158
Antimicrobial therapy
  for bacterial arthritis, 81–82
  for prosthetic joint infection, 89–90
Antinuclear antibodies, in scleroderma patients, 177t
Antinuclear antibody test, 3, 14, 39
  indications for, 4t, 176–177
  positive, 154, 193
    multisystem autoimmune diseases with, 14, 14t
    with negative rheumatoid factor, 39
Anti-P antibody, 1, 153
  diagnostic specificity, 9t
  levels of, with lupus psychosis, 10f
  prognostic value of, 10, 10f
  in systemic lupus erythematosus, 153t
Antiphospholipid antibody syndrome, differential diagnosis of, 179
Antiphospholipid antibody, 1
Antiphospholipid antibody test, indications for, 4t
Antiplatelet antibody, in systemic lupus erythematosus, 153t
Anti-PM-Scl antibody
  in polymyositis-scleroderma overlap syndrome, 164

  with scleroderma, 177t
Antirheumatic drugs, slow-acting. See Disease modifying antirheumatic drugs
Anti-RNP antibody, 1
  with scleroderma, 177t
  in systemic lupus erythematosus, 153t
Anti-Ro/La autoantibody, diagnostic specificity of, 9t
Anti-Ro/SS-A antibody, 153
  prognostic value of, 10
  in Sjögren's syndrome patients, 193
  in systemic lupus erythematosus, 153t
Anti-Ro/SS-A antibody test, indications for, 4t
Anti-Scl-70 antibody. See Anti-topo I antibody
Anti-Sm autoantibody
  diagnostic specificity of, 9t
  diagnostic value of, 9
  in systemic lupus erythematosus, 153t
Anti-Sm autoantibody test, 6
  indications for, 4t
Anti-ssDNA antibody, in systemic lupus erythematosus, 153t
Antistreptolysin-O test, indications for, 4t
Anti-topo antibody
  diagnostic value of, 14
  in systemic lupus erythematosus, 153t
Anti-topo I antibody
  diagnostic specificity, 9t
  with scleroderma, 177t
Anti-topo I antibody test, indications for, 4t
Anti-tRNA synthetase antibody, 1
  diagnostic specificity, 9t
Anti-U1 RNP antibody
  diagnostic specificity, 9t
  in systemic lupus erythematosus, 153t
Anti-U3 RNP antibody, with scleroderma, 177t
Aorta, giant cell arteritis of, 130, 130f
Arteparon, for osteoarthritis, 107
Arterial aneurysms, laboratory studies with, 3
Arterial insufficiency, 2
Arteriography, 3
  indications for, 5t
Arteritis
  giant cell, 127–131
    diagnosis of, 122t

  hepatitis B, 1
  Takayasu's, 127–128
Arthritis. See also Rheumatoid arthritis
  acute or persistent, parvovirus B19-induced, 28
  adjuvant, due to mycobacterial infection, 29–30
  bacterial. See Septic arthritis
  chronic
    differential diagnosis of, laboratory studies for, 5t
    induced by bacterial cell wall components, 29
  collagen type II, 30
  definition of, 155t
  due to rubella virus infection, 28
  fungal, clinical presentation of, 80
  gonococcal, 41, 80–82
  gouty, differential diagnosis of, 41
  hemophilus, 81, 81t
  hepatitis B, 1
  hydroxyapatite, acute, 148
  infectious, differential diagnosis of, 41–42
  laboratory studies for, 5t
  inflammatory
    hip, 213–215
    osteoarthritis after, 94t
    total hip replacement in patients with, 213–222
    with inflammatory bowel disease, 111
  juvenile. See also Juvenile rheumatoid arthritis
    systemic pattern, symptoms of, 2
  Lyme, 83–84, 86
  mycobacterial, clinical presentation of, 80
  mycoplasma, and arthritis in rodents, 26
  pathogenesis of, in rodents, 26
  polyarticular, chronic, with gout, 140
  post-diarrheal, 114
  psoriatic, 111
    differential diagnosis of, 33, 40–41
  reactive, 111–117
  traumatic, differential diagnosis of, 33
  viral, clinical presentation of, 80
Arthritis Foundation, The, 52
Arthrocentesis, with joint replacement infection, 89
Arthrocentesis fluid culture, sensitivity, 89, 89t
Arthrocentesis fluid gram stain, sensitivity, 89, 89t

Index

Arthrography, 3
  indications for, 5t
Arthropathy
  colitic, differential diagnosis of, 33, 41
  enteropathic, diagnosis of, 5t
  hepatitis, differential diagnosis of, laboratory studies for, 4t
  hepatitis B
    demographic characteristics, 2
    diagnosis of, 3
  hydroxyapatite, chronic, 148
  neuropathic, 1, 105–106
    complications of, 80
    osteoarthritis due to, 94t
  ochronotic, 104
  psoriatic, 2
Arthroplasty, total hip, 213, 215–221
  cemented
    alternatives to, 220–221
    long-term results of, 220
  complications of
    intraoperative, 218
    postoperative, 218–220
    trochanteric, 219
  contraindications to, 215
  general considerations for, 220
  hospital course for, 217–218
  indications for, 215–216
  long-term results of, 220–221
  medical considerations for, 216
  metal toxicity with, 220
  in patients with inflammatory arthritis, 213–222
  rehabilitation for, 217–218
    long-term protocol, 218
  reimplantation after infection, 219
  surgical considerations for, 216–217
Arthroscopic synovectomy, 52
Arthroscopy, 3
Articular cartilage
  age-related changes in, 94
  calcification of, with chondrocalcinosis, 146, 147f
Articular lesions, in rheumatoid joint, 20–21
Ascripton. See Aspirin, buffered
Aspirin
  buffered
    characteristics of, 59t
    preparation of, 59t
  enteric coated
    characteristics of, 59t
    preparation of, 59t
  plain
    characteristics of, 59t
    preparation of, 59t
  preparation of, 59t

time-release zero-order
  characteristics of, 59t
  preparation of, 59t
Assistive devices, ambulatory, 217
Asthma, NSAID-induced, 62
Atherosclerosis, with systemic sclerosis, 181
Auranofin, 65
Aurothioglucose, 65
Autoantibody, 7–8. See also specific antibody
  antigen-nonspecific actions of, 153
  biologic effects of, 7
  cell surface binding of, 12
  in clinical practice, 13–14
  definition of, 7
  diagnostic value of, 9
    with high degree of diagnostic specificity, 9t
  organ-specific, 13
  pathogenic roles for, 12
  production of, possible mechanisms of, 12–13
  prognostic value of, 9–10
  significance of, 8–9
  specificity of, 7–8
  in systemic lupus erythematosus, 153t, 153
  and tissue injury, 10–12
Autoantigens, 7
Autoimmune disease, 8
  idiopathic, etiology of, 13
  multisystem, 14
  organ-specific, 13
Autoimmune hemolytic anemia, with systemic lupus erythematosus, 156
  treatment of, 159
Autoimmunity
  mycobacterial and related antigens in, 30
  origins of, clues to, 12–13
Azathioprine, 19, 47, 49, 74–75, 205–206
  adverse reactions to, 75
  chemistry of, 74
  clinical efficacy of, 74
  contraindications to, 75, 205t
  cost of, 75
  for dermatomyositis and polymyositis, 169
  dosage, 75, 205t
  drug action of, 74
  drug interactions, 205t
  mechanism of action, 74
  metabolism of, 74
  oral, dosage and administration of, 159
  pharmacology of, 205t, 205

randomized trials of, 205t, 205
side effects of, surveillance for, 75
supply, 75
toxicity, 205t, 206
Azulfidine. See Sulfasalazine
Azulfidine EN-tabs. See Sulfasalazine

Bacteremia, differential diagnosis of, 124
Bacterial arthritis. See Septic arthritis
Bacterial cell wall components, 29
Bacterial culture, indications for, 5t
Bacterial disease, with myositis, 166
Bacterial endocarditis, differential diagnosis of, laboratory studies for, 5t
Bacterial synovitis, differential diagnosis of, laboratory studies for, 4t
Baker's cysts. See Popliteal cysts
Barium studies, indications for, 5t
Bartter's syndrome, association of CPPD deposition with, etiopathogenesis of, 137
Basic calcium phosphate crystals, formation of, 135, 138
  clinical factors affecting, 136t
Basic calcium phosphate–related joint inflammation, 148
  treatment of, 148
B cell(s)
  activation of
    stage I, 187
    stage II, 187
  activity of, 154
  function of, altered, in Sjögren's syndrome, 187
  hyperreactivity of, in Sjögren's syndrome, 186–187
  in synovial effusions, 22
B-cell lymphoma, and Sjögren's syndrome, 187
BCP crystals. See Basic calcium phosphate crystals
Bell's palsy, treatment of, 85
Benzothiazine series, 64t
Big toe, with gout, 142f
Biliary cirrhosis, primary, autoantibodies with high degree of diagnostic specificity for, 9t
Biologic fluids culture, indications for, 5t
Biopsy
  frozen, sensitivity, 89, 89t
  indications for, 5t, 126
  liver, with methotrexate, 78
  of minor salivary gland, 188

Biopsy *(continued)*
  renal, indications for, 5t, 156
  skin, indications for, 5t, 124
Bone marrow study, indications for, 5t
Bone marrow suppression, with allopurinol, 145
Bone scans, 3, 40, 89
  indications for, 5t
Borrelia burgdorferi infection. *See* Lyme disease
Bouchard's nodes, 99
Bronchiolitis, obliterative, with rheumatoid arthritis, 35
Bronchoalveolar lavage, sensitivity of, 180
Bufferin. *See* Aspirin, buffered
Bullous pemphigoid, autoantibodies with high degree of diagnostic specificity for, 9t
Bunions, management of, 236
Burkitt's lymphoma, etiology of, 29
Bursa, ruptured, diagnosis of, laboratory studies for, 5t
Bursitis, 2
  olecranon, 225–226
  shoulder, 3
  trochanteric, 231
Butazolidin. *See* Phenylbutazone

Calcific tendinitis, 225
Calcinosis
  with myositis, 163–164
  treatment of, 169
Calcium hydroxyapatite crystals, joint disorder induced by, differential diagnosis of, 41
Calcium oxalate monohydrate crystals, in inflamed joints, 139
Calcium pyrophosphate deposition disease. *See also* Pseudogout
  diagnostic criteria for, 146t, 146
  differential diagnosis of, 41
  hip arthritis with, 214
Calcium pyrophosphate dihydrate crystals
  formation of, 135–137
    clinical factors affecting, 136t
  in synovial fluids, 3
Capillary vasculitis
  course of, 122t
  diagnosis of, 122t
  differential diagnosis of, 119t
  underlying disease, 122t
Capsulitis, adhesive, shoulder, 225
Carcinoma
  metastatic, rheumatic manifestations of, laboratory studies of, 5t
  and myositis, 167
  nasopharyngeal, etiology of, 29
Cardiac disease, with rheumatoid arthritis, 36
  management of, 51
Carpal tunnel syndrome
  clinical presentation of, 226–227
  electrophysiologic findings in, 227
  physical examination with, 227
  radiographic findings in, 227
  with rheumatoid arthritis, 33
  treatment of, 227
Carpometacarpal joints, first, osteoarthritis of, 98–99
  radiographic features of, 99, 99f
Cartilage
  with aging, 96t, 96
  with osteoarthritis, 96t, 96
Cartilage matrix, formation and breakdown *in vitro*, factors influencing, 96, 98t
Cataracts, drug-induced, with rheumatoid arthritis, 36
Cefazolin, for joint prosthesis infection, 90
Ceftriaxone, for Lyme disease, 85–86
Cellular cytotoxicity, antibody-dependent, 12
Central nervous system, granulomatous vasculitis of, 131
Central nervous system lupus, management of, 160
Cerebrospinal fluid examination, indications for, 157
Cervical muscle spasm, 223
Cervical radiculopathy, 2, 223–224
Cervical spine disease
  atlantoaxial, 40
  with rheumatoid arthritis, treatment of, 51
  subaxial, 40
Charcot's joint, 105–106
Chemical profile, indications for, 4t
Chemotherapy
  combination, in treatment of joint and connective tissue disorders, 207
  for rheumatoid arthritis, 42
Chest percussion and postural drainage, differential diagnosis of, laboratory studies for, 5t
Chest radiograph
  indications for, 5t
  with methotrexate, 78
Childhood dermatomyositis, 161t. *See also* Dermatomyositis
  calcinosis with, 163
  genetics of, 166–167
  vasculopathy with, 164
Chlorambucil
  for dermatomyositis and polymyositis, 169
  efficacy of, 204
  pharmacology of, 204
  toxicity of, 204
Chloramphenicol, for Lyme disease, 85
Cholesterol crystals, in inflamed joints, 139
Choline magnesium salicylate
  characteristics of, 60t
  preparation of, 60t
Choline salicylate
  characteristics of, 59t
  preparation of, 59t
Chondrocalcinosis, 2, 41
  laboratory findings in, 3
Chondromalacia. *See* Patellofemoral pain syndrome
Chronology, 2
Cirrhosis, primary biliary, autoantibodies with high degree of diagnostic specificity for, 9t
Cisapride, 181
Claw toe deformity, 236
Clinoril. *See* Sulindac
Coagulation profile, indications for, 5t
Colchicine
  dosage and administration of, 144
  intravenous
    dosage and administration of, 143
    for pseudogout, 147
  oral
    for acute gout, 143
    prophylaxis, for pseudogout, 148
  prophylaxis, for gout, 143–144
Cold hemoglobinuria, paroxysmal, 8
Cold hemolytic anemia, autoantibodies with high degree of diagnostic specificity for, 9t
Colitis, ulcerative
  differential diagnosis of, laboratory studies for, 5t
  hip arthritis with, 214
Collagenase
  action of, 96
  in synovial fluid, 22
Collagen type II arthritis, 30
Colony stimulating factor, in synovial fluid, 22, 22t
Complete blood count, indications for, 4t

Index **243**

Computerized transaxial tomography, indications for, 40
Conjunctival staining, 188
Connective tissue-activating peptides, action of, 96
Connective tissue disease, mixed, hip arthritis with, 214
Connective tissue disorders
  pathogenesis of, mycobacterial and related antigens in, 30
  treatment of
    combination chemotherapy for, 209
    immunosuppressive therapy for, 201–211
Connective tissue syndromes
  causes of, 1
  mixed or undifferentiated, diagnosis of, laboratory studies for, 4t
  symptoms of, 2
Constipation, with systemic sclerosis, 181
Constipation/diarrhea cycle, with systemic sclerosis, 181
Coombs test
  indications for, 5t
  positive, with systemic lupus erythematosus, 156
Cornea, rose bengal staining of, 188
Corneal endothelium and epithelium, microscopic study of, 188
Corns, 236–237
Coronary vasculitis, with rheumatoid arthritis, 36
Corticosteroids, 2, 19, 49–50
  and cataracts, 36
  complications of, 168–169
  contraindications to, 49
  for dermatomyositis and polymyositis, 168–169
  for Felty's syndrome, 51
  for giant cell arteritis, 130–131
  indications for, 49
  injections, local, complications of, 50
  local, indications for, 50
  postinjection rest, 50
  side effects of, 49
  sparing agents for, DMARDs as, 48
  systemic, 50
  for systemic lupus erythematosus patient, 159
Coxarthrosis, 100
Coxsackie virus B infection, and polymyositis and dermatomyositis, 166

CPPD crystals. See Calcium pyrophosphate dihydrate crystals
Cranial arteritis. See Giant cell arteritis
Cranial vasculitis, 123
  isolated, 131
  diagnosis of, 122t
C-reactive protein, 38
Creatinine clearance test, indications for, 5t
CREST syndrome, 10
  autoantibodies with high degree of diagnostic specificity for, 9t
  clinical manifestations of, 177
  differential diagnosis of, laboratory studies for, 4t
Crohn's disease
  differential diagnosis of, laboratory studies for, 5t
  hip arthritis with, 214
Cryoglobulinemia, differential diagnosis of, laboratory studies for, 4t
Cryoglobulins test, indications for, 4t
Crystal(s). See also specific type
  arthritis caused by
    differential diagnosis of, 83
    osteoarthritis after, 94t
  disease caused by, differential diagnosis of, 33
  formation of, 135–138
    clinical factors affecting, 136t
  inflammation caused by, 138–139
  inflammatory joint disease caused by, 135–149
  pathophysiology of, 135–139
  joint disorders caused by, differential diagnosis of, 41
  release of, modes of, 138t, 138
Crystal arthropathies, 1
Crystal shedding. See Crystal(s), release of
Crystal traffic, 138
Cultures
  arthrocentesis fluid, sensitivity, 89, 89t
  indications for, 4t–5t
  operative, sensitivity, 89, 89t
Cuprimine. See D-Penicillamine
Cutaneous sinus drainage, with prosthetic joint infection, 87, 87t
Cyclophosphamide, 49, 202–204
  contraindications to, 203t
  for dermatomyositis and polymyositis, 169
  dosage and administration of, 202, 203t

  drug interactions, 203t
  efficacy of, 202–203
  long-term low-dose, 202
  oral, dosage and administration of, 159
  pharmacology of, 202, 203t
  for polyarteritis nodosa, 126
  randomized trials of, 203t, 203
  toxicity, 203t, 203–204
Cyclosporin A
  contraindications to, 208t
  dosage and administration of, 208t
  drug interactions, 208t
  pharmacology of, 208t
  randomized trials of, 208t, 208
  for Sjögren's syndrome patients, 194
  toxicity, 208t, 208–209
Cyclosporine, 49, 208–209
  for dermatomyositis and polymyositis, 169
  gout and, 146
  for lupus, 160
  mechanism of action, 208
  toxicity, 209
Cytokines
  inhibitors, for rheumatoid arthritis, 53
  for rheumatoid arthritis, 52–53
  in rheumatoid arthritis synovial fluid, 22t
  in synovial fluid, 22, 22t
Cytopenias, bases for, laboratory studies of, 5t
Cytotoxic agents
  for lupus nephritis, 159
  side effects of, 159

Deca-durabolin, for Sjögren's syndrome patients, 194
Deep vein thrombosis, after total hip arthroplasty, 218
Degenerative disk/joint disease
  complications of, 80
  treatment of, 224
Dementia, in Sjögren's syndrome, 190
Dendritic cells, in synovial effusions, 22
De-Pen. See D-Penicillamine
DeQuervain's stenosing tenosynovitis, 227
Dermatitis-arthritis syndromes, 80
Dermatomyositis, 161t, 161–173
  association with malignant disease, 167
  cardiac manifestations of, 163, 163t
  diagnosis of, 161
  laboratory findings in, 164

Dermatomyositis *(continued)*
  manifestations of, 2, 161–164
  muscle pathology with, 162
  pathogenesis of, 164–167
  prognosis for, 169–170
  pulmonary manifestations of, 163, 163t
  rash of, 162–163
    treatment of, 169
  treatment of, 168–169
    pharmacologic, 168–169
    physical measures for, 168
  vascular involvement, 164
Dermatomyositis vasculitis, 125
Desmoglein, diagnostic specificity, 9t
Diarrhea
  arthritis after, 114
  with systemic sclerosis, 181
Diet
  and arthritis, 52
  for rheumatoid arthritis patient, 52
Diffuse cutaneous systemic sclerosis
  cardiac involvement, 181–182
  clinical manifestations of, 176–177
  diagnostic test for, 177
  differential diagnosis of, 177, 180
  pattern of illness with, 177
  renal failure with, management of, 182
Diffuse fasciitis, 1
Diffuse idiopathic skeletal hyperostosis
  classification of, 94t, 98, 101
  differential diagnosis of, criteria for, 101
  laboratory findings in, 101
  manifestations of, 101
  osteophytes and syndesmophytes in, contrasting features of, 101, 101t
  radiographic findings in, 101, 101t, 102f
Diflunisal
  characteristics of, 60t
  preparation of, 60t
Dihydrate crystals, in inflamed joints, 139
Disease modifying antirheumatic drugs, 43, 47–49
  choice of, 48–49
  decision to use, 48
  indications for, 48
  NSAIDs in combination with, 46
  onset of action, 48
Disseminated tuberculosis, rheumatic manifestations of, laboratory studies of, 5t
Distal interphalangeal joint, osteoarthritis of, 98

Diuretics, 2
DNA
  double-stranded, antibody against. *See* Anti-dsDNA antibody
  single-stranded, antibody against. *See* Anti-ssDNA antibody
Dolobid. *See* Diflunisal
Double-crush syndrome, 224
Doxycycline, for Lyme disease, 85–86
DQ A gene, 24
DQ B gene, 24
DR A gene, 24
DR6 allele, association with rheumatoid arthritis, 24
DR beta 1 chains, sequenced from DR4 subtypes, first domain of, differences in amino acid composition in, 24t
DR B1 gene, 24
DR B3,4 gene, 24
DR1 haplotype, 24
DR4 haplotype, association with rheumatoid arthritis, 24
Drugs. *See also* Disease modifying antirheumatic drugs; Nonsteroidal antiinflammatory drugs; *specific drug*
  concomitant or antecedent use of, 2
  remittive, 19
Dry gland syndrome, 189
Dry mouth. *See* Xerostomia
Dw4 allele
  association with rheumatoid arthritis, 24
  first domain of, amino acid composition in, 24t
Dw14 allele
  association with rheumatoid arthritis, 24
  first domain of, amino acid composition in, 24t
Dw15 allele
  association with rheumatoid arthritis, 24
  first domain of, amino acid composition in, 24t
Dw16 allele, association with rheumatoid arthritis, 24
Dw10 allele, first domain of, amino acid composition in, 24t
Dw13 allele, first domain of, amino acid composition in, 24t
Dysentery, Reiter's syndrome after, 115
Dysphagia, 162
  in Sjögren's syndrome, 189

Easprin. *See* Salicylates, time-release enteric-coated

Ecotrin. *See* Aspirin, enteric coated
Eicosanoids, in synovial fluid, 22
Elbow, musculoskeletal disorders of, nonoperative treatment of, 225–226
Elderly
  achilles tendinitis in, 235
  heel pain in, 235
  NSAIDs for, 47
Electromyography, indications for, 5t
ELISA. *See* Enzyme-linked immunosorbent assay
Encephalopathy, in Sjögren's syndrome, 190
Endarteritis obliterans, in Sjögren's syndrome, 190
Endocarditis
  bacterial, differential diagnosis of, laboratory studies for, 5t
  infectious, leukocytoclastic vasculitis with, 123
  prophylaxis for, with joint prosthesis infection, 90
  verrucous, 151, 157
Enzyme-linked immunosorbent assay, 7
  false-positive, 85
  for Lyme disease, 85
Eosinophilia–myalgia syndrome, secondary to ingestion of contaminated tryptophan, 168
Eosinophilic fasciitis, myositis with, 168
Eosinophilic syndromes, myositis with, 168
Epicondylitis, 226
Episclerotis, with rheumatoid arthritis, 36
Epitope, 8f
Epstein–Barr virus, 29
  and muscle inflammation, 166
  in pathogenesis of rheumatoid arthritis, 29
Epstein–Barr virus infection, differential diagnosis of, laboratory studies for, 4t
Erythema infectiosum, 28
Erythrocyte sedimentation rate, 3
  elevated, 31, 38, 193
  indications for, 4t
Erythromycin, for Lyme disease, 85
Esophageal scintigraphy, quantitative, indications for, 180
Esophageal transit time, normal, 180
Esophagoscopy, indications for, 180
Esophagus
  dysmotility of
    diagnosis of, 5t

in Sjögren's syndrome, 189
systemic sclerosis, management of, 181
Ethylenediaminetetraacetic acid lead-mobilization test, indications for, 145
Exercise program, for rheumatoid arthritis patient, 45

Facet joints, osteoarthritis of, 101
Family education, about rheumatoid arthritis, 44–45
Fasciitis
  diffuse, 1
  eosinophilic, myositis with, 168
Fatigue, 31
Feldene. See Piroxicam
Felty's syndrome, 36–37
  diagnosis of, 37
  leukopenia with, 38
  thrombocytopenia with, 38
  treatment of, 50–51
Femur
  neck, stress fracture of, 233
  prosthetic head dislocation, after total hip arthroplasty, 219
  slipped epiphysis, osteoarthritis after, 94t
Fenoprofen
  characteristics of, 64t
  preparation of, 64t
Fever
  with prosthetic joint infection, 87, 87t
  rheumatic, pathogenesis of, 26
  with rheumatoid arthritis, 34
  with rigor, 2
  with systemic lupus erythematosus, 154
Fibrosis, pulmonary, with rheumatoid arthritis, 37f, 45
Fingers
  foreshortening of, with rheumatoid arthritis, 36f
  trigger, 227
Fish oil supplements, for rheumatoid arthritis patient, 52
Fluorescent treponemal antibody test, indications for, 4t
Folic acid antagonists, 206–208
Foot, musculoskeletal disorders of, nonoperative treatment of, 235–237
Fracture(s)
  osteoarthritis after, 94t
  osteoporotic compression, 230
  stress, of femoral neck, 233
Frozen biopsy, sensitivity, 89, 89t

Fungal arthritis, clinical presentation of, 80
Fungal culture, indications for, 5t

Gamma globulin, intravenous infusions of, for inflammatory myopathy, 169
Gamma-glutamyl transpeptidase, elevated, 39
Gammopathy, polyclonal, with rheumatoid arthritis, 38–39
Gangrene
  digital, management of, 179
  with systemic lupus erythematosus, 157
Gastrointestinal studies, indications for, 5t
Giant cell arteritis, 127–131
  angiography with, 130, 130f
  of aorta and great vessels, 130, 130f
  diagnosis of, 122t
  differential diagnosis of, 130
  laboratory studies for, 5t
  treatment of, 130–131
Glomerular basement membrane
  diagnostic specificity, 9t
  linear staining of, indications for, 13
Glomerulonephritis
  differential diagnosis of, laboratory studies for, 5t
  with wire loop lesions, 151
Glucocorticoids
  low-dose oral, for systemic lupus erythematosus patients, 158
  pulse dosing, 158
Glycocalyx, 87
Glycopeptide, 130kD and 85kD, diagnostic specificity, 9t
Glycoprotein, anti-myelin-associated, 12
Gold, 51
  cardiopulmonary reactions to, 68–69
  contraindications to, 69
  gastrointestinal reactions to, 68
  hematologic reactions to, 68
  injectable, mucocutaneous reactions to, 67–68
  intramuscular, 49
  mucocutaneous reactions to, 67–68
  musculoskeletal reactions to, 69
  ophthalmic reactions to, 69
  oral preparations, 43, 48–49
    adverse reactions to, 67
    chemistry of, 65
    clinical efficacy, 66

  cost of, 67
  distribution of, 65
  dosage, 67
  gastrointestinal reactions to, 68
  mechanism of action, 66
  pharmacokinetics of, 65
  side effects of, surveillance for, 69
  supply, 67
  parenteral preparations, 43, 48
    adverse reactions to, 67
    chemistry of, 65
    clinical efficacy, 66
    cost of, 67
    distribution of, 65
    dosage, 67
    gastrointestinal reactions to, 68
    mechanism of action, 66
    pharmacokinetics of, 65
    side effects of, surveillance for, 69
    supply, 66
  patient education about, 66
  reactions to, 69
  renal reactions to, 68
  retreatment with, 69
Gold salts, 47
  clinical-pharmacologic correlates, 66
  for rheumatoid arthritis, 65–69
  selection of compouond, 66
Gold sodium thiomalate, 65
Gonococcal arthritis
  clinical presentation of, 80
  differential diagnosis of, 41
  population at risk for, 81
  treatment of, 82
Gonococcal sepsis, symptoms of, 2
Gonococcemia, chronic, leukocytoclastic vasculitis with, 123
Goodpasture's syndrome, autoantibodies with high degree of diagnostic specificity, 9t
Gout, 2, 139–146
  acute, treatment of, 140–143
  chronic, 145
  clinical manifestations of, 139–140
  clinical pattern of, 2
  complications of, 80, 140
  and cyclosporine, 146
  demographic characteristics of, 2
  diagnosis of, 139–140
    laboratory studies for, 3, 4t
  diagnostic criteria for, 139, 140t
  differential diagnosis of, 83
  and drug use, 2
  factors that cause or worsen, 140

Gout (continued)
  hip arthritis with, 214
  idiopathic, 140
  joint involvement, 140, 142f
  osteoarthritis with, 105
  prophylaxis for, 143–145
  tophaceous, osteoarthritis with, 94t
  treatment of, 140–145
Gouty arthritis, differential diagnosis of, 41
Graft-vs-host-disease, chronic, differential diagnosis of, 188
Gram-negative bacillary joint sepsis, 81
  in prosthetic joint, 86–87, 87t
Gram-negative bacillary pyarthroses, population at risk for, 81
Gram-negative bacilli, septic arthritis caused by, therapeutic outcome, 82
Gram stain, indications for, 4t
Granulocyte–monocyte colony stimulating factor, in synovial fluid, 22, 22t
Granulocytopenia, with systemic lupus erythematosus, 156
Granulomatous vasculitis, of central nervous system, 131
Grave's disease, autoantibodies with high degree of diagnostic specificity for, 9t
Great vessels, giant cell arteritis of, 130, 130f
Groin, pulled, 229
Group B streptococci, joint sepsis caused by, 81

Hallux valgus, management of, 236
Hand, musculoskeletal disorders of, nonoperative treatment of, 226–227
Haptoglobin test, indications for, 5t
Hashimoto's thyroiditis, 8
  autoantibodies with high degree of diagnostic specificity for, 9t
Heat shock proteins, 30
Heat therapy
  for osteoarthritis, 106
  for rheumatoid arthritis patient, 45
Heberden's nodes, 99
  painful, 3
Heel pain, 235
Hemagglutination, 7
Hemarthrosis, 105
  and drugs, 2
Hematologic disorder, definition of, 155t

Hematologic studies, indications for, 5t
Hemidesmosome 230kD, diagnostic specificity, 9t
Hemochromatosis
  hip arthritis with, 214–215
  osteoarthritis with, 94t, 104
  pseudogout with, 146
Hemoglobinuria, paroxysmal cold, 8
Hemophilia, osteoarthritis with, 94t, 105
Hemophilus arthritis, 81, 81t
Hemophilus influenzae pyarthrosis, clinical presentations of, 80
Henoch-Schoenlein purpura
  childhood, 123
  distribution of lesions, 122
  leukocytoclastic vasculitis with, 123
Hepatitis, rheumatoid factors in, 26
Hepatitis arthropathy, differential diagnosis of, laboratory studies for, 4t
Hepatitis B antigen test, indications for, 4t
Hepatitis B arthritis/arteritis, 1
Hepatitis B arthropathy
  demographic characteristics, 2
  diagnosis of, 3
Hepatitis B infection
  differential diagnosis of, 42
  muscle inflammation with, 166
  synovitis with, 2
  vasculitis with, 123, 125
Herniated disk, lumbar, 229
Herpes virus infection, muscle inflammation with, 166
Hip
  dysplasia of, osteoarthritis after, 94t
  inflammatory arthritis of, 213–215
  total arthroplasty in treatment of, 213–222
  musculoskeletal disorders of, nonoperative treatment of, 231–233
  osteoarthritis of, 98–101, 232
  pain in, 101
  osteonecrosis of, 232–233
  rheumatoid arthritis of, 232
    clinical and radiographic features of, 215
    soft tissue contractures in, 216
    surgical treatment of, 215
  surgical reconstruction of, indications for, 213
  synovitis of, 231–232
  tendinitis in, 231
  total arthroplasty, 213, 215–221

  total replacement prosthesis, infected, radiographic evaluation of, 88, 88f
Hip joint disease, 2
Hip joint sepsis, diagnosis of, 80
Histopathologic disease, differential diagnosis of, laboratory studies for, 5t
HLA-B27, and sacroiliitis, 115
HLA-B$_8$ antigen, in Sjögren's syndrome patients, 193
HLA-B27-associated diseases, 111
HLA-B27 typing, 3
  indications for, 4t
HLA-DR2, association with systemic lupus erythematosus, 152
HLA-DR3, association with systemic lupus erythematosus, 152
HLA-DR$_3$ antigen, in Sjögren's syndrome patients, 193
HLA-DR5 histocompatibility complex, Lyme arthritis and, 84
HLA-DRw4, association with rheumatoid arthritis, 24
HLA-D$_{W52}$ antigen, in Sjögren's syndrome patients, 193
HLA typing, indications for, 66
Hospitalization, indications for, 45
Human immunodeficiency virus infection
  autoimmune-like disease with, 28
  demographic characteristics of, 2
  differential diagnosis of, 188
  pyomyositis with, 166
  rheumatic complications of, 1
Human T-cell leukemia virus-1 infection, 28
Humoral immunity, and antibodies to muscle components, 165
Hydralazine, 2
Hydroxyapatite, inflammation caused by, inhibitors of, 139
Hydroxyapatite arthritis, acute, 148
Hydroxyapatite arthropathy, chronic, 148
Hydroxyapatite crystals, joint inflammation caused by, 148
Hydroxyapatite deposition disease, of first metatarsophalangeal joint, 139
Hydroxyapatite osteoconductive prostheses, 220–221
Hydroxychloroquine, 48–49
  for Sjögren's syndrome patients, 194

Hydroxychloroquine sulfate, for rheumatoid arthritis, 43
Hyperglobulinemia, with rheumatoid arthritis, 38–39
Hyperlipidemia, rheumatic complications of, diagnosis of, laboratory studies for, 5t
Hypermyoglobinemia, with inflammatory muscle disease, 164
Hyperparathyroidism
 normocalcemic, with calcium pyrophosphate dihydrate, 136
 pseudogout with, 146
Hyperuricemia, 3, 4t
 asymptomatic
  definition of, 145
  treatment of, 145–146
 complications of, 140
 differential diagnosis of, laboratory studies for, 4t–5t
 with gout, 140
Hypocomplementemia, 3
Hypothyroid arthralgia syndrome, diagnosis of, laboratory studies for, 5t

Ibuprofen, 47
 characteristics of, 64t
 preparation of, 64t
Imipenem, for Lyme disease, 85
Immune complexes, with rheumatoid arthritis, 26–27
Immune complex glomerulonephritis, in Sjögren's syndrome, 190
Immune response
 antigen-derived, characteristics of, 13
 secondary, characteristics of, 13
Immunoconglutinis, pathogenic effects of, 12
Immunodeficiency states, differential diagnosis of, laboratory studies for, 4t
Immunoelectrophoresis, indications for, 4t
Immunofluorescense, indications for, 13
Immunogens, 7
Immunoglobulin G antibodies, 7
Immunoglobulin G immunoglobulin, 8f
Immunoglobulin G–immunoglobulin M cryoglobulinemia, leukocytoclastic vasculitis with, 123
Immunoglobulin M antibodies, 7
Immunoglobulin molecule, human, structure of, 27f

Immunoglobulin quantification, indications for, 4t
Immunoglobulin supergene family, with rheumatoid arthritis, 26–27
Immunologic disorder, definition of, 155t
Immunologic studies, 3–6
 indications for, 4t
Immunoregulatory disease, history of, 192
Immunosuppressives, 202–208
 indications for, 201–202
 in treatment of joint and connective tissue disorders, 201–211
Immunotherapy, for rheumatoid arthritis, 52–53
Impingement syndrome
 clinical presentations of, 224
 physical findings of, 224
 radiographic findings of, 224
 shoulder, 224–225
 treatment of, 224–225
Imuran. See Azathioprine
Inclusion body myositis, 161, 161t, 167
Indium-labeled leukocyte scans, 89
Indocin. See Indomethacin
Indoleacetic acid series, 63t–64t
Indomethacin
 characteristics of, 63t
 dosage and administration of, 141, 147
 preparation of, 63t
Infection(s), 2. See also specific agent
 after total hip arthroplasty, 218–219
 joint, radiographic signs of, 81
 prosthetic joint, 86–90
 treatment of, 219
Infectious agents, that cause muscle inflammation, 166
Infectious arthritis, differential diagnosis of, 41–42
 laboratory studies for, 5t
Infectious endocarditis, leukocytoclastic vasculitis with, 123
Inflammation
 crystal-induced, 138–139
 hydroxyapatite-induced, inhibitors of, 139
Inflammatory arthritis
 hip, 213–215
 osteoarthritis after, 94t
 total hip replacement in patients with, 213–222

Inflammatory bowel disease, arthritis with, 111
Inflammatory joint disease, crystal-induced, 135–149
Inflammatory muscle disease
 muscle pathology with, 162
 relationship to malignancy, 167
Inflammatory muscle disorders
 classification of, 161t
 connective tissue disorders associated with, 161
Inflammatory response
 in rheumatoid arthritis, 23, 23f
 therapy for, 42
 to vasculitis, 120
Inflammatory vascular disease
 mononuclear, 190
 neutrophilic, 190
Interdigital neuroma, 236
Interferon-gamma, for rheumatoid arthritis, 53
Interleukin-1
 action of, 96
 in synovial fluid, 22, 22t
Interleukin-6, in synovial fluid, 22, 22t
Interleukin-8, in synovial fluid, 22, 22t
Interleukin-1 receptor antagonist, 53
Interstitial lung disease
 diagnosis of, 179–180
 and pulmonary hypertension, 179
 in Sjögren's syndrome, 189
 treatment of, 194
Iron deficiency anemia, differential diagnosis of, laboratory studies for, 5t

Jaffe's rule, 72
Jarisch-Herxheimer reaction, 86
 treatment of, 86
Joint. See also specific joint
Joint(s)
 function of, alteration in, treatment of, 42
 fusion of, treatment of, 42
 infection of, radiographic signs of, 81
 inflammation of, basic calcium phosphate–related, 148
 radiograph of, indications for, 5t
 rheumatoid, pathology of, 20–22
 swollen, with rheumatoid arthritis, 31, 33f
Joint deformity, treatment of, 42
Joint disease
 neuropathic, 105–106
 in rheumatoid arthritis
  acute onset of, 31
  insidious onset of, 31
  intermediate onset of, 31

Joint disorders
  crystal-induced, differential
    diagnosis of, 41
  treatment of
    combination chemotherapy for,
      209
    immunosuppressive therapy in,
      201-211
Joint milk, with MSU crystals, 139
Joint prosthesis infection. See
    Prosthetic joint infection
Joint replacement infection. See
    Prosthetic joint infection
Joint space narrowing, with
    rheumatoid arthritis, 40
Joint stiffness, 31
  with osteoarthritis, 97
  treatment of, 42
Juvenile arthritis, systemic pattern,
    symptoms of, 2
Juvenile rheumatoid arthritis
  differential diagnosis of, 83
  hip, 214
    clinical and radiographic
      features of, 215
  immunity in, 24
  total hip arthroplasty in patients
    with, surgical considerations
    for, 216
  treatment of, considerations for, 214
Juxta-articular erosions, with
    rheumatoid arthritis, 40
Juxta-articular osteoporosis, with
    rheumatoid arthritis, 40

Kashin-Beck disease, 103-104
  classification of, 94t
Kawasaki disease, 1, 124
Kayser-Fleischer ring, 104
Keratoconjunctivitis
  diagnosis of, 188
  with rheumatoid arthritis,
    37f
  study of, 188
Keratoconjunctivitis sicca
  differential diagnosis of, 188
  with rheumatoid arthritis, 36
  in Sjögren's syndrome, 188
Ketoprofen
  characteristics of, 64t
  preparation of, 64t
Kidney stones
  with gout, 140
  with hyperuricemia, 140
Knee
  calcification of menisci and
    articular cartilage in, with
    chondrocalcinosis, 146, 147f

musculoskeletal disorders of,
    nonoperative treatment of,
    233-235
  osteoarthritis of, 98-100, 100f
  popliteal cysts of, diagnosis of, 40
  pseudogout of, 146
  synovitis of, 234
Knee ligament(s), injury to, 234-235

Laboratory studies, 3-6
LAMP antigen, anti-DNA antibody
    cross-reaction with, 12
Large airway obstructive disease, in
    Sjögren's syndrome, 189
Large vessel vasculitis, 126-131
  course of, 122t
  diagnosis of, 122t
  underlying disease, 122t
Latex agglutination test, 6, 39
Leg length discrepancy, after total
    hip arthroplasty, 220
Lentiviruses, 27-28
Leprosy, leukocytoclastic vasculitis
    with, 123
Leukemia, rheumatic manifestations
    of, laboratory studies of, 5t
Leukocytoclastic vasculitis, 121f,
    121-124
  with associated collagen disease,
    123
  complications of, 123
  diagnosis of, 122t
  differential diagnosis of, 119t,
    123-124
  with infection, 123
  lesions, 122, 124
    distribution of, 122
  midpregnancy, 123
  organ systems affected by, 122
  pathology of, 124
  secondary
    to allergic exposure, 123
    to malignancy, 123
  treatment of, 124
  without associated collagen
    disease, 122-123
Leukocytosis, with rheumatoid
    arthritis, 38
Leukopenia
  with Felty's syndrome, 38
  with rheumatoid arthritis, 38
  with systemic lupus
    erythematosus, 156
  treatment of, 159
Libman-Sacks endocarditis, 157
Limited cutaneous systemic
    sclerosis, 177
Lip biopsy, indications for, 5t
Lipid studies, indications for, 5t

Lipoproteinemia, differential
    diagnosis of, 188
Liquid lipid crystals, 139
Liver biopsy, with methotrexate, 78
Liver enzymes, salicylate therapy
    and, 3
Liver function tests, with
    methotrexate, 77-78
Löfgren's syndrome, diagnosis of, 3
  laboratory studies for, 5t
Long-acting thyroid stimulator
    (LATS) antibodies
  diagnostic specificity of, 9t
  and tissue injury, 10
Low back pain
  chronic, management of, 229
  physical examination of patient
    with, 228
  radiographic evaluation of, 228
  rehabilitation after, 228-229
  structures responsible for, 101
  treatment of, 228
Lumbar disk herniation, 229
Lumbar spine
  muscular and ligamentous strain
    of, 227-229
  musculoskeletal disorders of,
    nonoperative treatment of,
    227-230
  radiculopathy of, 2
  stenosis of, 229-230
Lupus
  acute cutaneous, 155
  drug-induced, 2, 151
    antinuclear antibodies assay of,
      14t
Lupus anticoagulant, 156
Lupus erythematosus. See also
    Systemic lupus erythematosus
  chronic cutaneous, treatment of, 158
  subacute cutaneous
    characteristics of, 155
    treatment of, 158
Lupus nephritis, 156
  treatment of, 159
Lupus pneumonitis, acute, 157
Lupus vasculitis, 125
  differential diagnosis of, 119t
Luschka joints, osteoarthritis of, 101
Lyme agent test, indications for, 4t
Lyme arthritis, 83
  and HLA-DR5 histocompatibility
    complex, 84
  treatment of, 86
Lyme disease, 1, 82-86
  associated with chronic neurologic
    dysfunction, 84-85
  cardiac involvement, 84
  treatment of, 85

clinical presentation of, 2, 80, 83–85, 84f
dermatologic manifestation of, chronic, 85
diagnosis of, 85
differential diagnosis of, 42, 83
early disseminated (stage 2), 83–84
early localized (stage 1), 83, 84f
geographic incidence of, 83
late persistent (stage 3), 84–85
neurologic symptoms of, 84
pathogenesis of, 83
prevention of, 86
similarity with syphilis, 86
treatment of, 85–86
Lymphadenopathy, reactive, with rheumatoid arthritis, 37f
Lymph node biopsy, indications for, 5t
Lymphoma
 B-cell, and Sjögren's syndrome, 187
 Burkitt's, etiology of, 29
 differential diagnosis of, laboratory studies for, 4t–5t
 leukocytoclastic vasculitis due to, differential diagnosis of, 119t
 non-Hodgkin's, and Sjögren's syndrome, 187
 rheumatic manifestations of, laboratory studies of, 5t
 in Sjögren's syndrome, 192
 treatment of, 195
Lymphophoresis, for rheumatoid arthritis, 19
Lymphoproliferative diseases, differential diagnosis of, laboratory studies for, 4t

Magnetic resonance imaging, 6
 indications for, 5t, 40
Major histocompatibility complex
 class II genes, 24, 25f
 class I molecule, 23–24
 class II molecule, 23–24
  in rheumatoid arthritis, 24
 in rheumatoid arthritis, 23–26
Malar rash, definition of, 155t
Male infertility, with sulfasalazine, 71
Mast cell growth factor, in synovial fluid, 22, 22t
McBride procedure, indications for, 236
Mechanical aberrations, osteoarthritis due to, 94t
Mechanical derangement, 2
 differential diagnosis of, 33
 laboratory studies of, 3

Mechanical disorders, diagnosis of, laboratory studies for, 5t
Meclofenamate sodium
 characteristics of, 64t
 preparation of, 64t
Meclomen. See Meclofenamate sodium
Medial collateral ligament, injury to, 234–235
Medical history
 general advice for, 1–2
 items of interest, 2
Medications, 45–50. See also Antibiotic therapy; Antimicrobial therapy; specific drug
 patient education about, 45
 uric acid–lowering, and acute gout, 143
Medium vessel vasculitis, 124–126
 course of, 122t
 diagnosis of, 122t
 underlying disease, 122t
Membranoproliferative nephritis, clinically silent, 156
Meningitis, aseptic, in Sjögren's syndrome, 190
Meningococcemia, chronic, leukocytoclastic vasculitis with, 123
Meniscal tears, 232
Meniscectomy, osteoarthritis after, 94t
Menisci, calcification of, with chondrocalcinosis, 146, 147f
6-Mercaptopurine, for dermatomyositis and polymyositis, 169
Metabolic bone disease, differential diagnosis of, laboratory studies for, 4t
Metabolic disease, osteoarthritis due to, 94t
Metacarpophalangeal joints
 osteoarthritis of, 99
 progressive changes in, with rheumatoid arthritis, 31, 34f
 subluxation of, 31, 33f, 36f
 swelling of, 31, 32f
Metal toxicity, with total hip arthroplasty, 220
Metatarsalgia, 236
Metatarsophalangeal joints, first
 arthritis of, 139
 osteoarthritis of, 98
Methotrexate, 19, 43, 47–49, 76–78, 206–208
 adverse reactions to, 77, 207
 clinical efficacy of, 76

contraindications to, 78, 207t
cost of, 77
for dermatomyositis and polymyositis, 169
dosage and administration of, 207t
drug interactions, 76, 207t
low-dose, 206
mechanism of action, 76, 206
metabolism and absorption of, 76
onset of action, 48
pharmacology of, 206, 207t
randomized trials with, 206–207, 207t
for Reiter's syndrome, 114–115
side effects of, surveillance for, 77–78
supply, 77
toxicity, 207t, 208
therapy for, 77
Methylprednisolone
 pulse dosing of, for lupus nephritis, 160
 for systemic lupus erythematosus patient, 158
Methylprednisolone acetate, for pseudogout, 147
Metoclopramide, 181
Microbiologic studies, indications for, 5t
Microcrystalline corticosteroid esters, intra-articular or intralesional injection of, 49
Milwaukee shoulder, 41, 148
Mitochondrial M2 protein complex, diagnostic specificity, 9t
Mode of onset, 2
Monoclonal antibody
 polyspecificity of, 7
 production of, 12
 specificity of, 7
Monocytes/macrophages
 role of, 154
 in synovial effusions, 22
Mononeuritis multiplex
 in Sjögren's syndrome, 190
 with vasculitis, 121
Mononuclear cells
 autosensitized, as instigator of inflammation, 165
 from patients with polymyositis and dermatomyositis, 165
Mononucleosis
 infectious, etiology of, 29
 synovitis with, 2
Monosodium urate crystals
 formation of, 135, 137–138
 clinical factors affecting, 136t
 inflammation caused by, 138
Mono test, indications for, 4t

Morning stiffness, 31, 97. *See also* Joint stiffness
Morphea, 175
Motor neuropathies, with rheumatoid arthritis, 36
Motrin. *See* Ibuprofen
Mseleni disease, 104
 classification of, 94t
MSU crystals. *See* Monosodium urate crystals
Mucocutaneous lymph node syndrome, 124
Muscle(s)
 atrophy of, with rheumatoid arthritis, 31, 33f
 biopsy of, indications for, 5t
 cervical spasm of, 223
 components of, antibodies to, 165
 wasting of, with rheumatoid arthritis, 37f
 weakness of, 155
  functional assessment of, 162, 162f
  quantification of, 161
Myasthenia gravis
 autoantibodies with high degree of diagnostic specificity for, 9t
 immune response to acetylcholine receptors with, 13
Mycobacterial arthritis, clinical presentation of, 80
Mycobacterial infection, atypical, leukocytoclastic vasculitis with, 123
Mycoplasma arthritidis, and arthritis in rodents, 26
Myelitis, transverse, in Sjögren's syndrome, 190
Myelopathy
 with rheumatoid arthritis, 36
 transverse, in Sjögren's syndrome, 190
Myocarditis, with rheumatoid arthritis, 36
Myochrysine. *See* Gold sodium thiomalate
Myoglobin levels, during myositis, 164
Myopathy
 with AIDS, 166
 antimalarial-induced, 155
 corticosteroid-induced, 155
 diagnosis of, laboratory studies for, 5t
 and drugs, 2
 granulomatous, 168
 low-grade, in Sjögren's syndrome, 191
Myositis
 allergic, experimental, 165
 antibody specificities with, 165
 antinuclear and anticellular reactions to, 164–165
 antinuclear antibodies assay of, 14t
 autoantibodies with high degree of diagnostic specificity for, 9t
 bacterial disease with, 166
 cardiac findings in, 163, 163t
 with connective tissue disorder, 161t
 diagnosis of, laboratory studies for, 4t–5t
 with eosinophilic fasciitis, 168
 immune mechanisms of patients with, 164–165
 laboratory findings in, 3
 with Lyme disease, 166
 with neoplasm, 161t
 pathogenesis of, 164
 risk of malignancy with, 167
 in Sjögren's syndrome, 191
 viruses associated with, 166

Nalfon. *See* Fenoprofen
Nandrolone decanoate, for Sjögren's syndrome patients, 194
Naprosyn
 characteristics of, 64t
 dosage and administration of, 141, 147
 preparation of, 64t
Naproxen. *See* Naprosyn
Nasopharyngeal carcinoma, etiology of, 29
Neck
 acute muscle spasm of, 223
 musculoskeletal disorders of, nonoperative treatment of, 223–224
Necrosis
 avascular, osteoarthritis after, 94t
 vascular, with vasculitis, 119–120
Neisseria gonorrhoeae
 pyarthrosis caused by, therapeutic outcome, 82
 septic arthritis due to, 81, 81t
Nephritis
 interstitial, in Sjögren's syndrome, 189–190
 lupus, 156
  treatment of, 159
Nerve biopsy, indications for, 5t
Nerve conduction studies, indications for, 5t
Neurologic disorder, definition of, 155t
Neuroma, interdigital, 236

Neuron(s), antibodies against, in systemic lupus erythematosus, 153t
Neuropathic joint disease, 105–106
Neuropathic syndromes, diagnosis of, laboratory studies for, 5t
Neuropathy
 with rheumatoid arthritis, treatment of, 51
 sensory, with rheumatoid arthritis, 36
Neutropenia, with rheumatoid arthritis, differential diagnosis of, 37
Neutrophil myeloperoxidase, diagnostic specificity, 9t
Nitrogen mustard alkylating agents, 202–204
Non-Hodgkin's lymphoma, and Sjögren's syndrome, 187
Nonsteroidal antiinflammatory drugs, 19, 43, 46–47, 60–63
 for acute gout, 141
 adverse effects of, 61
 allergic reactions and asthma with, 62
 auditory reactions to, 63
 cardiovascular reactions to, 62
 choice of, 46
 in combination with DMARDs, 46
 cost of, 47
 dosage, 46, 61
 for elderly patients, 47
 gastric effects of, 61
 gastrointestinal toxicity, 47
 hematologic and anticoagulant effects of, 61
 hepatic effects of, 61–62
 indications for, 60
 mucotaneous reactions to, 62
 neuropsychiatric reactions to, 62
 nonsalicylate, 63t–64t
 ocular reactions to, 62
 for osteoarthritis, 106
 patient compliance with, 46
 pharmacokinetics of, 60
 pregnancy and teratogenic reactions to, 63
 for pseudogout, 147
 for Reiter's syndrome/reactive arthritis, 114
 renal reactions to, 62
 response time, 46
 side effects of, 158
 for systemic lupus erythematosus patient, 158–159
 unresponsiveness to, 46
Nucleolar 4-6S RNA antibody, with scleroderma, 177t

Nucleoside triphosphate pyrophosphohydrolase, 137
5'-Nucleotidase, elevated, 39
Nuprin. *See* Ibuprofen

Obesity, and osteoarthritis, 95–96
Obstipation, with systemic sclerosis, 181
Ochronosis
  hip arthritis with, 214
  osteoarthritis with, 94t, 104
Ocular disease, with rheumatoid arthritis, 36
Olecranon bursitis, 225–226
Oligoarthritis, HLA-B27-positive, 114
Operative culture, sensitivity, 89, 89t
Oral ulcers, definition of, 155t
Orthopedics, nonoperative, 223–237
Orudis. *See* Ketoprofen
Ossification, heterotopic
  after total hip arthroplasty, 219–220
  diagnosis of, 219
Osteoarthritis. *See also specific joint involved*
  and age, 94–95
  biochemical monitoring with, 107
  cartilage features in, 96t, 96
  classification of, 94t
  clinical manifestations of, 2, 93, 97–98, 232
  differential diagnosis of, 41
  endemic, 103–104
    classification of, 94t, 98
  erosive inflammatory, 102
    classification of, 94t, 98
  generalized, 98–101
    classification of, 94t, 98
  and heredity, 94–95
  inflammatory component, crystal-associated, 97
  influence of sex hormones on, 95
  joints involved, 98
  localized, 98–101
    classification of, 94t, 98
  local metabolic and environmental factors, 93–94
  and mechanical force, 93–94
  metabolic disorders associated with, 104–105
  and obesity, 95–96
  occupation-related, classification of, 94t
  pain mechanisms in, 97–98
  pathogenesis of, 93, 95f
    current concepts, 93–97
    role of chondrocyte, inflammation, and immunologic and biochemical factors in, 96–97
  theories for, 93
  patient education about, 106
  physical examination with, 232
  primary (idiopathic)
    classification of, 94t, 98
    joints involved, 98
    racial and ethnic differences in, 94–95
    radiographic findings in, 93
  secondary
    classification of, 94t
    to metabolic derangement, 98
  of spine, 99, 101
  treatment of, 232
    general considerations, 106
    medical therapy for, 106–107
  types of, 98–106
Osteoarthropathy, pulmonary, differential diagnosis of, laboratory studies for, 5t
Osteoid osteoma, diagnosis of, laboratory studies for, 5t
Osteomyelitis, 86
  diagnosis of, laboratory studies for, 5t
  laboratory findings in, 3
Osteonecrosis, 232–233
  avascular
    diagnosis of, laboratory studies for, 5t
    and drugs, 2
    laboratory findings in, 3
    with systemic lupus erythematosus, 155–156
Osteoporosis
  and drugs, 2
  juxta-articular, with rheumatoid arthritis, 40
  management of, 230
  senile, of axial skeleton, 230
  with systemic lupus erythematosus, 155–156
Osteoporotic compression fractures, 230
Overuse syndromes, treatment of, 223
Oxacillin
  for joint prosthesis infection, 90
  for Lyme disease, 85
Oxypurinol, 145

Pain. *See also* Low back pain
  heel, 235
  hip, with osteoarthritis, 101
  with osteoarthritis, mechanism of, 97–98
  patellofemoral pain syndrome, 233
  with prosthetic joint infection, 87, 87t
  with synovitis, 2

Palindromic rheumatism, 31–32
Panniculitis, differential diagnosis of, laboratory studies for, 5t
Parotid gland enlargement, in Sjögren's syndrome. *See* Xerostomia
Paroxysmal cold hemoglobinuria, 8
Parvovirus(es), 28
Parvovirus B19 infection, 28
  differential diagnosis of, 42
Parvovirus RA-1, 28
Patellofemoral joint space narrowing, with pseudogout, 146
Patellofemoral pain syndrome, 233
Pathologic studies, 6
  indications for, 5t
Patient education
  about joint protection, 45
  about medications, 45
  about osteoarthritis, 106
  about Reiter's syndrome, 115
  about rheumatoid arthritis, 44–45
Pemphigus foliaceus, autoantibodies with high degree of diagnostic specificity for, 9t
Pemphigus vulgaris
  autoantibodies with high degree of diagnostic specificity for, 9t
  immunity in, 24
Penicillamine, 51
  side effects of, 69
D-Penicillamine, 49, 72–74
  adverse reactions to, 73
  autoimmune reactions to, 73
  chemistry and biochemical properties of, 72
  clinical efficacy of, 72
  contraindications to, 74
  cost of, 72
  dosage, 72–73
  gastrointestinal reactions to, 73
  hematologic reactions to, 73
  mechanism of action, 72
  mucocutaneous reactions to, 73
  pulmonary reactions to, 73
  renal reactions to, 73
  side effects of, surveillance for, 73–74
  supply, 72
Penicillin, 2
  for Lyme disease, 85–86
Pentosan polysulfate, for osteoarthritis, 107
Peptic ulcer disease, with rheumatoid arthritis, 38
Periarthritis, acute calcific, 148
Periarticular swelling, with prosthetic joint infection, 87, 87t

Pericardial effusions
  with rheumatoid arthritis, 37f
  with systemic sclerosis, 181
Pericarditis, with rheumatoid arthritis, 36
Peripheral nerve entrapment syndromes, in Sjögren's syndrome, 190
Peripheral neuropathy
  with rheumatoid arthritis, 37f
  severe, with vasculitis, 121
Pharyngeal dysmotility, diagnosis of, 5t
Phenylbutazone
  characteristics of, 64t
  preparation of, 64t
Phlebothrombosis, with systemic lupus erythematosus, 157
Photosensitivity, definition of, 155t
Physical examination, 2
Physical medicine, for rheumatoid arthritis, 45
Physical therapy, for osteoarthritis, 106
Picornavirus infection, muscle inflammation with, 166
Pigmented villonodular synovitis, hip arthritis with, 214–215
Piroxicam
  characteristics of, 64t
  preparation of, 64t
Plaquenil. See Hydroxychloroquine sulfate
Plasma cell dyscrasias, rheumatic manifestations of, laboratory studies of, 5t
Plasmapheresis
  for dermatomyositis and polymyositis, 169
  for lupus, 160
  for rheumatoid arthritis, 19
Platelet disorders, with rheumatoid arthritis, 38
Pleural disease, differential diagnosis of, laboratory studies for, 5t
Pleural effusions, with rheumatoid arthritis, 35, 37f
Pleuritis, with systemic lupus erythematosus, 157
Pneumococcus pneumoniae infection, arthritis caused by, therapeutic outcome, 82
Pneumoconiosis, rheumatoid, with rheumatoid arthritis, 35
Pneumonitis
  acute lupus, 157
  interstitial
    differential diagnosis of, laboratory studies for, 5t
    with rheumatoid arthritis, 35
Polarized light microscopy, indications for, 4t
Polyarteritis, differential diagnosis of, 3
Polyarteritis nodosa, 124–126, 125f
  arteriography with, 126, 127f–128f
  with associated collagen disease, 125–126
  Churg-Strauss type, 124
  diagnosis of, 119, 122t, 125–126
  differential diagnosis of, 119t, 126, 179
  pathology of, 126
  treatment of, 126
  variants of, 124
  without associated collagen disease, 124–125
Polyarthritis
  acute, induced by bacterial cell wall components, 29
  symmetric, with involvement of small joints of hand and feet, 31
  viral, differential diagnosis of, 42
Polyarticular arthritis, chronic, with gout, 140
Polychondritis, diagnosis of, 122t
Polyclonal gammopathy, with rheumatoid arthritis, 38–39
Polymethylmethacrylate cement, and infection, 87
Polymyalgia rheumatica, diagnosis of, 32
Polymyositis, 161t, 161–173
  association with malignant disease, 167
  autoantibodies in patient with, 12
  autoantibodies with high degree of diagnostic specificity for, 9t
  cardiac manifestations of, 163, 163t
  clinical manifestations of, 161–164
  course of, 162f
  diagnosis of, 161
  differential diagnosis of, laboratory studies for, 4t
  genetics of, 166–167
  humoral factors, 164–165
  inflammatory cell infiltrate in muscle of patients with, 165
  laboratory findings in, 164
  muscle pathology with, 162
  pathogenesis of, 164–167
  prognosis for, 169–170
  pulmonary manifestations of, 163, 163t
  treatment of
    pharmacologic, 168–169
    physical measures for, 168
  vascular involvement, 164
Polymyositis-scleroderma overlap syndrome, 164
Polyneuropathy, sensory, in Sjögren's syndrome, 190
Polypharmacy, contraindications to, 47
Popliteal cysts, of knee joints, diagnosis of, 40
Postjejunoileal bypass syndrome, 113–114
Prednisone
  dosage and administration of, 50
  oral, for lupus nephritis, 160
Probenecid
  dosage and administration of, 144
  prophylaxis, for gout, 144
Procainamide, 2
Progressive systemic sclerosis
  antibody specificity with, 165
  differential diagnosis of, laboratory studies for, 5t
  inflammatory muscle disease with, 161
  myositis with, 161t
  with Sjögren's syndrome, 191–192
Proprionic acids, for rheumatoid arthritis, 64t
Prostaglandin E$_2$, action of, 96
Prostheses
  femoral head, dislocation of, after total hip arthroplasty, 219
  hydroxyapatite osteoconductive, 220–221
  microstructured or porous-ingrowth, 220–221
  press-fit, 220
  total hip replacement, infected, radiographic evaluation of, 88, 88f
Prosthetic joint infection
  bacteriology of, 86–87, 87t
  clinical manifestations of, 87
  diagnosis of, 87–89
    examinations to establish, 89, 89t
  pathogenesis of, 86–87
  prevention of, 90
  radiographic evaluation of, 88, 88f
  suppressive antibiotic therapy for, 90
    indications for, 90
  symptoms of, 87, 87t
  treatment of, 89–90
Prosthetic joint sepsis. See Prosthetic joint infection
Proteinuria, gold-induced, 66

Index

Proteoglycan monomers, 96, 97f
Protrusio deformity, 215
Proximal interphalangeal joint(s)
　osteoarthritis of, 98
　swelling of, in early rheumatoid arthritis, 31, 32f
Pseudogout, 2, 146–148. *See also* Calcium pyrophosphate deposition disease
　clinical manifestations of, 146–147
　complications of, 80
　diagnosis of, 146–147
　diagnostic criteria for, 146t, 146
　differential diagnosis of, 41, 83
　laboratory studies for, 4t
　of first metatarsophalangeal joint, 139
　hip arthritis with, 214
　joint distribution of, 146
　prophylaxis for, 147–148
　treatment of, 147
Pseudolymphoma, treatment of, 195
Pseudo-obstruction syndrome, management of, 181
Pseudosepsis, with rheumatoid arthritis, 34
Psoriasis, hip arthritis with, 214
Psoriatic arthritis, 111
　differential diagnosis of, 33, 40–41
Psoriatic arthropathy, 2
Psychiatric dysfunction, with systemic lupus erythematosus, 156–157
Pulled groin, 231
Pulmonary disease
　with myositis, 163
　with rheumatoid arthritis, management of, 51
Pulmonary embolism, after total hip arthroplasty, 218
Pulmonary fibrosis, with rheumatoid arthritis, 37f, 45
Pulmonary hypertension
　and interstitial lung disease, 179
　with rheumatoid arthritis, 35
Pulmonary infection, recurrent, in Sjögren's syndrome, 189
Pulmonary lesions, with rheumatoid arthritis, 35
Pulmonary nodules, with rheumatoid arthritis, 35, 37f
Pulmonary osteoarthropathy, differential diagnosis of, laboratory studies for, 5t
Pulmonary scleroderma, 179
Pulmonary vasculitis, with polymyositis, 163
Purine analogs, 204–206
　mechanism of action, 204–205

Purpura, palpable, diagnosis of, 124
Pyarthrosis
　clinical presentations of, 80
　gram-negative bacillary, population at risk for, 81
　Hemophilus influenzae, clinical presentations of, 80
　laboratory findings in, 3
　Neisseria gonorrhoeae, therapeutic outcome, 82
Pyomyositis, 166
Pyrazoles, 64t
Pyrophosphate, inorganic
　disordered metabolism of, in CPPD-containing cartilage, 136–137
　high concentrations of, 137

Quinacrine, side effects of, 158

Radiation
　total lymphoid, for lupus, 160
　total nodal, for rheumatoid arthritis, 19
Radiation synovectomy, 52
Radiculopathy
　cervical, 2, 223–224
　lumbar, 2
Radiographic studies, 6
　indications for, 5t
　with methotrexate, 78
Radioimmunoassay, 7
Radioisotopic scans, with technetium diphosphonate, 89
Radionuclide bone scan, 3
　indications for, 5t
Rash
　of dermatomyositis, 162–163
　treatment of, 169
　discoid, 155
　definition of, 155t
　treatment of, 158
　malar, definition of, 155t
Rat-bite fever, 80
Raynaud's phenomenon
　capillary-negative, differential diagnosis of, 176
　capillary-positive HEp-2 ANA-positive patient, 176
　clinical manifestations of, 175–176
　diagnostic test for, 176
　with systemic lupus erythematosus, 157
Reactive arthritis
　antecedent infections, 113
　clinical manifestations of, 111–112
　differential diagnosis of, 33, 114
　HLA-B27-positive precondition, 113

　laboratory findings in, 112
　organisms that cause, 112–113
　pathogenesis of, current concepts, 112–114
　prognosis for, 115
　synovitis in, 113–114
　treatment of, 114–115
Rectal biopsy, indications for, 5t
Reflex sympathetic dystrophy
　radiographic changes with, 225
　shoulder, 225
　treatment of, 225
Reiter's disease, hip arthritis with, 214
Reiter's syndrome, 111–117
　Chlamydia-related, 113
　clinical manifestations of, 111–112
　clinical pattern of, 2
　demographic characteristics of, 2
　diagnosis of, criteria for, 111
　differential diagnosis of, 33, 41, 83, 114
　extra-articular features of, 112
　of first metatarsophalangeal joint, 139
　HLA-B27-positive precondition, 113
　incomplete, 111
　laboratory findings in, 112
　natural history of, 115
　organisms that cause, 112–113
　pathogenesis of, current concepts, 112–114
　patient education about, 115
　postdysenteric, 115
　postvenereal, 115
　prognosis for, 115
　treatment of, 114–115
Remittive drugs, 19
Renal biopsy, indications for, 5t, 156
Renal disease
　diagnosis of, laboratory studies for, 5t
　in Sjögren's syndrome, 189–190
　treatment of, 194
Renal disorder, definition of, 155t
Renal impairment, with systemic sclerosis, 182
Renal tubular acidosis, in Sjögren's syndrome, 190
Reticulocytes test, indications for, 5t
Retinal disease, drug-induced, with rheumatoid arthritis, 36
Rheumatic disease, malignant, treatment of, 51
Rheumatic disorders
　demographic characteristics of, 2
　diagnosis of, clinical formulation of, 3

Rheumatic disorders *(continued)*
  differential diagnosis of, elements of, 1–6
  functional alterations with, 2
  scope of, 1
  symptoms of, aggravation or amelioration of, 2
Rheumatic syndromes, nonarticular, 2
Rheumatism, palindromic, 31–32
Rheumatoid arthritis, 19–58
  acute, clinical picture of, 2
  animal models of, 29–30
  characteristic patient, 31
  clinical presentation of, 2, 19, 31, 215
    early symptoms, 31
    unusual, 31–33
  combination chemotherapy for, 209
  constitutional features of, treatment of, 51
  demographic characteristics of, 2
  diagnosis of, laboratory studies for, 3, 4t
  diagnostic and clinical aspects of, 31–33
  differential diagnosis of, 33, 40–42
  early events in, 21, 21f
  epidemiology of, 20
  extraarticular manifestations of, 34–37
    treatment of, 51
  of first metatarsophalangeal joint, 139
  hematologic and serologic abnormalities with, 38–40
  hepatobiliary disorders with, 39
  of hip, 213–214, 232
  histopathologic changes characteristic of, 21, 21f
  humoral and cellular immunity in, 23–27
  impact of, 20
  incidence of, 20
  infectious agents of, 27–29
  infectious etiology of, 19
  inflammatory muscle disease with, 161
  inflammatory response to, 23, 23f
  joint disease in, onset of, 31
  joint involvement, 31
  laboratory manifestations of, 38–42
  leukocytoclastic vasculitis with, 123
  malignant. *See* Rheumatoid vasculitis
  management of, goals of, 44
  microbial products and, 29–30
  monoarticular onset of, 33
  with multiple joint involvement, total hip arthroplasty in patients with, surgical considerations, 216–217
  myositis with, 161t
  nutritional factors, 35
  osteoarthritis after, 94t
  pathogenesis of, 19–31
    model for, 26
  patient and family education about, 44–45
  physical examination with, 230
  polymyalgia rheumatica-type presentation of, 32
  premature death with, 20
  prevalence of, 20
  prodromal features of, 31
  prognostic factors, 20
  radiographic findings in, 40, 215
  with Sjögren's syndrome, 191
  socioeconomic factors related to, 20
  treatment of, 19, 232
    approaches to, 42–43, 43t
      traditional, 42, 43t
    basic concepts, 42
    general concepts, 42–44
    goals of, 44
    hospitalization in, 45
    immunotherapy for, 52–53
    medications for, 45–50
      general concepts, 45–46
    multi-DMARD stepwise approach, 43t, 44
    physical medicine for, 45
    surgical, 51–52
    systemic and articular rest for, 45
    traditional approach, 43t
    two-DMARD combination, 43t, 43–44
Rheumatoid arthritis mutilans, 36f
Rheumatoid disease, organs involved in, 37f
Rheumatoid factor(s), 39
  production of, 12, 26–27
    agents responsible for, 27
  in rheumatoid arthritis, 26–27
  specificity of, 8, 26
Rheumatoid factor test, 3, 6
  indications for, 4t
  low titers, 39
  negative, with positive ANA test, 39
  positive, 31
Rheumatoid nodules
  with rheumatoid arthritis, 35, 35f
  treatment of, 51
  valvular disease and conduction abnormalities due to, 36
Rheumatoid vasculitis, 37, 125
  diagnosis of, 119
  differential diagnosis of, 119t
  treatment of, 51
Rheumatrex. *See* Methotrexate
Ridaura. *See* Auranofin
RNA polymerase 1 antibody, with scleroderma, 177t
7-2 RNA protein complex antibody, with scleroderma, 177t
Rocky Mountain spotted fever, differential diagnosis of, 125
Rose bengal corneal staining, 188
Rubella virus infection, 28
  arthritis induced by, 28
  differential diagnosis of, 42
  synovitis with, 2
Rumalon, for osteoarthritis, 107

Sacroiliitis, HLA-B27 and, 115
S-adenosylmethionine, for osteoarthritis, 107
Salicylates, 3, 46, 59t–60t
  acetylated, 59t
  nonacetylated, 46, 59t–60t
  for osteoarthritis, 106
  time-release enteric-coated
    characteristics of, 59t
    preparation of, 59t
Salivary flow rates, measurement of, 188
Salivary gland, minor, biopsy of, 188
Salivary scintigraphy, with ^{99}MTc sodium pertechnetate, 188
Sarcoiditis, differential diagnosis of, laboratory studies for, 5t
Sarcoidosis
  differential diagnosis of, 188
  laboratory studies for, 5t
  inflammatory muscle disease with, 161
  myositis with, 161t
Schirmer's test, 188
  positive, 187
Schmorl's nodes, 101
Scintigraphy
  esophageal, quantitative, indications for, 180
  salivary, with ^{99}MTc sodium pertechnetate, 188
Scleritis, with rheumatoid arthritis, 36, 37f
Scleroderma, 175–183
  antinuclear antibodies assay of, 14t
  autoantibodies observed in patients with, 177t

autoantibodies with high degree of
diagnostic specificity for, 9t
cardiac involvement, 181–182
classification of, 175
clinical manifestations of, 175–177
diagnosis of, 179–182
differential diagnosis of, 179
early detection of, 175–176
environmental triggers for, 178t, 178
gastrointestinal features of, management of, 180–181
immune response to topoisomerase with, 13
linear, 175
localized. See Morphea
management of, 179–182
pathogenesis of, 177–178
pathology of, autoantibodies in, 12
pulmonary, 179
management of, 179–180
renal impairment with, 182
subsets of, 176–177
vascular impairment with, management of, 179
Scleromalacia perforans, with rheumatoid arthritis, 36
Sclerosis. See Systemic sclerosis
Scurvy, differential diagnosis of, 125
Seizure, with systemic lupus erythematosus, 156
Senile osteoporosis, of axial skeleton, 230
Sensory neuropathies, with rheumatoid arthritis, 36
Sensory polyneuropathy, in Sjögren's syndrome, 190
Sepsis
gonococcal, symptoms of, 2
gram-negative bacillary joint, 81
in prosthetic joint, 86–87, 87t
group B streptococcal joint, 81
hip joint, diagnosis of, 80
Septic arthritis, 79–82
bacteriology of, 81
age-related, 81t, 81
clinical manifestations and diagnosis of, 80–81
drainage procedures, 82
osteoarthritis after, 94t
pathogenesis of, 79
predisposing factors, 79–80
prognosis for, 82
routes of infection in, 79
treatment of, 81–82
incomplete recovery after, related factors, 82
Septicemia, differential diagnosis of, 124

Serologic test for syphilis
false-positive, 154, 156
indications for, 4t
Serositis, definition of, 155t
Serum calcium measurement, 4t
Serum complement measurement, 6
indications for, 4t
Serum enzyme levels
increased, 3
during myositis, 164
Serum immunoelectrophoresis, indications for, 4t
Serum iron test, indications for, 5t
Serum sickness, drug-induced, 2
Serum uric acid concentrations, medications aimed at lowering, acute gout with, 143
Shoulder
adhesive capsulitis of, 225
bursitis of, 3
calcific tendinitis of, 225
musculoskeletal disorders of, nonoperative treatment of, 224–225
reflex sympathetic dystrophy of, 225
Shoulder impingement syndrome, 224–225
Sialochemical measurements, indications for, 188
Sialography, with radiocontrast, 188
Sicca complex, 37
Sicca syndrome, antinuclear antibodies assay of, 14t
Sjögren's syndrome, 36–37, 185–198
autoantibodies with high degree of diagnostic specificity for, 9t
autoimmune hallmarks of, 185
cellular antigens in, 186–187
clinical manifestations of, 187
course of, 185
diagnostic criteria for, 187
differential diagnosis of, laboratory studies for, 4t–5t
epidemiology of, 185–186
extraglandular disease in, 189
treatment of, 194
eye involvement, 188
gastrointestinal involvement, 189
glandular manifestations of, 188
treatment of, 193–194
hepatobiliary disorders with, 39
humoral studies with, 186
inflammatory muscle disease with, 161
laboratory tests with, 193
leukocytoclastic vasculitis with, 123
differential diagnosis of, 119t

malignancy in, 192
myositis with, 161t
oral manifestations of, 188
treatment of, 194
pathogenesis of, 186–192
prevalence of, 185
primary, 185
clinical manifestations of, 187
pathogenesis of, 186
with progressive systemic sclerosis, 191–192
renal disease in, 189–190
treatment of, 194
respiratory system involvement, 189
with rheumatoid arthritis, 191
rheumatoid factors in, 26
secondary, 185
clinical manifestations of, 187
treatment of, 193–195
vaginal manifestation of, 194
vasculitis in, 190–191
treatment of, 194
Skin
biopsy of, indications for, 5t, 124
lesions of, 2
thinning of, with rheumatoid arthritis, 37f
Slime, 87
Small airway disease, in Sjögren's syndrome, 189
Small vessel vasculitis, 121f, 121–124
course of, 122t
diagnosis of, 122t
with systemic lupus erythematosus, 157
underlying disease, 122t
Sodium salicylate
characteristics of, 59t
preparation of, 59t
Soft tissue contractures, in rheumatoid hip, 216
Soft tissue swelling, with rheumatoid arthritis, 40
Solganal. See Aurothioglucose
Spinal stenosis, lumbar, 229–230
Spine, osteoarthritis of, 99, 101
Spleen, onion skin lesions in, 151
Splenectomy, 51
Splenomegaly, with rheumatoid arthritis, 37f
differential diagnosis of, 37
Splinting, for rheumatoid arthritis patient, 45
Spondyloarthropathies
diagnosis of, laboratory studies for, 3, 4t
seronegative
characteristics of, 111

Spondyloarthropathies *(continued)*
  differential diagnosis of, 33, 40–41
Spondylosis, radiographic findings in, 101, 103f
Staphylococcus aureus
  in prosthetic joint, 86–87, 87t
  septic arthritis caused by, 81, 81t
  therapeutic outcome, 82
Staphylococcus epidermidis, in prosthetic joint, 86–87, 87t
Steroid psychosis, 157
Steroids
  intra-articular, 50
    for osteoarthritis, 106
  intralesional, 50
  intravenous, very-high-dose, 50
  liposome-entrapped, 50
  local injection of, for acute gout, 143
  oral
    high-dose, 50
    low-dose, 50
  topical, 49–50
Stool guaiac, indications for, 4t
Streptococci
  beta-hemolytic. *See also* Group B streptococci
    differential diagnosis of, laboratory studies for, 4t
    in prosthetic joint, 86–87, 87t
    septic arthritis caused by, 81, 81t
    therapeutic outcome, 82
  viridans, in prosthetic joint, 86–87, 87t
Stress fracture, of femoral neck, 233
Stromelysin, in synovial fluid, 22
Subacute cutaneous lupus erythematosus
  characteristics of, 155
  treatment of, 158
Submandibular gland enlargement, in Sjögren's syndrome. *See* Xerostomia
Sugar therapy, for osteoarthritis, 107
Sulfasalazine, 43, 48–49, 70–71
  absorption, metabolism and distribution of, 70
  adverse reactions to, 71
  autoimmune reactions to, 71
  central nervous system reactions to, 71
  chemistry of, 70
  clinical efficacy of, 70
  contraindications to, 48–49, 71
  cost of, 70
  dosage, 70–71
  gastrointestinal and hepatic reactions to, 71

hematologic reactions to, 71
male infertility with, 71
mechanism of action, 70
mucocutaneous reactions to, 71
pulmonary reactions to, 71
side effects of, surveillance for, 71
supply, 70
teratogenicity of, 71
Sulfinpyrazone
  dosage and administration of, 144
  prophylaxis, for gout, 144
Sulindac
  characteristics of, 64t
  dosage and administration of, 141
  preparation of, 64t
Superantigens, in rheumatoid arthritis, 26
Surgery, for rheumatoid arthritis patient, 51–52
Synovectomy
  arthroscopic, 52
  radiation, 52
Synovial biopsy, indications for, 5t, 39–40
Synovial fluid
  cell content of, 22
  cytokines in, 22t, 22
  osteoarthritic, 97
  in rheumatoid joint, 22
Synovial fluid analysis, 3, 39, 80t
  indications for, 4t
Synovial tissue evaluation, 39–40
Synovitis
  bacterial, differential diagnosis of, laboratory studies for, 4t
  diagnosis of, 231
  of hip, 231–232
  of knee, 234
  mild to moderate, with osteoarthritis, 98
  monoarticular, differential diagnosis of, 33, 41
  pain with, 2
  physical examination with, 231
  pigmented villonodular, hip arthritis with, 214–215
  recent-onset, 2
  traumatic, 3
  treatment of, 232, 234
  x-ray findings in, 231, 234
Syphilis
  diagnosis of, 122t
  serologic test for
    false-positive, 154, 156
    indications for, 4t
  similarity with Lyme disease, 86
Systemic cutaneous lupus erythematosus
  prognosis for, 160

treatment of, 158
Systemic lupus erythematosus, 8, 151–160
  antibody specificity with, 165
  antinuclear antibodies assay of, 14t
  autoantibodies in, 153t, 153
  autoantibodies with high degree of diagnostic specificity for, 9t
  cardiovascular manifestations of, 157
  clinical presentation of, 2, 40, 154–157
  complications of, 80
  congenital, differential diagnosis of, laboratory studies for, 4t
  constitutional manifestations of, 154
  course and prognosis, 160
  cutaneous manifestations of, 155
  death with, causes of, 160
  definition of, 151
  demographic characteristics of, 2
  diagnosis of, 154
  diagnostic criteria for, 154, 155t
  differential diagnosis of, 3, 40
    laboratory studies for, 3, 4t–5t
  distribution of lesions, 122
  drug-induced, differential diagnosis of, laboratory studies for, 4t
  epidemiology of, 152
  etiology of, 151–152
  gastrointestinal manifestations of, 157
  hematologic manifestations of, 156
  hip arthritis with, 212
  inflammatory muscle disease with, 161
  leukocytoclastic vasculitis with, 123
  major organ involvement in, treatment of, 158
  management of, 157–160
    considerations for, 158
  morbidity in, cause of, 157
  musculoskeletal manifestations of, 155–156
  myositis with, 161t
  nervous system manifestations of, 156–157
  palindromic rheumatism with, 32
  pathogenesis of, 152–154
  pattern of manifestations, 154
  prevalence of, 152
  pulmonary manifestations of, 157
  renal manifestations of, 156
  rheumatoid factors in, 26
  serologic features of, 3

Systemic sclerosis, 175
  cardiac features of, 181–182
  clinical manifestations of, 2, 176
  constipation with, 181
  demographic characteristics of, 2
  differential diagnosis of, 180
  diffuse. See also Diffuse cutaneous systemic sclerosis
    differential diagnosis of, laboratory studies for, 4t
  endothelial cell studies with, 178
  environmental triggers for, 178t, 178
  etiology of, 178
  fibroblast studies with, 178
  gastrointestinal features of, 180–181
  immune studies with, 178
  limited cutaneous, 177
  management of, 182
  pathogenesis of, 177–178
  pathophysiology of, 178
  pattern of illness with, 177
  progressive. See Progressive systemic sclerosis
  pulmonary involvement, 179–180
  renal impairment with, 182
  vascular impairment with, 179

Takayasu's arteritis
  aortic arch arteriography with, 127, 129f
  clinical presentations of, 127
  diagnosis of, 119, 122t
  differential diagnosis of, 119t, 127–128, 130f
  treatment of, 128
T cell(s)
  altered function of, in Sjögren's syndrome, 187
  effector, in pathogenesis of systemic lupus erythematosus, 154
  suppressor, altered activity of, in systemic lupus erythematosus patients, 154
  in synovial effusions, 22
T cell CD4/CD8 (helper/cytotoxic) ratio, in synovial effusions, 22
T-cell receptor
  in rheumatoid arthritis, 26
  specificity of, 26
Tear(s)
  chemistry of, study of, 188
  slow-release, 194
Tear break-up time, 188
Technetium diphosphonate scans, 89

Technetium-gallium scans, sequential, 89
Telangiectasia, periungual, diagnosis of, 122t
Temporal arteritis. See Giant cell arteritis
Temporal artery biopsy, indications for, 5t
Tendinitis, 2
  of Achilles tendon, 235
  calcific, 225
  in hip, 231
  physical examination with, 231
  treatment of, 231
Tenosynovitis, 3
  DeQuervain's, 227
  with rheumatoid arthritis, 33
Tetracycline, for Lyme disease, 85
Thoracic duct drainage, for rheumatoid arthritis, 19
Thromboangiitis, differential diagnosis of, 179
Thrombocytopenia
  with Felty's syndrome, 38
  gold-induced, 66
  with systemic lupus erythematosus, 156
  treatment of, 159
Thrombocytosis
  reactive, 38
  with rheumatoid arthritis, 37f
Thrombosis, deep vein, after total hip arthroplasty, 218
Thumb, trigger, 227
Thyroglobulin, diagnostic specificity, 9t
Thyroid chemistry, indications for, 5t
Thyroiditis, Hashimoto's, 8, 9t
Thyrotoxicosis, autoantibody-mediated, mechanism of, 10
Tissue culture, indications for, 5t
Tissue injury, autoantibody-mediated, 10–12
  mechanism of, 10–12, 11f
Toe
  big, with gout, 142f
  claw deformity, 236
Tolmetin
  characteristics of, 64t
  preparation of, 64t
Total iron binding capacity test, indications for, 5t
Total lymphoid irradiation, for lupus, 160
Total nodal irradiation, for rheumatoid arthritis, 19
Total parenteral nutrition, 181
Toxoplasmosis
  with myositis, 166

  treatment of, 169
Transforming growth factor beta, in synovial fluid, 22, 22t
Trapezioscaphoid joint, osteoarthritis of, 98–99
Trauma, 2
Trigeminal neuropathy, in Sjögren's syndrome, 190
Trigger finger or thumb, 227
Trilisate. See Choline magnesium salicylate
Trochanteric bursitis, 231
Trochanteric nonunion, after total hip arthroplasty, 219
Tuberculosis
  diagnosis of, 122t
  leukocytoclastic vasculitis with, 123
Tumor necrosis factor
  in synovial effusions, 22
  in synovial fluid, 22, 22t
Tumor necrosis factor inhibitors, 53

Ulcerative colitis
  differential diagnosis of, laboratory studies for, 5t
  hip arthritis with, 214
Ulcers
  oral, definition of, 155t
  with rheumatoid arthritis, 37f
Ulnar deviation, with rheumatoid arthritis, 31, 33f
Ultrasound, of knee joint, 40
Urate, in synovial fluids, 3
Urate crystals, polarized light microscopy of, 139, 141f
Uric acid
  24-hour excretion test, indications for, 5t
  serum levels, 3
    medications aimed at lowering, acute gout with, 143
Uricosuric prophylaxis, for gout, 144
Urinalysis, indications for, 4t
Urine immunoelectrophoresis, indications for, 4t
Urine protein, 24-hour test, indications for, 5t

Vancomycin, for joint prosthesis infection, 90
Vascular necrosis, with vasculitis, 119–120
Vascular spasm, with vasculitis, 121
Vasculitis, 4t, 119–134, 122t
  classification of, 119t
  coronary, 36

Vasculitis *(continued)*
  cutaneous, manifestations of, 190
  definition of, 119–121, 120t
  dermatologic definition of, 120t
  diagnosis of, laboratory studies for, 4t–5t
  HB-associated, diagnosis of, laboratory studies for, 4t
  laboratory findings in, 3
  leukoclastic, 190
  lymphocytic, 190
  neurologic definition of, 120t, 121
  pathologic definition of, 120t, 120–121
  pulmonary, with polymyositis, 163
  radiologic definition of, 120t, 121
  rheumatoid, 37, 125
    diagnosis of, 119
    differential diagnosis of, 119t
    treatment of, 51
  rheumatologic definition of, 119–120, 120t
  in Sjögren's syndrome, 190–191
    treatment of, 194
  symptoms of, 2
  systemic, palindromic rheumatism with, 32

VDRL. *See* Serologic test for syphilis
Venereal disease, Reiter's syndrome after, 115
Verrucous endocarditis, 151, 157
Viral arthritis, clinical presentation of, 80
Viral polyarthritis, differential diagnosis of, 42
Viruses, that cause muscle inflammation, 166

Waldenström's macroglobulinemia, and Sjögren's syndrome, 187
Walker, with platforms, for total hip arthroplasty patient, 217
Wassermann test, false-positive, 4t
Weakness, with myositis, 161–162
Wegener's granulomatosis, 126
  autoantibodies with high degree of diagnostic specificity for, 9t
  differential diagnosis of, laboratory studies for, 5t
  leukocytoclastic vasculitis with, 123
Weight loss, with rheumatoid arthritis, 35

Westergren sedimentation rate. *See* Erythrocyte sedimentation rate
White blood cell counts, 39
Widefield nailfold capillary microscopy, 176–177
Wilson's disease, osteoarthritis with, 94t, 104–105
Wound drainage, with prosthetic joint infection, 87, 87t
Wrist
  musculoskeletal disorders of, nonoperative treatment of, 226–227
  osteoarthritis of, 99

Xerophthalmia, in Sjögren's syndrome, 189
Xerostomia
  differential diagnosis of, 188
  in Sjögren's syndrome, 188–189
Xerotrachea, in Sjögren's syndrome, 189

Zorprin. *See* Aspirin, time-release zero-order